The Essential
Hoof Book

The Essential
Hoof Book

The Complete Modern Guide to Horse Feet:

Anatomy, Care and Health,
Disease Diagnosis and Treatment

Susan Kauffmann and Christina Cline

Foreword by Gene Ovnicek

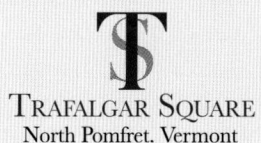

TRAFALGAR SQUARE
North Pomfret. Vermont

First published in 2017 by
Trafalgar Square Books
North Pomfret, Vermont 05053

Disclaimer of Liability

The authors and publisher shall have neither liability nor responsibility to any person or entity with respect to any loss or damage caused or alleged to be caused directly or indirectly by the information contained in this book. While the book is as accurate as the authors can make it, there may be errors, omissions, and inaccuracies.

Trafalgar Square Books encourages the use of approved safety helmets in all equestrian sports and activities.

Library of Congress Cataloging-in-Publication Data

Names: Kauffmann, Susan, 1965- author. | Cline, Christina, author.
Title: The essential hoof book : the complete modern guide to horse feet --
    anatomy, care and health, disease diagnosis and treatment / Susan
    Kauffmann and Christina Cline ; foreword by Gene Ovnicek.
Description: North Pomfret, Vermont : Trafalgar Square Books, 2017. |
    Includes bibliographical references and index.
Identifiers: LCCN 2017011524| ISBN 9781570767326 (hb concealed wiro) | ISBN
    9781570768538 (ebook)
Subjects: LCSH: Hoofs--Care and hygiene. | Horses--Health.
Classification: LCC SF907 .K38 2017 | DDC 636.1--dc23 LC record available at
https://lccn.loc.gov/2017011524

Book design by Lauryl Eddlemon
Cover design by RM Didier
Front cover photograph by Heike Bean
Back cover: Top photo by Jill Willis, AANHCP; bottom photos by (clockwise starting with top left) Susan Kauffmann and The Glass Horse; Susan Kauffmann; Susan Kauffmann; April Raine; The Laminitis Site; Wallace Liberman, DVM; Susan Kauffmann; Patricia Stiller
Typeface: Open Sans

Printed in China

10 9 8

This book is dedicated to everyone who strives
to make this world a better place for horses—
and to the horses, for the depth of their mystery,
and for all they continue to teach us.

Contents

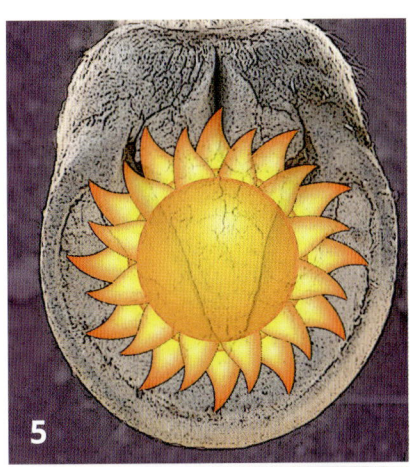

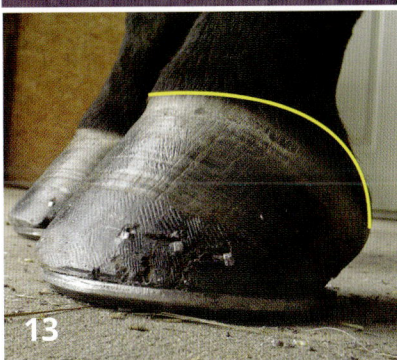

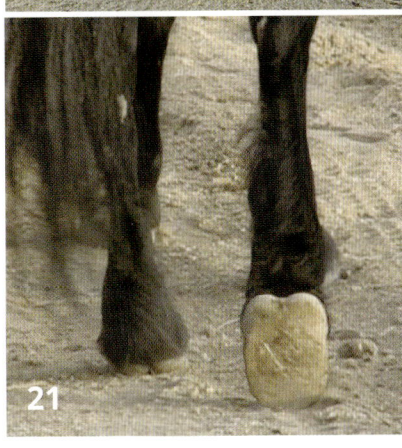

Section Two: Recognizing Healthy and Unhealthy Feet

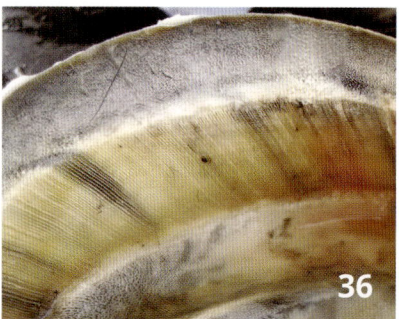

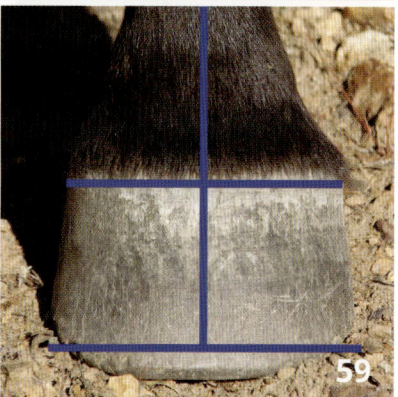

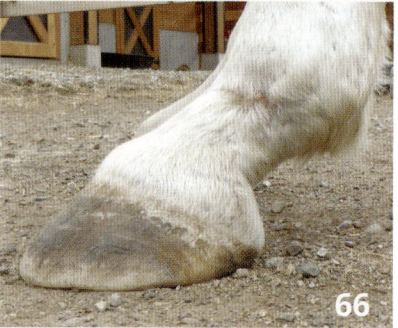

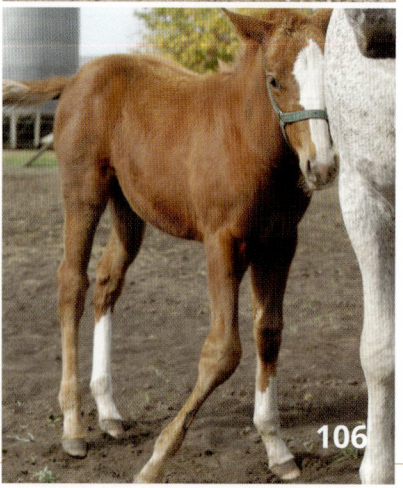

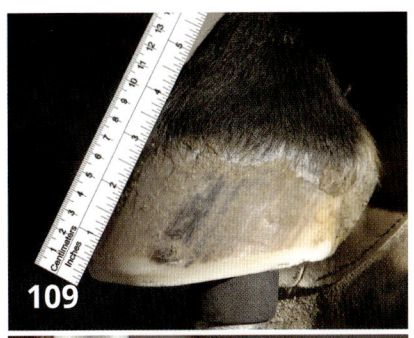

109

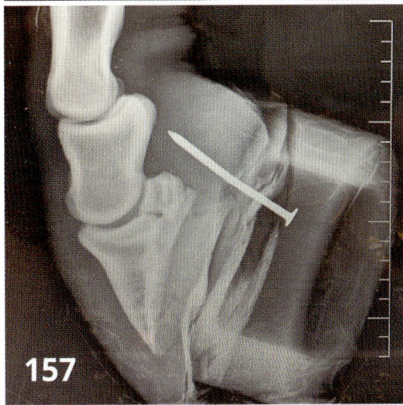

157

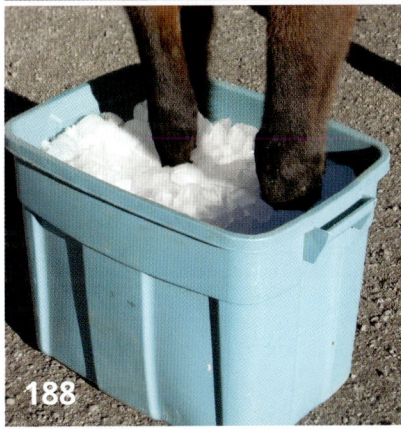

188

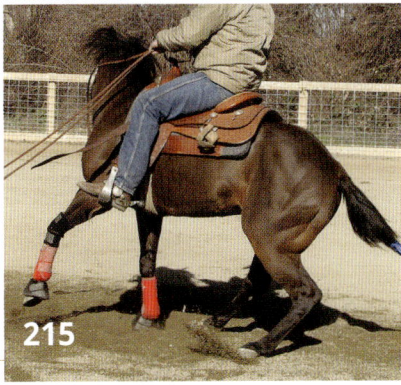

215

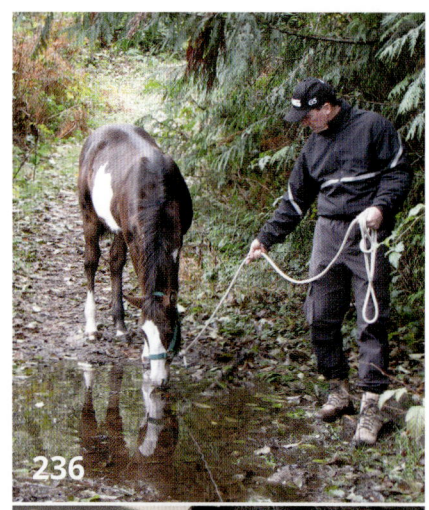

236

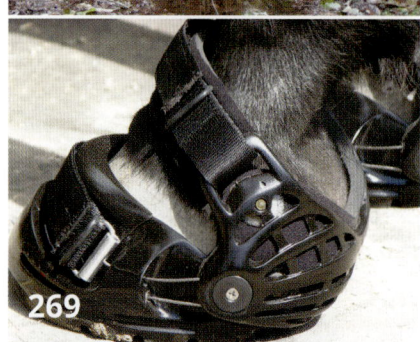

269

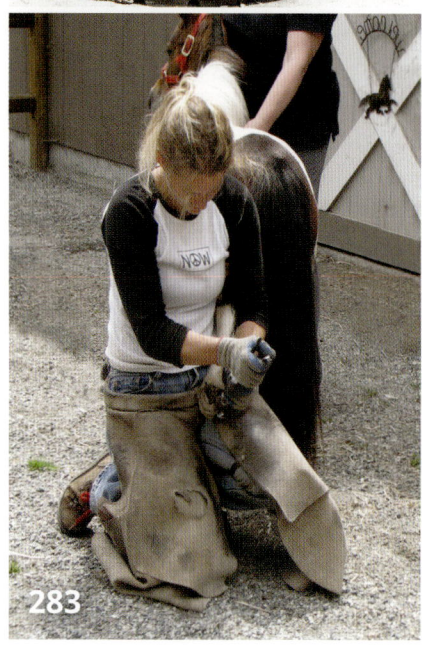

283

Foreword

I have studied and worked with the horse's foot for more than 50 years, and I continue to participate in research projects focused on treating and preventing equine lameness. Through the articles and book chapters I've had published over the years, and via clinics and seminars I have given, I have sought to share as much of my knowledge as possible with both hoof care professionals and horse people in general. Always the intention has been to improve the life of the domestic horse through educated care of the hoof.

But there has remained a need for a complete resource for those who have not spent years studying the equine foot, whether they be horse owners, trainers, veterinary or farriery students, or anyone else who wants an easy-to-grasp guide to hoof management, anatomy, function, and the many things that can, for one reason or another, go wrong with the equine foot. *The Essential Hoof Book* fulfills that need, bringing the most up-to-date understanding and research to every horse person, in a practical and highly readable format clarified with hundreds of enlightening photographs and illustrations. Once you've read *The Essential Hoof Book*, you will have a much deeper understanding of the horse's hoof and how to keep it healthy and sound in ways you perhaps never thought of—or thought possible.

Between the covers of this book, you will also find in-depth discussion of two important issues (among many others) that have been debated for years, until now providing little clarity. First is the issue of mismatched feet and how to *manage* them rather than change them. Second is long-toe/low-heel syndrome, which is present in an alarming number of domestic horses, with devastating health and performance consequences.

The book also provides a clear and concise mapping system that you can use as a guideline for recognizing hoof distortions or abnormalities, as well as information on how to deal with them. This hoof mapping protocol was developed by the Equine Lameness Prevention Organization (ELPO), a progressive group that collectively reviews hoof-related issues from a scientific approach.

During the course of my career, I have witnessed and experienced many changes in the hoof-care industry—some have been helpful, many not. Often traditionally accepted ideas related to hoof biomechanics and hoof management have, in fact, stymied progress. Luckily now, with the use of better imaging and communication, we can see the equine foot more clearly.

Susan Kauffmann and Christina Cline have recognized a need for us all to see the equine foot more clearly. They have done a tremendous amount of work, assembling information that will undoubtedly help many horses by creating clarity and understanding for those who care for them. They have included a number of highly regarded contributors in this book—all seasoned practitioners who have a passion to move forward in finding answers to consistent problems that have plagued the equine industry. *The Essential Hoof Book* will be an extremely useful addition to any horse person's library. I applaud the authors.

Gene Ovnicek

GPF-RMF (Guild of Professional Farriers - Registered Master Farrier)
CNBBT, CNBF, CLS, CE, CI

Introduction

The equine hoof is a complex marvel of natural engineering, built to withstand tremendous forces and able to adapt to an astonishing range of environmental conditions. It may look like a hard, fixed structure, but in truth, it is surprisingly plastic, changing daily—for better or for worse—in response to a continual flux of external and internal factors. We, as horse owners, have the ability to control most of those factors, but as few of us have had the opportunity to acquire a deep understanding of the hoof, we tend to turn that control over to others—to our vets, farriers, trainers, and barn managers. They make decisions about what is best for our horses' feet, and we write the checks. Sometimes, that arrangement works just fine, but given that an alarmingly high percentage of domestic horses are walking around on distorted feet with varying degrees of dysfunction, it clearly isn't working well enough.

The fact that you have picked up this book means that you want something more. You want to understand what is going on with your horse's feet so that you can be a stronger advocate and make informed decisions about his hoof health. The authors of *The Essential Hoof Book* share that goal. Like you, we want the very best for your horse, so we have done our utmost to bring you the most current and useful information available, gleaned from the research and wisdom of top hoof experts around the world.

We'll get you started by orienting you with some basic terms and anatomy, then move into the main section of the book, which will show you the differences between healthy and unhealthy feet, and help you understand how those feet got to be that way. You will learn about the biomechanics and importance of good hoof balance, as well as the causes, treatments, and prevention of commonly encountered problems like laminitis, white line disease, and thrush. Best of all, the book's easy-to-follow language, clear illustrations, and hands-on exercises will enable you to get out there and start really assessing your own horse's feet.

As you read through these pages and look at the examples presented, there are just a few things we would like you to keep in mind. One is that while most of our photographs show horses without shoes, this was done for the simple reason that it is easier to see the features on a bare foot, not because we wish to push any particular agenda in the bare versus shod debate. It is our belief that the equine foot can be healthy both shod and unshod, and it can also be unhealthy either way. Whether it trends one way or another depends on a multitude of influences, many of which are at least as important as what is or isn't on the bottom of the foot.

We would also like you to understand that there is no perfect model for how every hoof should be, so we have not presented one. As R.F. (Ric) Redden, DVM, the father of modern equine podiatry puts it, "Although certain generalities can be made, there is a range for normal hoof characteristics, which is influenced by the horse's breed, age, environment, and use. Considering the variability imposed by these factors, the range of normal can be very broad." And, just as there is no one ideal for how a hoof should look, there is also no universally right answer when it comes to how a given hoof problem is best approached. It would certainly make life easier if there was some reliable standard, some set of absolute truths that would apply to every hoof in every circumstance, but the more you deal with the equine foot, the more you come to realize that what may be true most of the time is almost never true all of the time. Perhaps it is that very variability that makes the hoof such a fascinating subject, and which makes it so important—indeed essential— that we learn to understand its ever-changing form.

Section One:
Anatomy

I f you've ever felt like your vet or farrier lapsed into Swahili when talking about your horse's feet, you're not alone. Few horse owners are entirely at ease with the avalanche of anatomical terms used to talk about the equine hoof, and trying to keep them all straight is about as easy as herding cats. But, learning a few key terms can go a long way toward deciphering all that "hoof speak," and will ultimately help you take better care of your horse's feet. Not only will you be able to have more meaningful conversations with your vet and hoof-care provider, you will also have a solid foundation to really understand how the hoof works. Anatomy gives you the keys to the kingdom, and we're about to unlock the door (figs. I–IV).

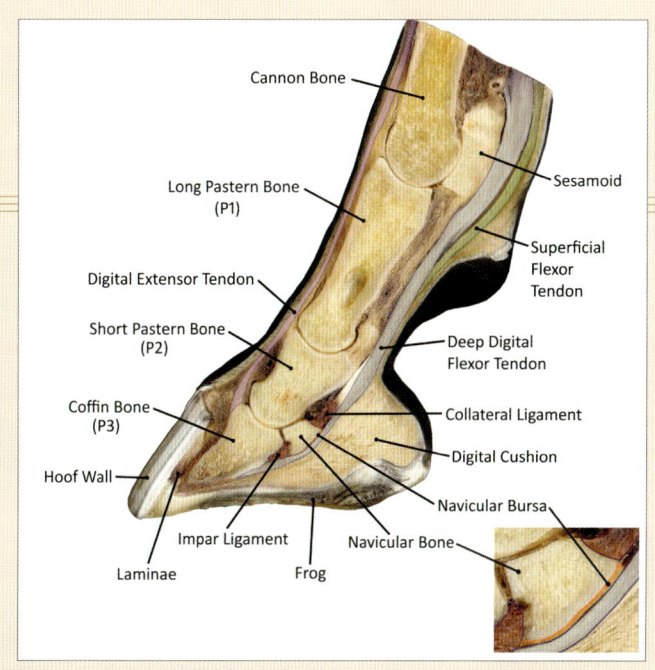

I Structures of the distal limb with navicular inset.

Cannon Bone
Sesamoid
Long Pastern Bone (P1)
Superficial Flexor Tendon
Digital Extensor Tendon
Short Pastern Bone (P2)
Deep Digital Flexor Tendon
Coffin Bone (P3)
Collateral Ligament
Hoof Wall
Digital Cushion
Navicular Bursa
Impar Ligament
Navicular Bone
Laminae
Frog

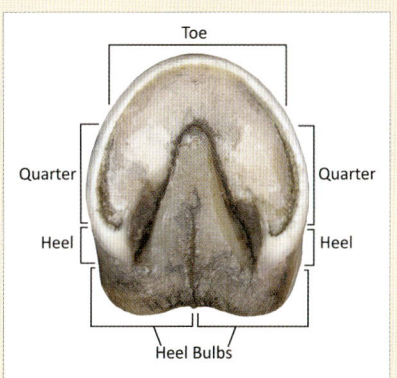

Toe
Quarter
Quarter
Heel
Heel
Heel Bulbs

II Regions of the hoof, solar view.

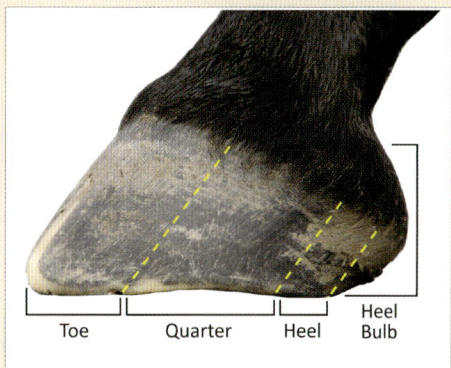

Toe
Quarter
Heel
Heel Bulb

III Regions of the hoof, side view.

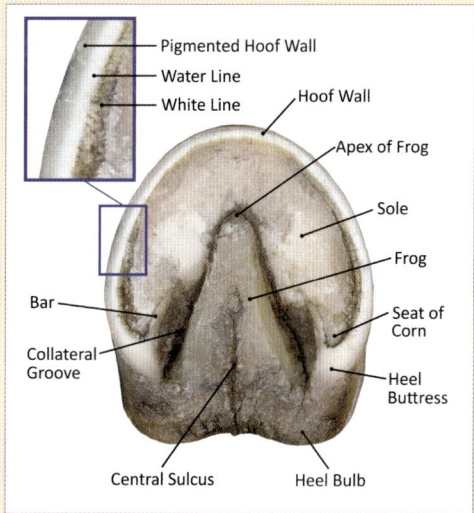

Pigmented Hoof Wall
Water Line
White Line
Hoof Wall
Apex of Frog
Sole
Frog
Bar
Seat of Corn
Collateral Groove
Heel Buttress
Central Sulcus
Heel Bulb

IV Solar view.

Useful Anatomical Terms

1

Anatomists like to name stuff—it gives them something to do. Not only do they name specific parts, but they have also come up with a system of words to tell us the location of the parts they are talking about. Here are a few key terms used to reference different locations on the hoof. Each is followed by its definition, then used in a sentence.

Solar: When it comes to the horse's foot, the term "solar" has nothing to do with the sun. Instead, it refers to the surface of the hoof that faces the ground, like the soles of our own feet. Example: The

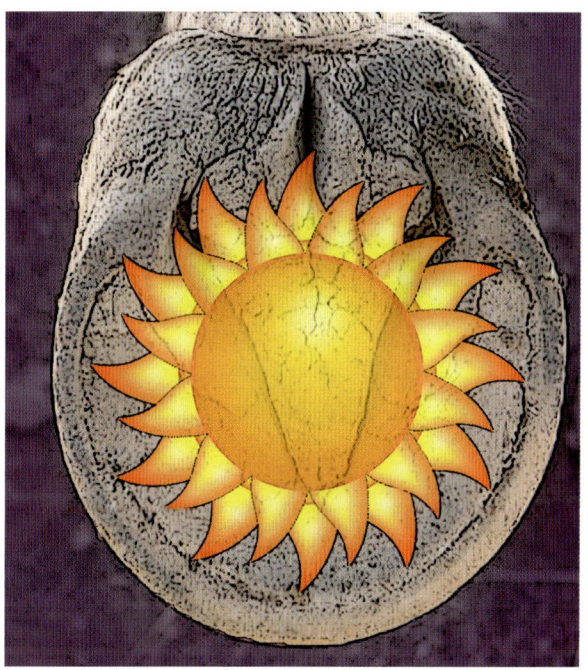

1.1 The solar surface may have nothing to do with the sun, but it is a good way to remember what to call it.

degree of curvature of the solar surface is related to the size and shape of the coffin bone (fig. 1.1).

Caudal: This word is used to talk about anything in the back part of the foot, both inside and out. The heels, navicular bone, most of the frog, and the majority of the digital cushion are all in the caudal region of the foot. Example: Several structures in

Alphabetical List of Useful Terms

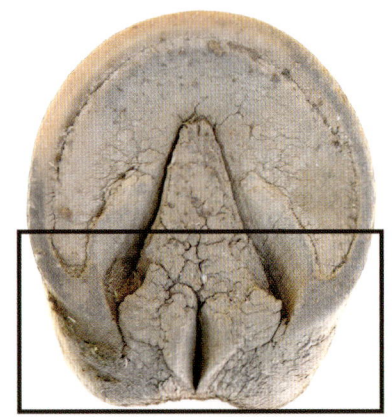

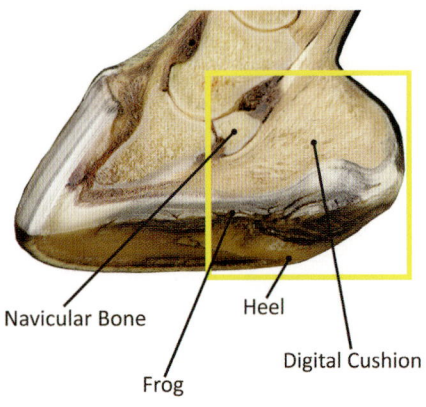

Navicular Bone

Heel

Frog

Digital Cushion

1.2 A & B The caudal area consists of all the structures in the back of the foot.

the caudal area of the hoof work together to absorb shock (figs. 1.2 A & B). Sometimes, you will hear vets and farriers talk about "caudal heel pain." If this seems redundant to you, that's because it is! It's just one of the many examples of common usage that don't always make sense; "caudal hoof pain" would be more correct.

Dorsal: In general anatomy, "dorsal" refers to the upper or top surface, often along the back of an animal, like when we talk about the dorsal fin of a shark. When talking about the hoof, however, dorsal refers to the front surface of the hoof wall. Still, if you picture a dorsal fin coming out of the front of the hoof, you will likely remember this term forever. Example: The dorsal wall should be free of any dishing or rippling (fig. 1.3).

Palmar: "Palmar" technically refers to anything down the back of the leg below the knee and wrapping around to include the back portion of the bottom of the *front* feet only. In actual use, it is used to talk about the caudal area of the front feet, though it is also often used interchangeably with "solar" to refer

to the entire bottom of the foot. Therefore, when your vet/farrier uses this term and you are not sure if they mean the whole solar surface or just something in the back of the foot, ask them to clarify. Example: Large pincers called hoof testers are often used to diagnose palmar pain in the hoof.

Plantar: The word "plantar" is used exactly like "palmar" except that it refers to the *hind* feet. This term is useful for photographs and X-rays, as it allows you to know if you are looking at the front or hind feet in the image. Example: Palmar heel pain is more common than plantar heel pain.

Medial: The medial side of the hoof is the one closest to the midline of the horse's body. The medial wall, therefore, is the inside wall. Example: In most horses, the medial wall is slightly more upright than the lateral wall.

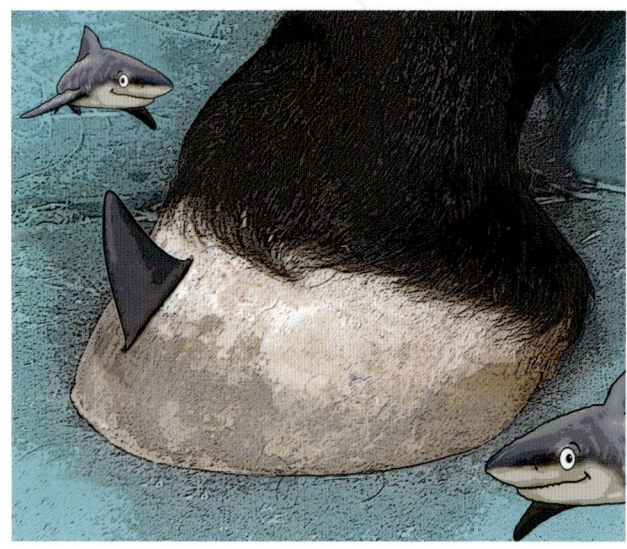

1.3 The dorsal wall is the front surface of the hoof, but thinking of a shark's dorsal fin helps the term stick for some people.

Remembering Palmar and Plantar

Bipeds and quadrupeds share a lot of anatomical terminology. We human bipeds have palms on our hands, and the ground surface of our feet is referred to as plantar (hence the pain-in-the-foot disorder called "plantar fasciitis"). Even so, it is easy to forget which is which when it comes to palmar and plantar in the horse. If you picture someone doing a "bear crawl" with palms on the ground and feet planted behind, that might keep it clear that palmar is the front feet, and plantar is the hind (fig. 1.4).

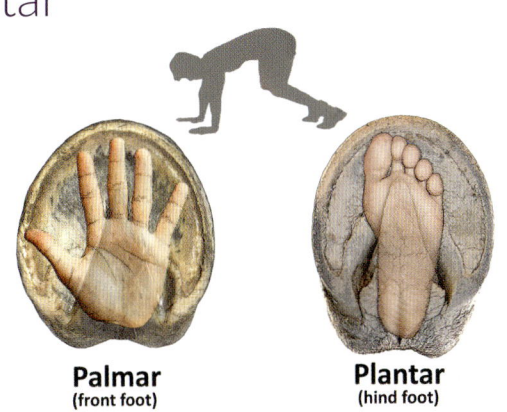

Palmar
(front foot)

Plantar
(hind foot)

1.4 A man doing a "bear crawl" has his palmar surfaces in front and his plantar surfaces behind—just like a horse.

Lateral: The lateral side is the one farthest away from the midline of the body. When talking about the lateral wall, we mean the outside wall (fig. 1.5). Example: A study of wild horses in New Zealand showed that 85% of them had lateral wall flares.

Dorsopalmar and Mediolateral Balance: Hoof-care providers and veterinarians talk a lot about "hoof balance," and you are likely to hear them use the terms "dorsopalmar balance" and "mediolateral balance" in that context.

"Dorsopalmar balance" refers to how the front half of the foot relates to the back half. You can look at dorsopalmar balance two ways, one being from the side, where you are observing how the height, length, and angle of the heels relate to the height, length, and angle of the dorsal wall (fig. 1.6). You can also assess dorsopalmar balance in terms of what

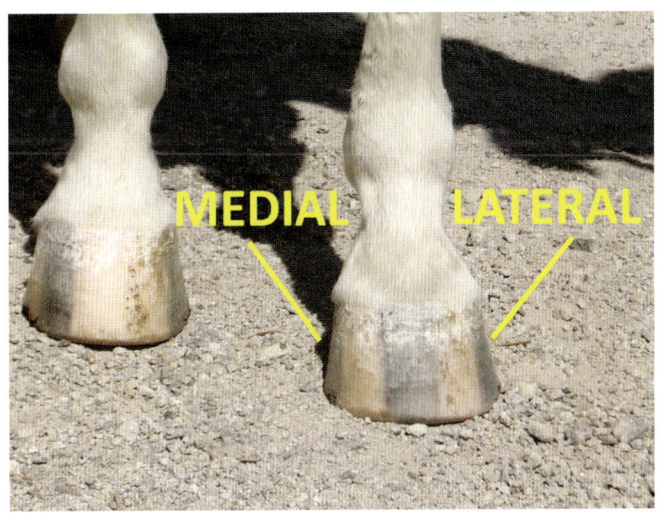

MEDIAL   LATERAL

1.5 Like most normal hooves, this one has a medial wall that is slightly more upright than the lateral wall.

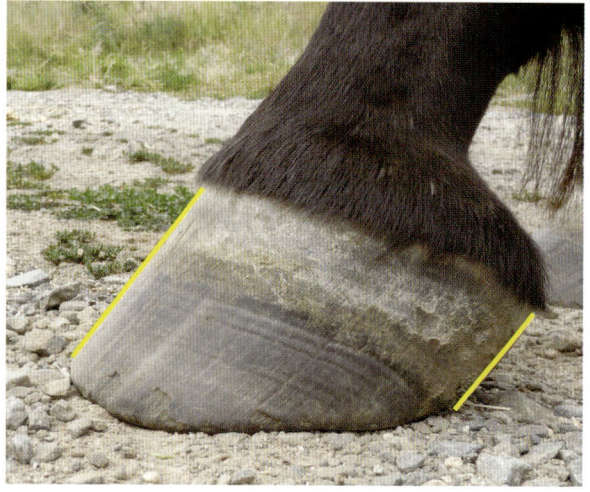

1.6 This foot has good dorsopalmar balance as viewed from the side, with the heel angle closely matching the toe angle, and neither being too high or too low.

1.8 Looking at the hairline on the front of this foot, you can see that it is much higher on the medial (inside) side than on the lateral side. This is a prime example of mediolateral imbalance.

you see on the bottom of the foot. A hoof that has good dorsopalmar balance will have approximately 50% of its mass ahead of the center of articulation, which corresponds with the widest part of the foot, and 50% behind that point (fig. 1.7).

"Mediolateral balance" refers to how the medial (inside) half of the hoof matches up with the lateral (outside) half of the hoof. If one-half is taller or significantly wider than the other when looking at the foot from the front or the back, or one-half

is noticeably wider or shaped differently than the other when looking at the sole of the foot, you have a mediolateral imbalance (fig. 1.8).

Proximal: When talking about the limb or the foot, something that is "proximal" is closer to the body than it is to the ground. If you are talking about the coffin bone, for instance, the proximal surface would be the top surface. Example: The proximal surface of the coffin bone interfaces with the short pastern bone (see fig. I, p. 3).

Distal: Something in the limb or foot that is "distal" is closer to the ground than it is to the body. The word derives from the word "distant," so just think of it as distant from the body. Example: The distal limb of the horse includes everything below the knee. The words "distal" and "proximal" are often used to say where one structure is in relation to another. Example: The coffin bone is distal to the short pastern bone.

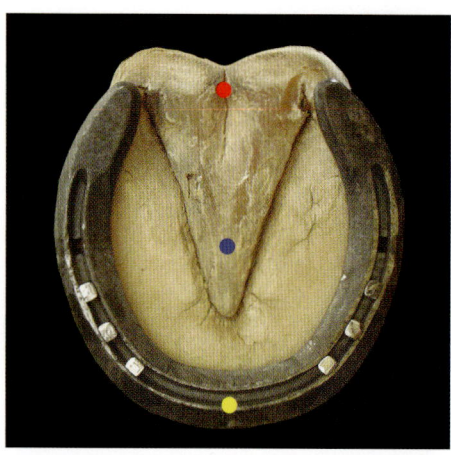

1.7 If you look at how much mass is behind the center of articulation on this foot (blue dot to red dot), then look at how much mass is ahead of it (blue dot to yellow dot—the latter being placed at the point of breakover, see *Understanding Breakover,* p. 95), you can see that it is split almost exactly 50/50, meaning this foot has very good dorsopalmar balance. It also has excellent mediolateral balance, as the inside and outside halves of the foot are nearly identical.

Exterior Hoof Anatomy—Coronary Band and Hoof Wall

The Coronary Band

When looking at the dorsal view of the hoof, you see several features. Wrapping around the top, where the skin of the limb meets the top of the hoof wall, is the *coronary band*, also called the *coronet*. The inside of the coronary band is made up of highly vascular tissue that provides nourishment to the hoof wall, called the *coronary corium* (see *The Corium*, p. 37), and a layer of *germinal cells* (cells from which other cells proliferate), which produce most of the material that makes up the hoof wall. (Corium is a type of specialized tissue rich in blood vessels.) From the outside, the coronary band should have a plump, firm feel to it, without dips or depressions.

The Hoof Wall

Below the coronary band is the hoof wall, which should form a sloping line from the coronet all the way to the ground free from dips, flares, or bulges (fig. 2.1).

The hoof wall has three layers, two of which you can see at least parts of. The outer layer, which is entirely visible, is made up of the *periople* and the *stratum externum*, also called the *stratum tectorium*.

The *periople* is the transition between the hoof horn to the skin above it, similar to the cuticle on your own nails. It is somewhat rough in appearance in a dry environment, and softer and plumper in wet regions (fig. 2.2). It extends only a short way down the hoof wall, although it is wider where it caps the heel bulbs.

The *stratum externum,* which starts below the periople, is a thin layer of hard cells that forms the

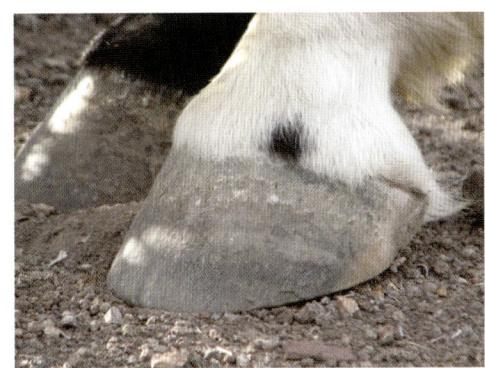

2.1 The wall on this healthy foot flows down from the coronet to the ground in a virtually perfect, sloping line.

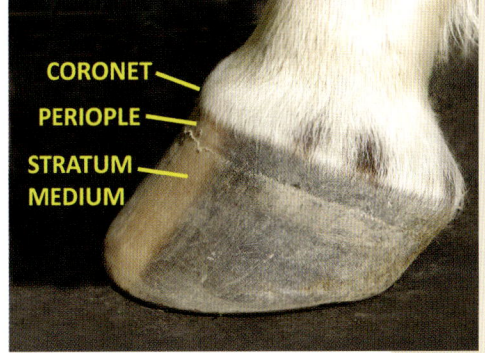

CORONET
PERIOPLE
STRATUM MEDIUM

2.2 The periople, which starts just below the coronet, is similar to the cuticle on your own fingernails.

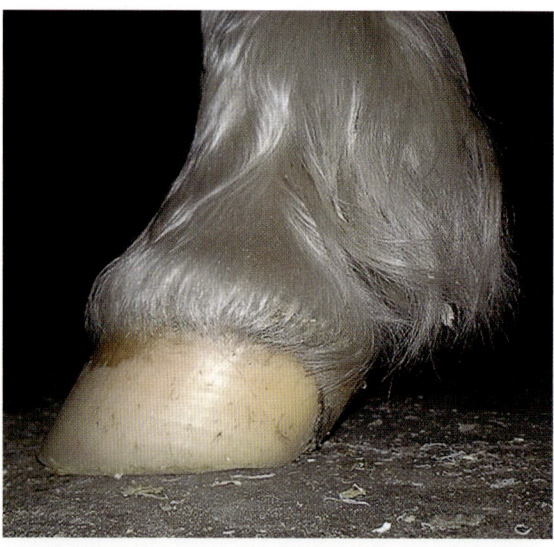

2.3 The stratum externum creates the lovely shine on this foot, but if this horse were to live in a dry, abrasive environment, that thin layer of cells would wear away.

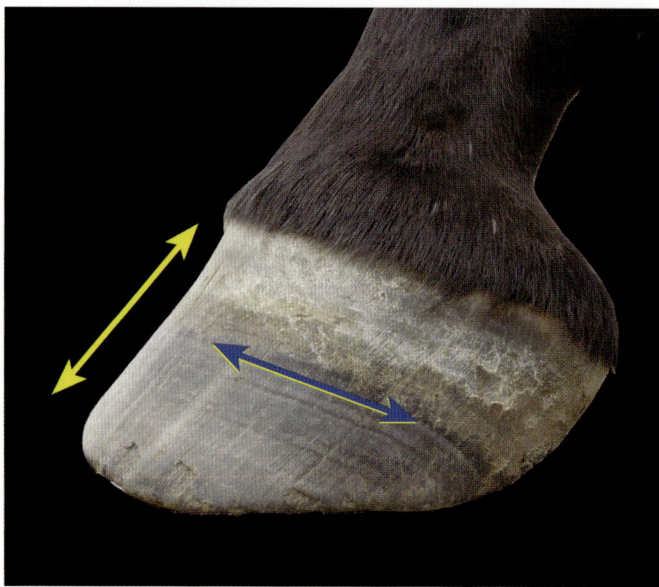

2.4 The horn tubules run down the face of the hoof wall (yellow line), while the growth rings, if they are visible, run across it (blue line). The barely visible growth rings in this hoof are a sign of good health.

smooth, shiny coating on the exterior of the wall (fig. 2.3). This coating acts as a moisture barrier, its most important function being to keep moisture from the environment out. Moisture can actually be damaging to the equine hoof, which is well adapted to dry conditions. In abrasive terrain, the stratum externum and sometimes even the periople can wear away, leaving the hoof with a dull and sometimes rough appearance. While this may not look "pretty," it does not generally cause problems for the foot, as there doesn't tend to be much moisture in environments where this happens.

Also visible when you look at the hoof wall is the outer surface of the middle layer of the wall. This middle layer, called the *stratum medium*, contains straw-shaped *horn tubules* that form long, thin, vertical lines all the way down to the ground. The tubules, along with the *intertubular horn* that fills in the spaces between them, are made of keratinized cells arranged to form an incredibly strong but flexible matrix. The lines made by the tubules should not be confused with *growth rings*, which are horizontal lines that will be indistinguishable or only slightly visible in a normal foot, but can become more pronounced in response to some kind of systemic stress in the body or inflammation in the hoof at the time when that part of the hoof wall was being produced (fig. 2.4). The outer zone of the stratum medium can be pigmented, making the hoof brown, gray, or almost black, or unpigmented in "white" feet (see sidebar on p. 11 for more on the *stratum medium*).

The innermost layer of the hoof wall, the *stratum internum* or *stratum lamellatum*, is not visible externally except for where it shows as the *white line* on the bottom of the foot. For this reason, we will talk about it more in the internal anatomy section (p. 34). For now,

Delving Deeper:
The Stratum Medium

The stratum medium contains three zones of tubules that differ in both density and moisture content. The outermost zone is the driest and most dense, while the inner one contains the most water and is the least dense. This arrangement helps dampen the transfer of energy as it passes into the foot, diminishing the threat of wall cracks and aiding in the protection of the coffin bone. The higher moisture content of the inner zones also helps ensure that when cracks do occur, they are more likely to run up and down in the drier, more brittle outer zone, and not inward toward the critical inner structures of the hoof.

This beneficial tendency for cracks to run vertically and remain superficial also has to do with the characteristics of the intertubular horn. Containing microscopic, reinforcing fibers, the composite material of the intertubular horn forms right angles with the tubules. The hoof wall is stronger and more rigid along this plane, having nearly three times the fracture resistance of the tubules. For this reason, the tubules are more likely to crack than the intertubular horn, with the drier exterior tubules being the most likely to fracture. This is the hoof's way of trying to keep cracks on the surface, where they do the least damage. Anything that compromises the health of the hoof wall (for example, nutritional deficits,

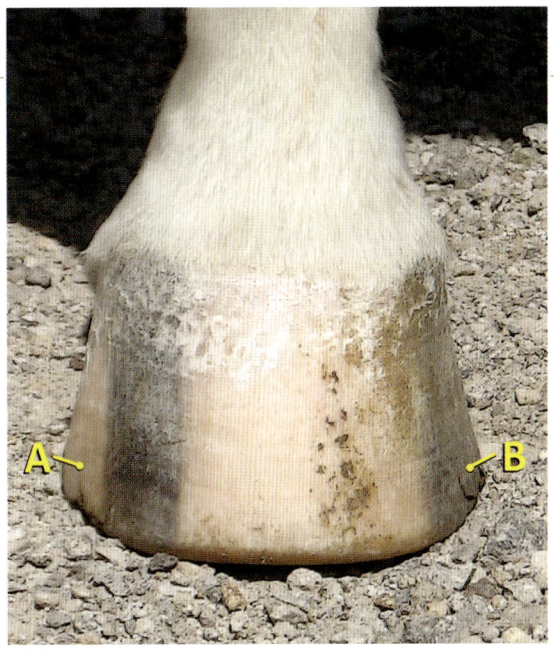

2.5 This rocky terrain striped foot, due for a trim, has minor but equal chipping in the white lateral quarter (A) and the black medial quarter (B)—see fig. 2.7 for location of hoof regions. If the old myth about white horn being weaker were true, it would be chipping and wearing more in the white sections.

metabolic problems, hoof imbalance) can weaken the hoof wall, leaving it more vulnerable to deeper, more serious cracks.

One thing that does *not* make the stratum medium weaker is being white in color. While many people still believe that white feet are softer and poorer quality than black feet, scientific studies have proven otherwise. White feet have exactly the same structure and strength as their black counterparts. The only difference is pigmentation, which has no influence on moisture content, rigidity, or how much force the wall can withstand. Add to this the fact that almost all horse hooves become white or mostly white about halfway through the stratum medium, and you can see that the myth of white horn being weaker simply doesn't hold up to scrutiny (fig. 2.5). It is true, though, that hoof wall blemishes such as cracks and bruises are more visible on white hooves than on dark ones, so this may be why this myth gets perpetuated.

Stratum tectorium
(periople remnant)

Stratum medium (outer zone)

Stratum medium (middle zone)

Stratum medium (inner zone)

Stratum internum
(epidermal lamellae)

2.6 The hoof horn becomes less pigmented and less dense as it gets closer to the coffin bone (see fig. I, p. 3).

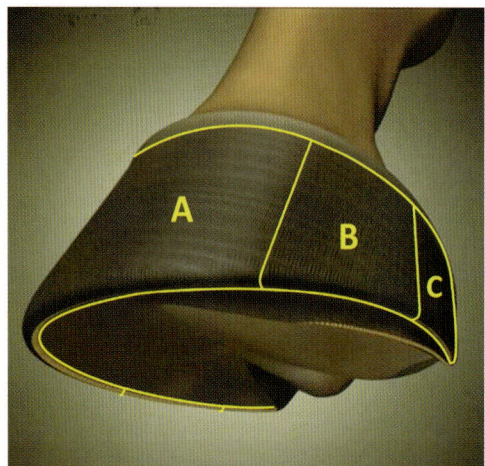

2.7 Knowing the names for the regions of the wall is helpful when communicating with vets and hoof-care professionals. In this illustration, (A) is the toe, (B) is the quarter, and (C) is the heel.

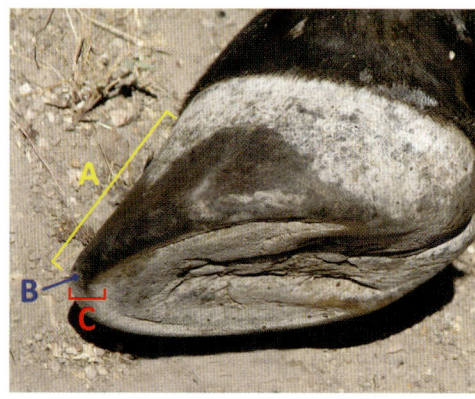

2.8 This wild horse's foot shows the shorter toe (A) and beveled edge (B) that is produced by a very active life on rough terrain. Note the thickness of the toe wall (C), despite the continual wear.

take a look at this cross-section of the hoof horn and see how the various layers differ in both color and structure (fig. 2.6).

Hoof Wall Regions

The hoof wall is often spoken of with reference to three distinct regions: the toe, the quarters, and the heels. Each region spans the entire height of the wall from the periople down, then wraps around to include the bottom edge of the wall that touches the ground (fig. 2.7).

The Toe

The toe region has the starring role in the process of *breakover*, where the heel lifts off the ground and the whole foot rotates over the toe, which digs in and pushes to propel the horse forward (see *Understanding Breakover*, p. 95). The toe is, therefore,

subject to a unique set of stresses, but is well equipped to cope with them.

The horn in this region is thicker than in any other part of the wall and has a dense arrangement of horn tubules, characteristics that provide stiffness and allow the toe to resist wear. Even so, the toes on an active, barefoot horse may wear to be relatively short and take on a beveled or rounded edge, more so in abrasive terrain. This may seem alarming if you are used to the sharp, flat edge and long toes often seen in the feet of shod horses, but it is very rarely cause for alarm (fig. 2.8).

The Quarters

The quarters of the wall tend to differ a little from one another, even in the healthiest feet. Like the toe, the medial quarter has a dense arrangement of tubules, while the lateral quarter tubules are slightly less dense than either the toe or the medial quarter. The medial quarter also tends to be thicker and a

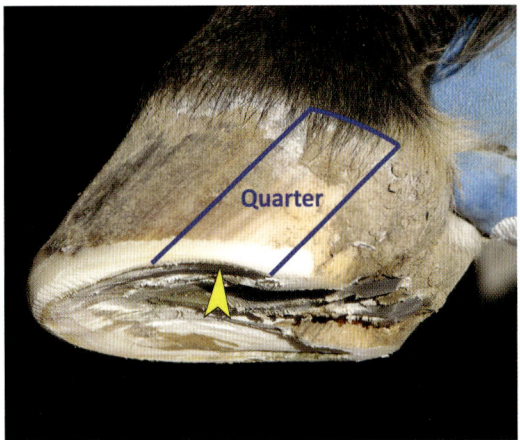

2.9 The natural scoop (yellow arrow) in the quarters of this foot adds to its flexibility and shock-absorbing capabilities. You can see that the arch along the bottom of the wall follows the arch that is present in the sole.

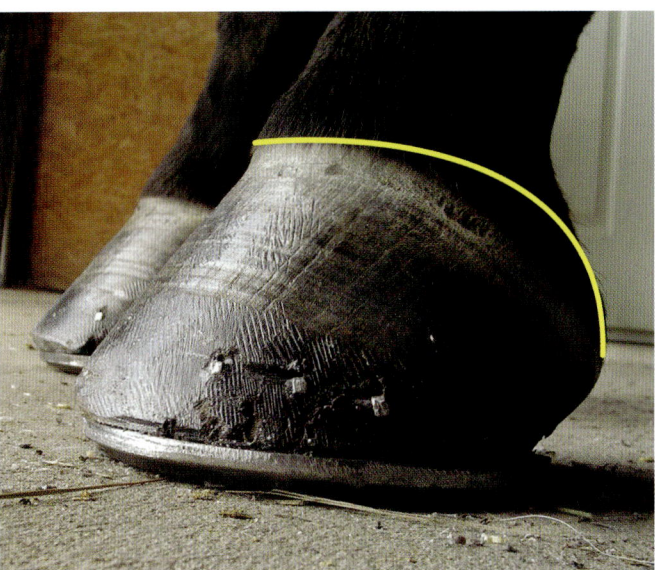

2.10 While the quarters on this foot are trimmed flat to sit flush with the shoe, they are a healthy height, which is reflected by the very gentle curve in the hairline. Quarters that are left too long will push upward or "jam," thus distorting the hairline upward and leaving it shaped more like the yellow line in this photo. Heels that have migrated forward can also cause an upward curve in the hairline. Either way, too much curve is indicative of a problem.

bit more upright than its counterpart, giving it more load-carrying capacity. This reflects the fact that most horses bear more weight on the medial sides of their limbs and hooves.

The quarters on healthy bare feet often have what is called a "scoop" to them, meaning that there is a bit of an upward curve in the quarters when viewed from the side (fig. 2.9). This front-to-back arch is part of the natural shape of many optimally functioning feet, allowing the foot to flex more when weighted than if the foot is flat along the bottom of the quarters. Though it may not look significant, having scooped quarters increases the shock-absorbing capacity of the foot, offering some additional protection for the coffin bone, and is thus considered a positive feature.

However, it is a big mistake to try to force the walls to take on this shape if the sole doesn't allow for it. The trimming of the hoof wall, including the quarters, should be a reflection of what the sole

dictates, not the other way around. If the live sole has a scoop in the area adjacent to the quarters, follow that shape and you will have a scoop in the quarters. But carving a "fake" scoop into a foot with a flat sole will only thin the sole in that area, which is not going to improve function and could make the horse sore.

Feet that are shod are generally rasped flat across the quarters in order for the wall to fit flush against the shoe. However, it is important that the quarters not be allowed to get too long (tall), as this may cause them to "jam" upward, a common problem that shows up most often as a significant curve or bulge upward in the hairline above the quarters (fig. 2.10). An upward bulge in the hairline can also be caused by heels that have been allowed to migrate forward or "underrun," which causes the hairline to push upward.

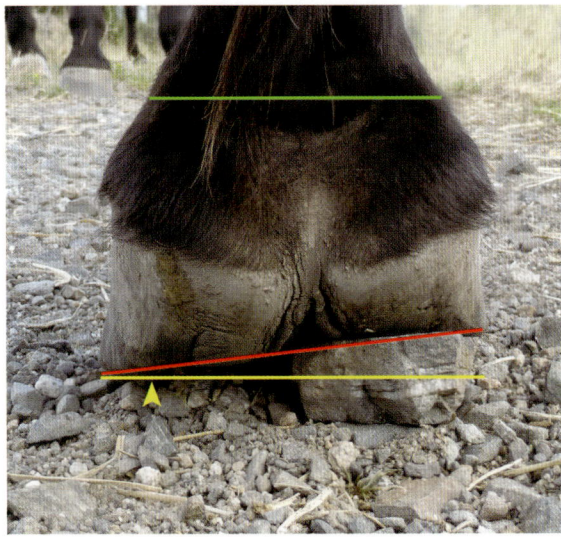

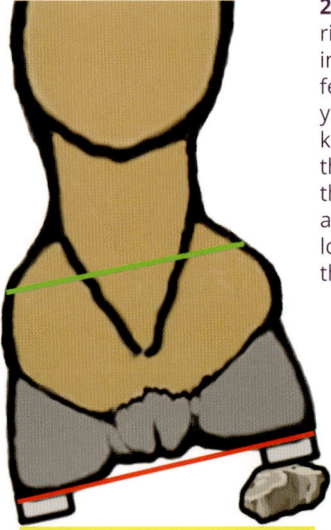

2.12 Typical steel shoes are too rigid to allow the heels to flex independently. Think of what it feels like to twist your ankle, and you'll get the idea of what this kind of torque might be doing to the horse's joints. Notice that in this image, the angle of the joint above the foot (green line) is no longer in parallel alignment with the ground (yellow line).

2.11 The heels of the horse are designed to flex and compress independently of one another, as seen here. While the right heel is lifted and compressed by the rock, the left heel is still in contact with the ground (yellow arrow). When the heels can flex independently like this, the joints and bones of the entire distal limb are best able to maintain good alignment on uneven ground. Note that the angle of the joint above the foot (green line) remains parallel with the ground (yellow line) in correct alignment, despite the divergent angle of the heels (red line).

The Heels

The heels, aided by the frog, are designed to bear the brunt of the impact forces generated when the hoof makes contact with the ground. You would think the heels, therefore, are the thickest part of the wall, but they actually have thinner wall horn than the toe or the quarters. This allows this region to flex in and out, as well as up and down, when the hoof lands, thus acting as an important component of the shock-absorption system of the foot. The heels of a barefoot horse can also flex independently of one another, which helps prevent torque on the joints on uneven ground (fig. 2.11), when doing lateral movements, or when circling. This independent flexion is greatly inhibited by rigid shoes, which could contribute to joint damage over time (fig. 2.12). Plastic shoes do allow the heels to flex independently, which may provide some health advantages over steel shoes.

Exterior Hoof Anatomy—
Solar View

The solar view of the hoof shows us a feast of features designed to share in the jobs of weight bearing, energy dissipation, and protection of the interior of the foot (fig. 3.1 A).

The Water Line

In the toe cross-section in figure 3.1 B, you can see the pigmented horn of the outer wall, and the unpigmented inner horn, which is usually fairly white when it is not stained from ground contact. On the bottom of the foot, this strip of inner horn is referred to as the *water line*, which is appropriate given that the inner zones of the wall contain more moisture, which also makes them softer. However, the pigmented part of the wall does not always end in a nice, even line. In some feet, it is patchy or wavers in and out, making the water line look very irregular.

Occasionally, a foot will be black all the way through, while white feet have no pigment at all in

3.1 B This cross-section gives a clear view of the pigmented wall and the unpigmented "water line." It also shows that black feet are almost always white under the surface, so the old myth about black feet being stronger than white feet just doesn't make a whole lot of sense.

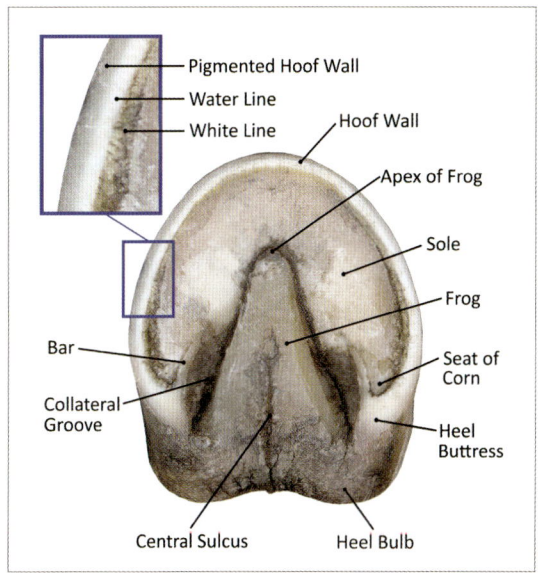

3.1 A The features visible here all play key roles in helping the foot cope with the enormous forces generated when the hoof is in contact with the ground.

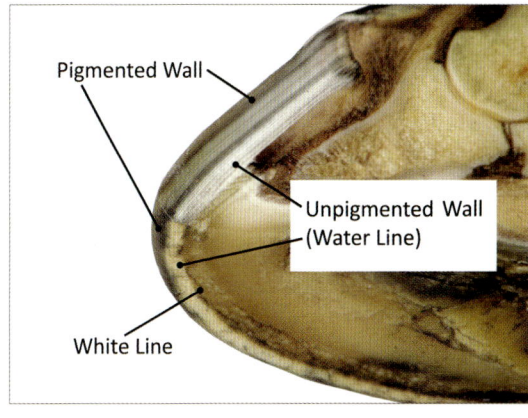

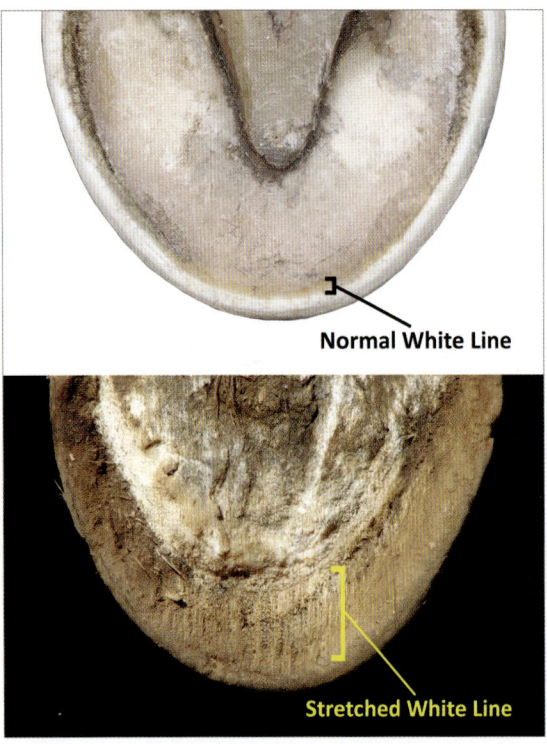

3.2 The foot in the upper photo has a normal white line, forming a tight seam between the wall and the sole. The Miniature Horse foot in the bottom photo shows dramatic widening of the white line, which is called "stretching." In this Mini mare's case, the stretching was caused by chronic laminitis.

Normal White Line

Stretched White Line

the outer wall, which can make it harder to see the transition between the outer wall and the water line. Typically, the outer wall horn on white feet will be more yellowish or ivory colored, while the water line will appear whiter. Some hooves will have a thin water line in relation to the pigmented wall; others will have the exact opposite. So, while some barefoot trimmers talk about using the water line as a guide for where to begin the bevel or rolling of the toe, trying to figure out where that "line" actually is can be a challenge.

The White Line

To the inside of the water line is the junction where the wall meets the sole, which is called the *white line*.

Yes, it is definitely confusing that the white line *isn't* white (it is yellowish or grayish depending on the pigmentation), while the water line usually *is*. What is important to know is that the white line is the only externally visible part of the *laminae*, the fabulously strong connective tissues that attach the hoof wall to the bone inside the foot (see *The Laminae*, p. 34).

Even more important is to get really familiar with your own horse's white lines, because the appearance of these structures provides important clues about what is going on inside the feet. A healthy white line will look like a tight seam, as you see in figures 3.1 A and 3.1 B. Any widening of the white line, called "stretching," indicates some degree of failure in the attachment of the hoof wall to the coffin bone. When the white line stretches, you can often see part of the epidermal laminae, which look a bit like the gills on the underside of a mushroom (fig. 3.2). We'll talk more about the implications of stretched white lines later (see *Laminitis*, p. 163).

The Heel Buttresses, Bars, and Seat of Corn

At the back of the foot, the wall angles back on itself to form the *heel buttresses*, then continues on to form the *bars*. These structures are designed to share in weight bearing, energy dissipation, and support. The heel buttresses should be widely spaced and well back, lining up with the widest part of the frog. The farther forward they are of this position, the less able they are to support the bony column of the leg. Ideally, the heel buttresses are relatively thick, so they are less likely to crush.

The bars are ideally straight and upright, but many perfectly sound horses show variation in the shape of their bars without any apparent issues. As for weight bearing, the bars may be partially or totally passive if the horse is on flat, hard ground, but this is changed when the foot is on a more pliable surface. The relative position of the bars to the ground also changes when the foot is loaded during active use. Under load, the walls flex outward and the sole flattens to a degree, moving the bars toward the ground. They are actually meant to "bottom out," as that is when they can play their part in helping to keep the coffin bone suspended.

The area of sole where the hoof wall angles back to form the bars is called the *seat of corn*. It gets its name from the fact that this is where horses can get "corns," which is just the old-time but still-in-use name for bruises in that area. Hoof-care professionals often use the level of the live sole at the seat of corn to determine the correct height of the heels.

The Sole

The *sole*, like the wall, is composed of both tubular and intertubular horn, though it is less dense, more porous, and more flexible than the wall horn. The sole horn is produced by the *solar corium*, which lines the surface of the bottom of the coffin bone.

In a healthy hoof, the live sole will have a fairly uniform thickness ranging from a little over ½ inch to about ¾ inch across the entire foot. Healthy live sole has a smooth, waxy appearance, while exfoliating or "dead" sole has a rough, sometimes chalky appearance (fig. 3.3).

The horse's sole is similar to your skin in the sense that the cells grow to a certain point, and then they become non-functional and slough off. In a dry climate, the exfoliating material on the sole will tend

to accumulate and won't abrade away as easily as it does in wet environments. If the foot has been dry for a while, built up some dead sole, then suddenly gets wet, the exfoliating sole will tend to start falling out at a rapid rate—often in rough chunks or big flakes. This can look alarming, almost like the bottom of the foot is falling off, but it is a normal reaction to a changing environment.

In most cases, exfoliating sole can be left alone, and it may even provide some extra protection for the foot. It will tend to flake off or pop out on its own when the foot no longer needs it. Occasionally, however, a horse will get a buildup of dense, exfoliating sole that causes problems for the foot and will need to be removed (see *Retained Sole,* p. 126).

Should the Sole Be Weight Bearing?

Hoof-care experts differ in their opinions about whether or not the sole is designed to be weight bearing. One long-held view is that the walls are

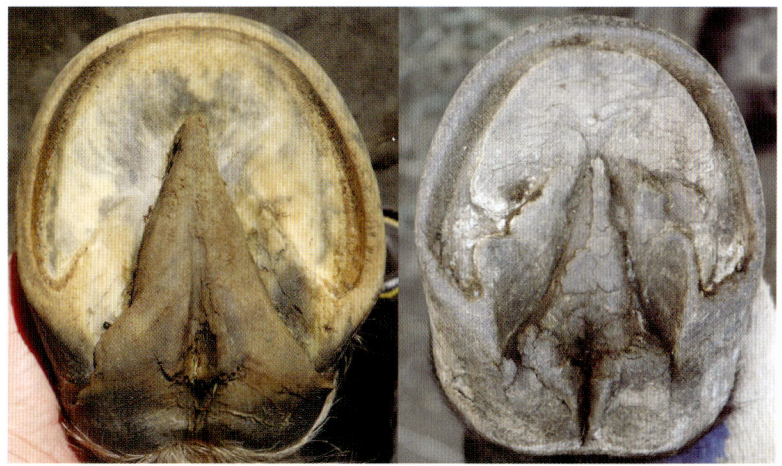

3.3 The foot on the left shows the smooth, waxy appearance of live sole, while the one on the right has a dry, chalky layer of exfoliating sole that is starting to peel off. Note that the frog on the right is peeling as well—a normal process at certain times of the year.

pretty much exclusive in the weight-bearing department, but many no longer agree with this theory. Some, like Robert Bowker, VMD, PhD (see sidebar below), now say that trimming or shoeing the hoof so that the walls are the exclusive weight-bearing structure is damaging, as they believe the hoof was never designed to "hang" from the laminae. Simple observation tells us that a healthy hoof on a hard, inflexible surface (for example, concrete) will be standing on its walls with the sole lifted off the ground to some degree due to the natural concavity of the foot. But, move the same horse onto a conformable surface like grass, dirt, or sand, and the sole will be sharing the load. Since modern horses evolved in grassland areas with mostly conformable surfaces, it seems logical that the soles are meant

Delving Deeper: Four on the Floor

Professor Emeritus Robert Bowker, VMD, PhD, former director of the Equine Foot Laboratory at the College of Veterinary Medicine at Michigan State University, has done research that shows that the frog plays an important role in the development and protection of the internal structures of the foot. But, in order to do this, it must be in contact with the ground. As Dr. Bowker explains:

"It is critical to have the frog on the ground, not only because this stimulates the development of the structures inside the foot designed to support and protect the bones, but also because the frog itself dissipates part of the energy of impact through its fibrocartilaginous inner mass, if the frog has been allowed to develop properly. That fibrocartilage contains a lot of proteoglycans—which are compounds that bind water—and it's that fluid that dissipates the energy. Think of the gel pads used in many high-end running shoes, and you'll get some idea of how this helps the frog."

The contact the frog makes with the ground is also critical for another reason: it is the main way the horse feels the characteristics of the surface it is moving on. This process, called *proprioception*, allows the horse to orient his feet properly to respond to changes in the ground. Pressure on the frog is transmitted to specialized nerves called proprioceptors, located mostly within the digital cushion. Through these proprioceptors, the horse can tell when the ground becomes harder or softer, when he has stepped on a rock, or that the ground has started to slope downward or upward. Strong proprioception and the ability to respond to those signals help prevent injury and make a horse "sure-footed."

And, as if those things weren't important enough, pressure on the frog is a big part of Dr. Bowker's theory of *hemodynamic flow*, in which the hoof moves extra blood into the back of the foot on impact, where the fluid then assists in energy dissipation. The next moment, when pressure on the frog is released, the blood gets boosted back up the leg. In this way, the hooves assist circulation through the whole body, acting like four extra hearts.

to share in the work of supporting the weight of the horse. Barefoot hoof-care expert Pete Ramey puts it this way: "Nature would not and did not put anything on the bottom of the horse that was not intended to bear weight. The wall, sole, bars, and frog should be sharing the load."

Master Farrier Gene Ovnicek also endorses this concept. "This may sound odd from someone who puts shoes on horses, but I agree that the sole is designed to share in weight bearing. In light of that, we encourage that dirt packed into the bottom of the shoe not be cleaned out, as it helps to maintain that sole support function." He notes, however, that muck and manure should be cleaned out from the bottom of the foot, and it is okay to clean out the feet before a competition. "At other times, leave

None of this amazing stuff can happen the way it is supposed to when the frog is lifted off the ground by long hoof walls and/or shoes, something Dr. Bowker calls *peripheral loading* (figs. 3.4 A & B). Dr. Bowker believes that peripheral loading is a major factor in many kinds of hoof problems, particularly those involving pain in the back of the foot.

However, it is extremely important to distinguish between a healthy frog on a healthy foot making ground contact, and a prolapsed frog on a weak foot making ground contact. You also have to take into account factors like what kind of footing the horse spends the majority of his time on, as a frog that is slightly off the ground on a hard, flat surface may be well in contact with the ground when the footing is soft. (For more on these factors, see *Physiologically Correct Hoof Care,* p. 247.)

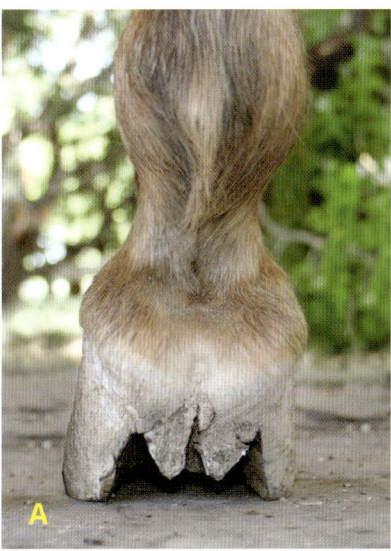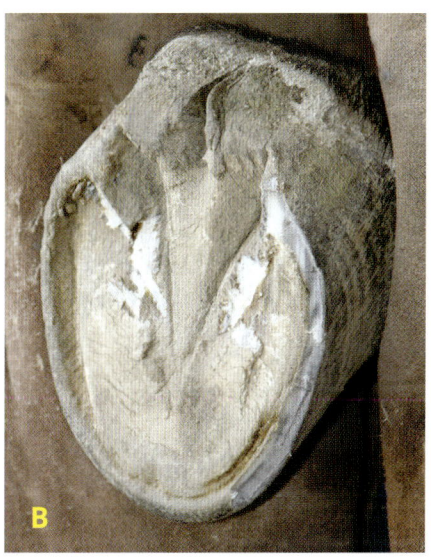

3.4 A & B When the walls of the foot grow too long, they can lift the frog right off the ground, compromising the health and function of the entire foot (A). Even though the frog on this foot has grown very thick and the shoe has been pulled, the frog still can't touch the ground to support the back of the foot. Peripheral loading is common among shod horses, but it can also occur in barefoot horses (B). This foot is mid trim, with the right side having been lowered to eliminate the peripheral loading caused by the slightly long wall seen on the left side.

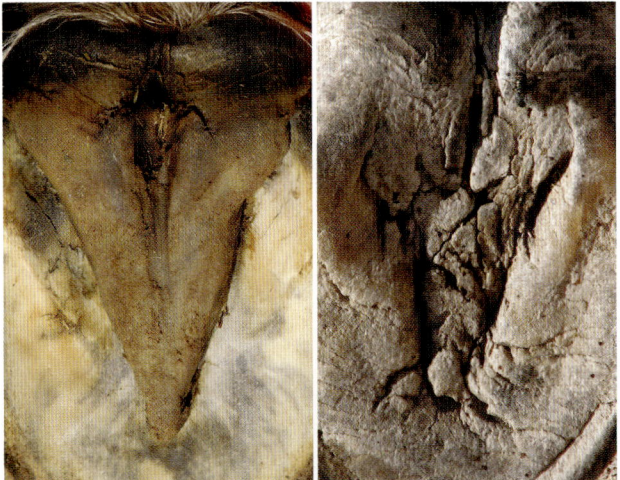

3.5 The appearance of the frog will vary tremendously depending on how much moisture is in the environment. The frog on the left has the smooth, full, rubbery look typical of a wet climate. The frog on the right is from a dry, rocky area.

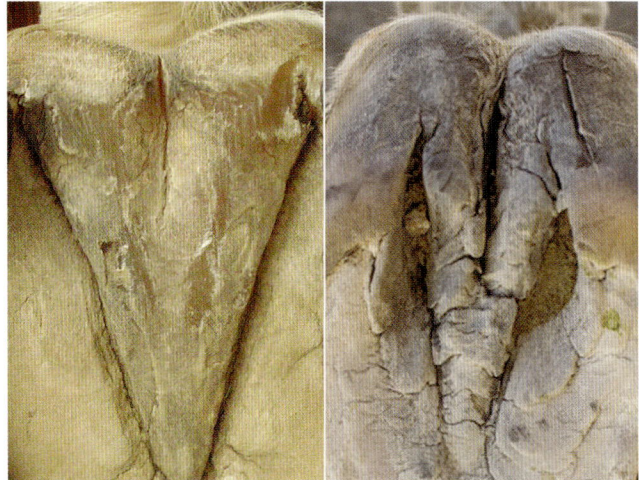

3.6 On the left is a central sulcus with the wide, shallow look of good health. The sulcus on the right is narrow and deep, indicating disease.

the dirt packed in nice and firm" (see more in the sidebar, p. 21).

The Frog

The arrow-shaped structure on the bottom of the foot is called the *frog*, and it is truly a multipurpose wonder. It provides traction, helps the foot to read the ground, provides cushioning, and helps move blood through the foot as it compresses and decompresses with each step. In a climate with reasonable moisture, a healthy frog will be wide and plump with a rubbery feel to it. In low-moisture, rough-terrain areas, the frog may become drier, harder, narrower, and more vaulted as it adapts to the environment (fig. 3.5).

And here is a little known fact: the frog actually has *apocrine sweat glands*, like those found in our

armpits. They secrete an odorless film that can get a bit smelly when it is broken down by bacteria. However, this odor is different from the noxious, rotting stench of the frog infection known as "thrush" (see *Thrush*, p. 115). While people might give you a look for sniffing around your horse's feet, it is a good idea to get familiar with the normal odors of the frog and other parts of the foot, as this can help you clue in when something is going wrong.

Central Sulcus

Toward the rear of the frog is an indentation called the *central sulcus*, also known as the *central cleft*. In a healthy foot, this feature is no more than a shallow depression, looking somewhat like the impression a thumb would make when pressed into firm clay. Unfortunately, the central sulci of many domestic horses often show evidence of disease, forming deep cracks that can run far up between the heel bulbs and penetrate far into the sensitive tissues of the frog (fig. 3.6).

The Collateral Grooves

On either side of the frog lie the *collateral grooves*, which are the juncture between the frog, the bars, and the sole. These clefts act like expansion joints, allowing the sole to flex to a

much greater degree than it would be able to if it were one solid mass. They also increase traction, providing extra grip like the ridges on the sole of a hiking boot. Like the central sulcus, the part of the frog that lies within the collateral grooves is vulnerable to thrush.

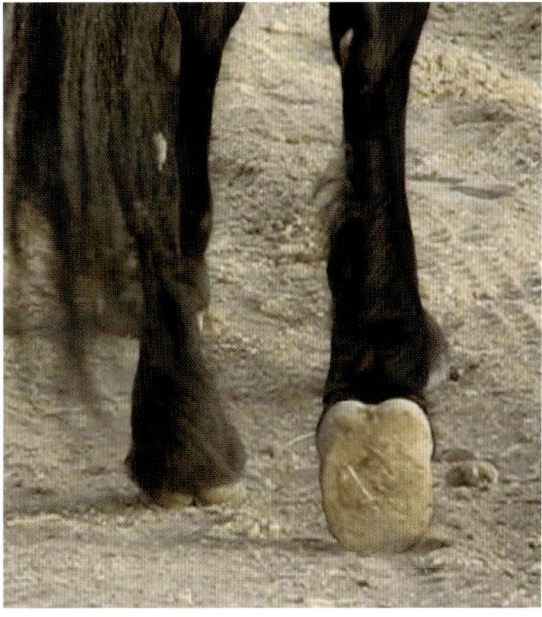

3.7 This free-roaming horse may be getting extra foot protection from the moist dirt packed into the bottom of his foot.

Good, Clean Dirt

There are times when dirt will pack into the collateral grooves, and even the entire bottom of the foot, especially when the ground is soft and moist. Some experts, like Master Farrier Gene Ovnicek, now believe that the hoof is *designed* for this to happen, as the compressed dirt provides a bit of extra protection and support, similar to a man-made hoof pad. This would be most useful to the hoof when the ground is soft and moist. Why? Because at such times, the sole absorbs moisture from the environment and becomes softer itself, and is thus less protective and supportive than when it is hard and dry. The packed-in dirt may be just the thing to compensate for the more moist sole.

Does this mean we should not clean out the dirt that collects in the feet of our horses? That depends. In horses living a free-roaming lifestyle in large areas, the soil packed into the foot is likely to be "clean" dirt,

free of manure and urine (fig. 3.7). This type of dirt may provide benefit to the horse. But, most domestic horses live in much smaller spaces and often walk through manure and urine-soaked dirt, which can create the perfect breeding ground for bacteria and fungi harmful to the hoof. If the dirt in the foot is likely to contain any manure or urine, it should be cleaned out as often as possible.

4 Interior Hoof Anatomy

The Coffin Bone

The hoof is the foundation of the horse, and the *coffin bone*, located inside the hoof, is the foundation of the horse's skeleton (see fig. I, p. 3). Small but incredibly strong, this little bone sports five commonly used names: *coffin bone*, *pedal bone*, *third phalanx*, *P3*, and *distal phalanx*. For the purposes of this book, we will refer to it as either the coffin bone or P3.

Whatever you call it, the coffin bone is a remarkable structure. Its shape alone shows us that Mother Nature is one heck of an engineer. With its roughly cone-shaped outer surface and its curved bottom, the coffin bone works a lot like the arches seen in Roman bridges and similar structures, spreading compression forces through the entire bone and reducing the effects of tension on the underside (fig. 4.1). This natural arch gives a tiny bone the ability to hold up to the whopping loads created by a large, heavy animal running at speed. Of course, any structure that has to deal with the continual stresses that the coffin bone experiences is bound to have its problems, so it's not surprising that the coffin bone is often involved in foot-related lameness.

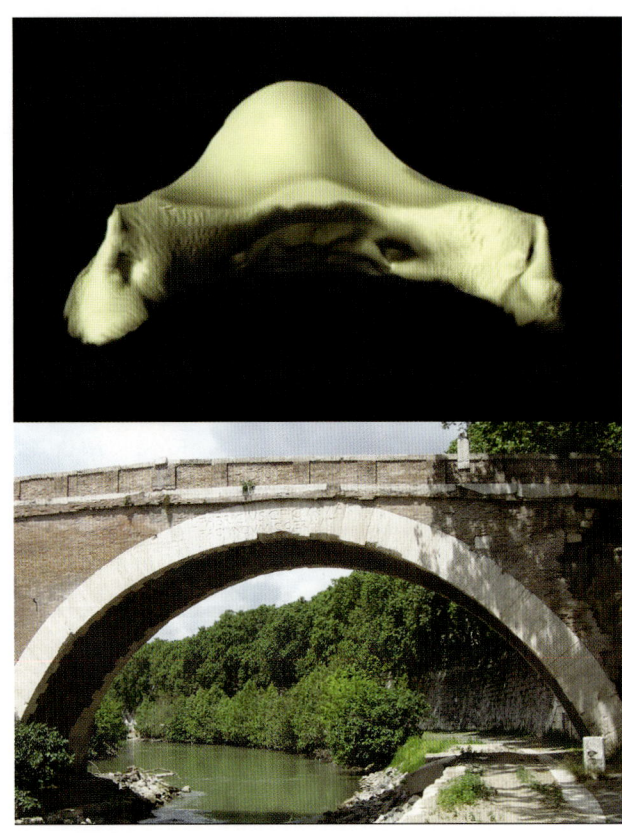

4.1 Viewed from the back, it is easy to see the natural vault on the bottom surface of the coffin bone (top), which is similar to the sturdy arch of a Roman bridge (bottom).

What It Should Look Like

The coffin bones of the front feet are shaped a little differently than those of the hind. The front bones are usually a little more rounded and the hind bones are slightly more pointed, which is reflected by the shapes of the feet. The front bones also have a lower angle than the hind, which is reflected in the angles of the feet (figs. 4.2 & 4.3).

The edge around the bottom of a healthy coffin bone (called the *distal border* or the *solar margin*, for you technical types) is crisp and almost sharp (fig. 4.4). Bone loss and damage from various conditions such as laminitis can make the edge change shape or become ragged. In the worst cases, the whole front portion of the bone may dissolve away (see *Laminitis*, p. 163).

Some coffin bones have a small notch in the

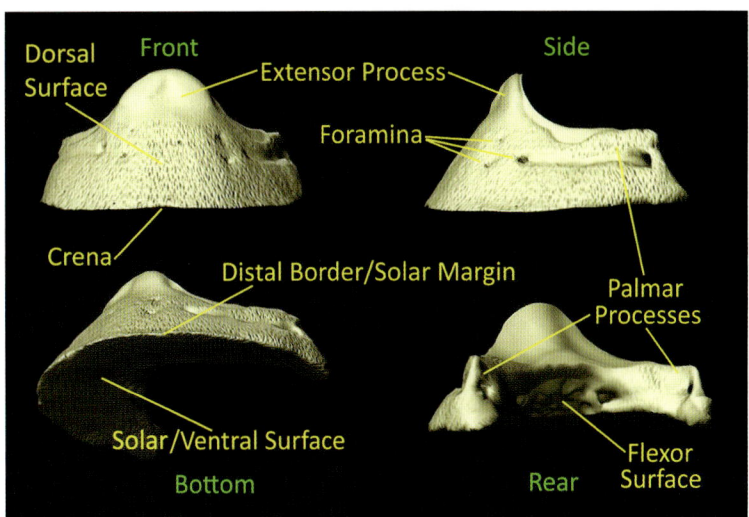

4.2 Coffin bone: four views—front, side, bottom, and rear.

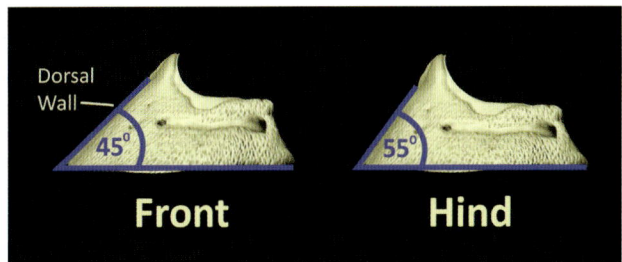

4.3 When comparing the front and hind coffin bones, it is normal for the angle of the dorsal (front) surface to be shallower on the bones of the front feet and more upright on the hind feet, as seen here. Front feet generally range from about 45–50 degrees, while the hind feet usually fall in the range of 50–60 degrees.

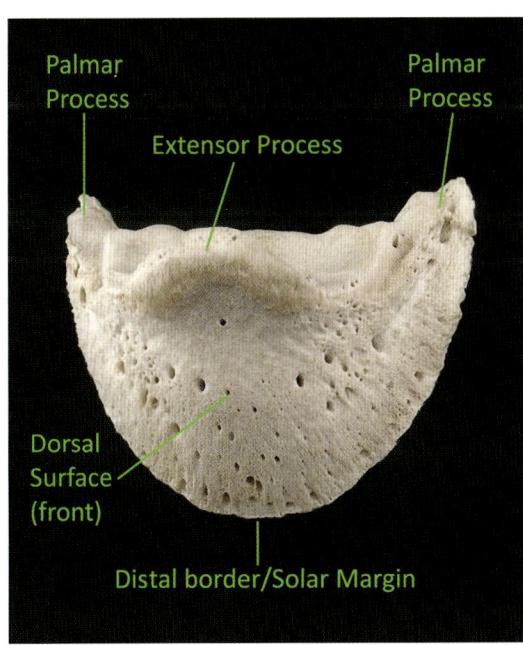

4.4 A healthy coffin bone has a crisp, relatively smooth distal border.

center of the bottom edge called a *crena*. When it is very small, the crena is considered a normal feature, but it is sometimes relatively large, in which case it may be reflected by the presence of a visible notch in the center toe of the sole and/or white line. This notched area will fill in with material that is not as strong and organized as regular wall horn, but even so, the presence of a crena is normally not anything to worry about. Though it might make a horse a little more susceptible to a toe crack or white line

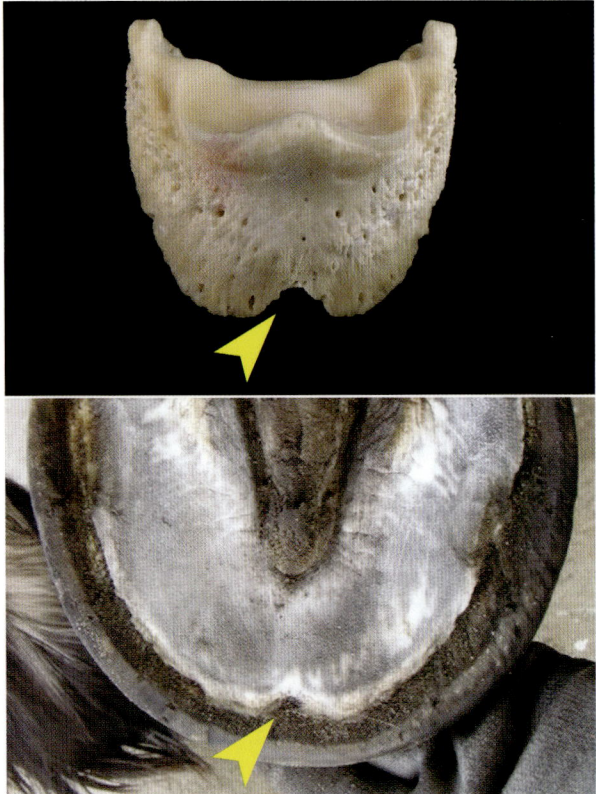

4.5 When the coffin bone has a larger than normal indentation or "crena" at the center of the solar margin (yellow arrow above), it will often be reflected externally in the sole/wall junction (yellow arrow below). This can make the foot more vulnerable to toe cracks.

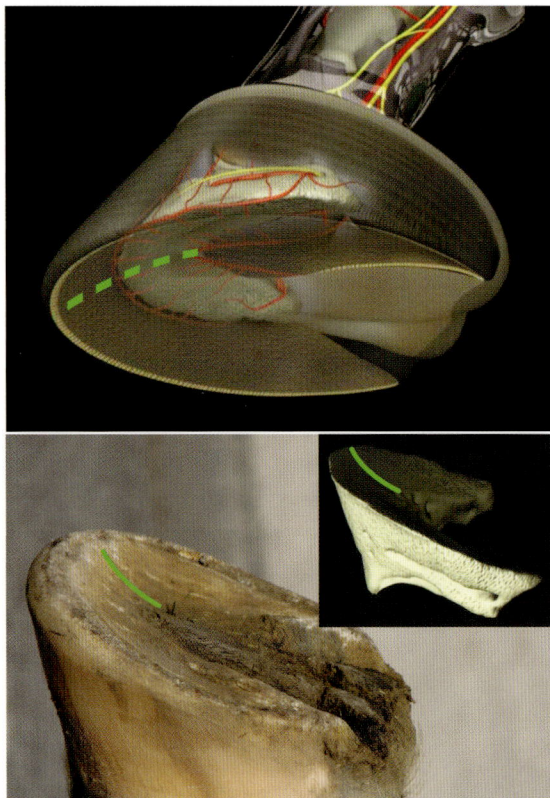

4.6 The dashed green line in the top image shows how the cup of the sole echoes the shape of the bottom of the coffin bone. On a real foot like the one in the bottom photo, you can't see the coffin bone, but if you could, it would generally show a similar degree of concavity as the sole (green lines), unless the sole had a buildup of exfoliating material.

disease (see pp. 134 and 55), it should not be a problem with regular, good farrier care (fig. 4.5).

A normal coffin bone is somewhat porous and also has a number of small perforations that pass all the way through. These little inlets, called *foramina*, allow blood vessels to pass through the bone. If the coffin bone is more porous than usual, however, you are looking at bone loss.

The solar (palmar/plantar) surface of the coffin bone is concave or "vaulted," but the degree of concavity is more pronounced in some horses than in

others. In a healthy hoof, the sole echoes the vault of the bone (fig. 4.6).

How It Attaches to Other Parts

The coffin bone is anchored to the hoof capsule (the "shell" formed by the entire hoof wall) by the interlocking laminae (see *The Laminae,* p. 34). The strength of this attachment keeps the coffin bone suspended within the hoof capsule, preventing it from crushing the blood vessels and other tissues that lie between the bone and the sole. If the

The "Correct" Palmar/Plantar Angle of the Coffin Bone

There are two schools of thought on what the "correct" angle of the coffin bone should be. Some argue that the bottom (palmar for the fronts, plantar for the hinds) edges of the sides of the bone should be parallel to the ground, while others believe they should have a "positive palmar/plantar angle," which is just a fancy way of saying they should be slightly higher in the back.

The "ground parallel" camp believes that lining up the bone with the ground when the horse is standing still (stance phase) allows the best distribution of load forces around the entire bone when the horse is in motion. They say that if the bone were higher in the back, there would be unnatural stresses on various parts of the bone and connecting tissues during loading.

The "positive palmar/plantar angle" folks argue that at peak loading, when the distribution of forces is most critical, the heels expand and effectively "squish down," allowing the back of the coffin bone to drop. This results in a ground parallel position when it is actually needed, whereas if you start out with a bone that is ground parallel during the stance phase, it will actually be in a negative palmar/plantar angle during peak loading. When you add in the fact that sound horses typically land heel first when traveling at any pace above an average walk, this argument becomes hard to ignore (fig. 4.7). Most experts agree that a

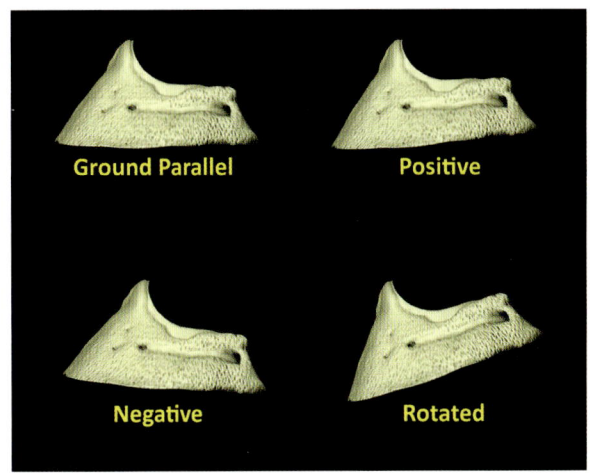

4.7 While there is still some debate over whether a healthy coffin bone should be "ground parallel" or have a "slightly positive angle," most experts believe the latter.

slightly positive palmar/plantar angle of approximately 2–5 degrees is correct.

What everyone agrees on is that a negative palmar/plantar angle is a problem, as it indicates serious issues with hoof balance, mechanics, disease, or all of them. It will also place the important structures in the back of the foot under a great amount of pressure and strain. There is also no argument that a coffin bone tipped or rotated too far forward is harmful. Not only can this damage the bone itself, but it can also harm the solar corium (see p. 37) as the tip of the bone pushes down into it.

Reminder: If you're being technically correct, you would use "palmar angle" to refer to the front feet, and "plantar angle" to refer to the hind. However, in common parlance, many people use "palmar angle" to talk about both.

laminae become damaged, as they do in the disease process called *laminitis* (commonly called "founder"), they can pull apart, allowing the coffin bone to move within the hoof capsule.

Another important area of attachment is the *extensor process* (see fig. 4.2, p. 23), which forms the bump at the top center of the dorsal surface. It is cleverly called the extensor process because the *digital extensor tendon* (see p. 28) attaches to the coffin bone in this spot. These parts are named for their function, which—surprise, surprise—is to extend or swing the toe forward when the extensor muscles contract. Viewed in a side view X-ray, the top of the extensor process should be close to level with the coronet band. In cases where the coffin bone has "sunk" or rotated due to chronic laminitis, the extensor process will be significantly lower than the coronet (see *Laminitis*, p. 163).

On either side at the rear of the coffin bone are the *palmar processes*, also known as the "wings" of the coffin bone (see fig. 4.2, p. 23). These wedges of bone are not present at birth, but develop over time as the horse matures. The palmar processes help give the back of the foot its shape and also serve

as an attachment point for the collateral cartilages, which are small sheets of fibrous cartilage that give form, support, and flexibility to the back of the foot. On the central bottom surface of the coffin bone, about where the palmar processes begin, is the *flexor surface* (see fig. 4.2, p. 23). This is where the *deep digital flexor tendon* (DDFT) attaches to the coffin bone. The DDFT pulls the foot backward and up (see p. 28).

The Navicular Bone, aka the Distal Sesamoid

The terms "navicular disease" or "navicular syndrome" strike fear into the heart of horse owners, as a diagnosis of either one has often meant progressive disability for the horse. However, we now know that what is called navicular disease or navicular syndrome may actually be one or more of a number of different problems that all cause pain in the back part of the foot, though most of them have nothing to do with the *navicular bone*. Still, it is important to understand what the navicular bone is and what it does, as it is so commonly discussed as a possible source of heel pain.

Where It Is

The navicular bone, also called the *distal sesamoid*, is an unassuming little wedge of bone sometimes described as being shaped like a boat or a flying saucer (fig. 4.8). It is located at the back of the coffin bone, between the palmar processes (fig. 4.9). It is held in place by two *collateral ligaments*, which attach it to the short pastern bone (P2), and by the *impar ligament*, which attaches it to the coffin bone. It is protected by several different kinds of tissue,

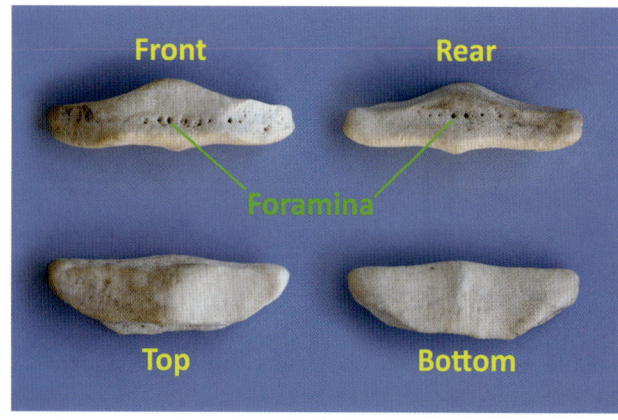

4.8 The navicular bone gets its name from the Latin word *navicula,* which means "little ship." It does look a bit like a boat when viewed from the top or bottom. Note the foramina that pass through from front to rear.

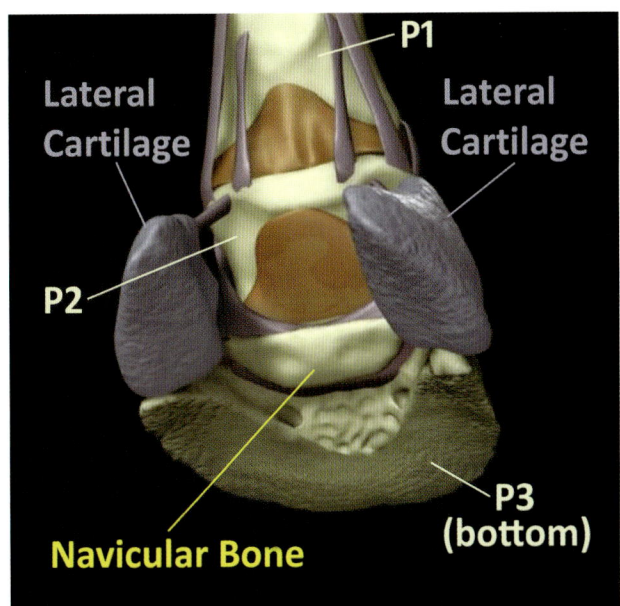

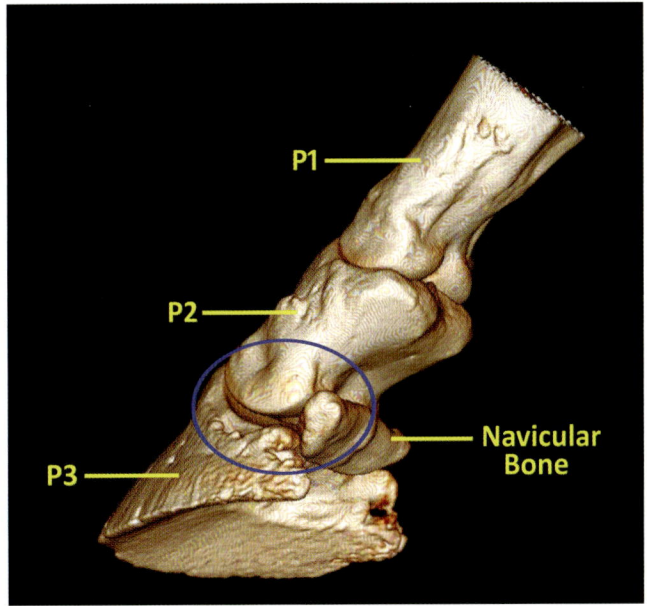

4.9 This view of the navicular bone shows its location tucked up against the back of the coffin bone. In real life, it would be covered with bursa, ligaments, and the DDFT (deep digital flexor tendon).

4.10 The coffin joint, circled in blue, is formed by the coffin bone (P3), the short pastern bone (P2), and the navicular bone. In the foot, this joint is surrounded by ligaments, tendons, nerves, and blood vessels.

one of which is the *navicular bursa*—a tiny pouch filled with synovial fluid. The navicular bursa helps the deep digital flexor tendon glide over the navicular bone, and provides a bit of cushioning. The navicular bone, together with the coffin bone (P3) and the short pastern bone (P2) form the *coffin joint* (fig. 4.10), also called the *distal interphalangeal joint*, or the *DIP joint* (P1 is the long pastern bone, see 4.10).

The navicular bone is also shielded from impact by the digital cushion (see p. 32) and the frog. Some researchers and hoof-care professionals believe that inadequate development of one or both of these protective structures—an unfortunately common observation in the feet of domestic horses—may be a contributing factor in the development of pain issues in the back of the foot. Certain hoof

forms and loading patterns can also wreak all sorts of havoc with the navicular bone; we'll talk more about these problems a bit later (see p. 207).

What It Does

The main purpose of the navicular bone is not to bear weight, but to assist the function of the deep digital flexor tendon. It essentially serves as a pulley for the DDFT as it wraps around the bones when the muscles cause the DDFT to contract. Other structures form additional pulleys, and when all these are working together, the navicular bone, short pastern bone, and the fetlock create a long, swooping arc when the muscles contract to reduce the acute angles that would have to occur without the pulleys. This system helps mitigate strain on the deep digital flexor tendon.

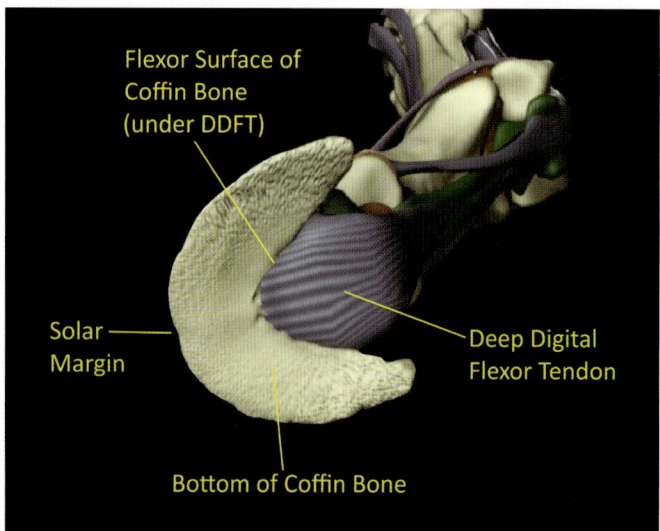

Flexor Surface of
Coffin Bone
(under DDFT)

Solar
Margin

Deep Digital
Flexor Tendon

Bottom of Coffin Bone

4.11 In this view looking up from underneath the coffin bone, you can see how the deep digital flexor tendon attaches to the flexor surface of the bone.

4.12 The digital extensor tendon (DET) moves the toe forward and upward by pulling on the extensor process of the coffin bone.

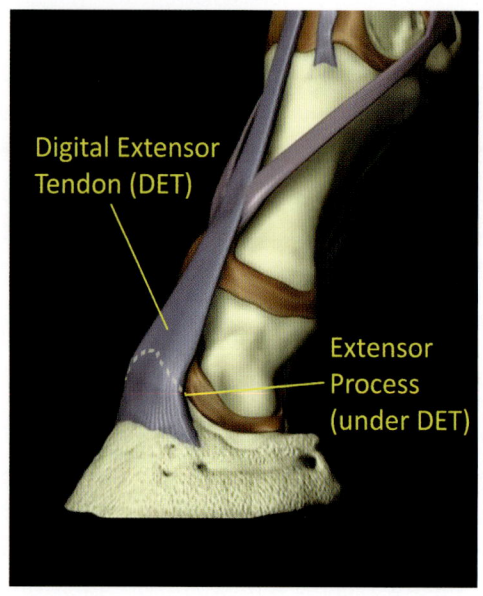

Digital Extensor
Tendon (DET)

Extensor
Process
(under DET)

The Deep Digital Flexor Tendon

The *deep digital flexor tendon* (*DDFT*) runs down the back of the horse's foreleg from the knee down, and on the hind limb, from the hock down. It curves around the navicular bone, and attaches to the underside of the coffin bone (fig. 4.11). The DDFT, operated by its associated muscle, is responsible for flexing the hoof by pulling the toe backward. When the hoof is weight bearing, the DDFT acts like a sling, supporting the navicular bone so that the bone is not over-flexed downward. If it has to deal with abnormal or excessive forces and strain, the DDFT can develop tendonitis, often right around the area where it makes contact with the navicular bone.

The Digital Extensor Tendon

We already talked a little about the *digital extensor tendon* (DET) and how it connects to the coffin bone (p. 26), but just to clarify, the DET is the counterbalance to the DDFT. Like the DDFT, its related muscles lie above the knee and hock, but the tendon itself attaches to that little bump at the top-front-center of the coffin bone called the extensor process. The extensor muscle/tendon unit is responsible for flicking the hoof forward (fig. 4.12).

The Impar Ligament

The *impar ligament* is a short but tough little piece of connective tissue that holds the navicular bone to the back of the coffin bone (fig. 4.13). Diagnostic techniques utilizing MRI have shown us that lesions in this ligament are the cause of lameness in a significant number of cases where horses present with palmar heel pain that would previously have been labeled as navicular syndrome. Anything that places abnormal strain on the back of the foot, whether from something like hoof imbalance or an activity that involves high impact, a lot of turning, or quick movements, can injure the impar ligament and cause lameness.

The Collateral ("Lateral") Cartilages

The coffin bone gives a fairly rigid structure to the front half of the hoof. The back part of the foot, however, is much more dynamic. To function, it needs a framework that is rigid enough to keep its shape, but flexible enough to allow for the expansion and contraction that takes place in the back of the foot when the horse moves. Fortunately, nature came up with the perfect compromise—the *collateral cartilages*. Now, if you want to get technical, there is actually a medial (inside) and a lateral (outside) collateral cartilage, and if you want to be a real snooty pants, you can call them the *ungular cartilages*. Most people just refer to both as "lateral cartilages," and that will do just fine.

The lateral cartilages (LCs) are rhomboid-shaped sheets of cartilage that attach to the palmar processes of the coffin bone, then fan upward like the half-raised wings of a territorial swan (fig. 4.14). When a horse is young, the LCs are made up of hyaline cartilage, which is almost see-through and not very fibrous. With healthy development, this cartilage becomes stronger and much more fibrous, yet it remains elastic. Poorly developed LCs may be only about ¼ inch thick where you can palpate them at the hairline, while robust LCs may be closer to an inch thick.

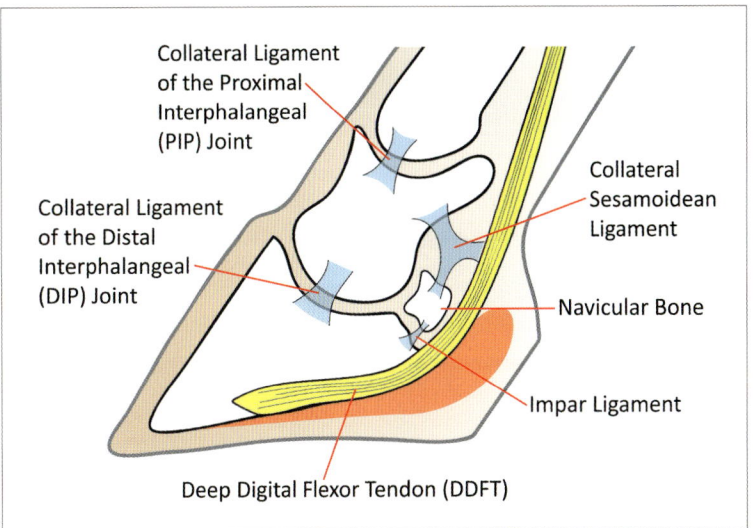

4.13 The impar ligament is a tiny thing, but it can cause big trouble if it gets sore or injured. It is sometimes responsible for pain that can be mistaken for navicular bone issues.

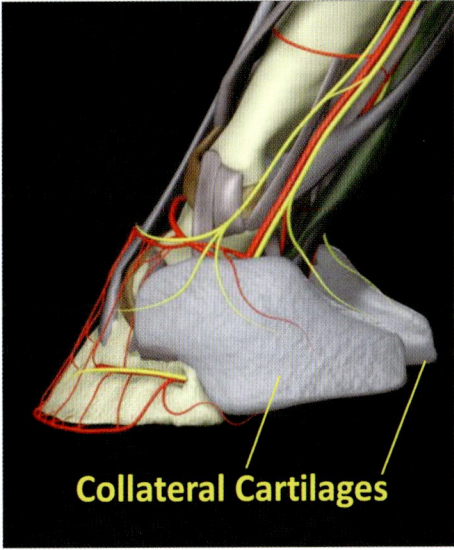

4.14 The wing-like lateral cartilages toughen dramatically over a horse's lifetime—if the horse is afforded plenty of movement on varied terrain.

The elasticity of the LCs is important for the hoof to work properly. First, it allows the back part of the horse's foot to expand and contract during weight bearing, which lessens shock to protect the bones, tendons, and ligaments of the hoof and leg.

This same in-and-out movement also acts like a blood pump within the hoof, helping blood to get into the tissues of the foot and aiding circulation in the legs and the entire body. Lastly, the LCs act as sort of a booster, returning the energy created in the weight-bearing phase back to the leg during the "lift-off" phase. Put on a new, springy pair of athletic shoes that add a little bounce to your step and you'll get a sense of what this does for the horse.

The bulk of the lateral cartilages lie inside the hoof capsule, but you can feel the uppermost edge of the cartilages above the coronet band, from the quarters rearward. If pressed gently, healthy LCs feel firm but have a bit of give. If they feel hard, like bone, they have likely become calcified, a condition called *sidebone* (see *Sidebone,* p. 220).

The Blood Supply

While the lower limb of the horse has a limited blood supply (one reason why leg injuries below the knee do not always heal well), the interior of the hoof actually has a rich supply of blood vessels that form a mind-boggling system of arteries, veins, and capillaries (fig. 4.16).

It all starts above the hoof, where the *medial palmar artery* splits to form the *medial and lateral palmar digital arteries*. These then pass around the sesamoid bones and continue downward into the pastern area, where they branch again, and come together to form a circle around the bone. More arteries branch off this circle, some providing blood to the lateral cartilages, while others go to the heels, and on from there to the digital cushion, frog, and various parts of the corium.

At the level of the short pastern bone (P2), the digital arteries branch again then reconnect to form another circle around both that bone and the coronary band. This circle is called the *coronal circumflex artery*, and it supplies the digital extensor tendon and a number of other parts of the hoof with many branches that feed into the coronary corium and the laminae (the interlocking structures that attach the hoof wall to the coffin bone, see p. 34) of the dorsal area.

Various branches of the arteries also pass through the coffin bone in several places, traveling through foramina and grooves that prevent crushing of the arteries. Below the coffin bone,

Hands-On Activity

I f your horse will stand quietly, try palpating (assessing through feel) your horse's lateral cartilages, which can't really be seen but can be easily felt above the quarters (fig. 4.15). They should have some give to them, but if they feel like bone, talk to your vet or hoof-care professional and get them assessed for sidebone. If they do feel pliable, monitor them occasionally to keep track of any changes.

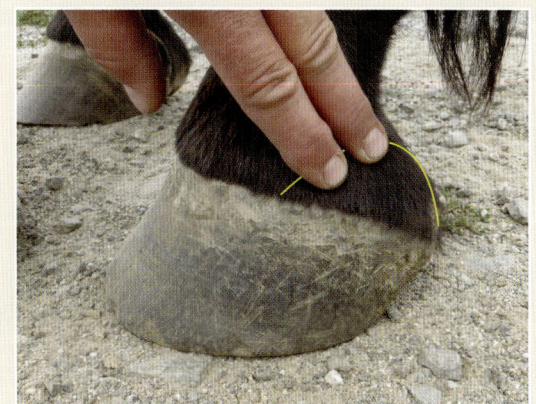

4.15 Palpating the lateral cartilages can help you determine if your horse has—or is developing—sidebone.

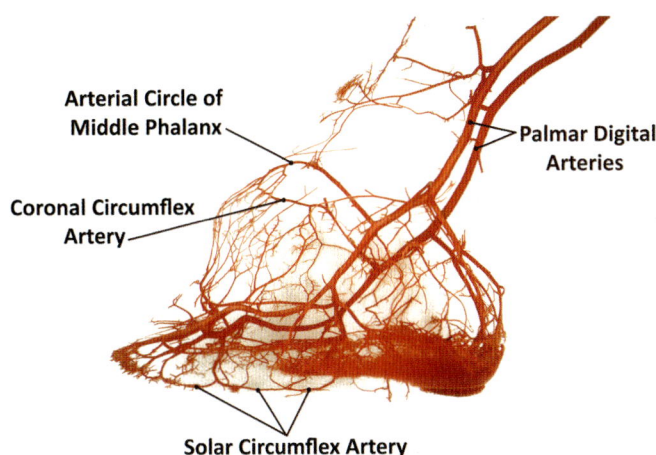

Arterial Circle of
Middle Phalanx

Coronal Circumflex
Artery

Palmar Digital
Arteries

Solar Circumflex Artery

4.16 The arteries in the hoof wrap around and pass through the bones, carrying blood to a vast network of smaller vessels.

they supply the heel and quarter portions of the blood-vessel rich layer of tissue called the *corria*, then join (anastomose) with other branches to form the *solar circumflex artery*. This final arterial loop provides the blood supply for the solar corium.

The finest branches from all of the arteries, called *arterioles*, are involved in microcirculation within the tissues of the structures of the hoof. These terminate in the capillaries, the even smaller blood vessels, which move the "used" or deoxygenated blood into the venous system, where it is returned to the heart.

Blood flow and perfusion in the foot is critical to hoof health. Unfortunately, it can be compromised by disease (for example, laminitis), poor development of the internal structures of the hoof, peripheral loading of the hoof wall, or by mechanical problems brought on by poor shoeing or trimming.

The Difference Between
Arteries, Capillaries, and Veins

There are **three** main types of blood vessels, all of which are present within the hoof:

- *Arteries* are large bore blood vessels that take blood from the heart and send it out to the organs and tissues. Arterial walls are thick and strong so that they can stand up to the high pressure of the pumping heart.

- *Capillaries* are tiny vessels with thin walls. They form complex networks to perfuse blood through the organs and tissues.

- *Veins* collect the "used" blood from the capillaries and send it back to the heart. Veins contain little one-way valves that prevent blood from flowing backward. The walls of the veins are not as thick as those of the arteries, as blood pressure is much lower on the return trip.

The Digital Cushion

The *digital cushion* is a wedged-shaped pad located between the lateral cartilages, below the DDFT and the back part of the coffin bone, and above the frog (fig. 4.17). This extremely important little pillow does several important things for the hoof, if it is properly developed:

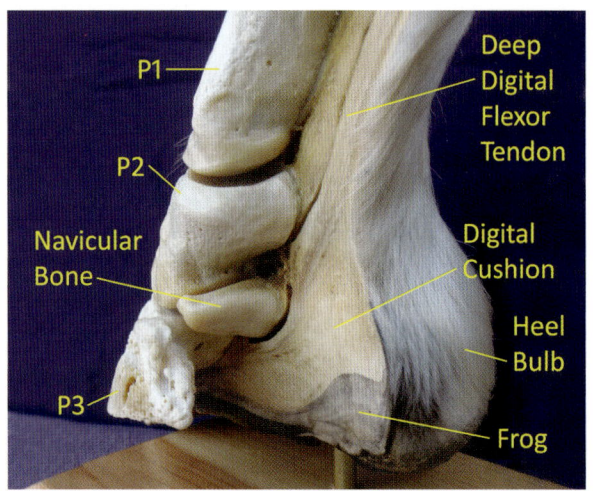

P1

Deep
Digital
Flexor
Tendon

P2

Navicular
Bone

Digital
Cushion

Heel
Bulb

P3

Frog

4.17 This preserved hoof specimen gives you a good view of the digital cushion. You can see how it sits in relation to the navicular bone, frog, and deep digital flexor tendon.

Hands-On Activity:
Palpating the Digital Cushion

How can you tell if your horse has well-developed digital cushions? To start with, if your horse has contracted heels, heel pain, contracted frogs, chronic thrush, or if he lands toe first, chances are that his digital cushions are not as robust as they should be. Another thing to look for is how "full" the heel bulbs are. In horses with good, thick digital cushions, the bulbs will be full and rounded. If they look flatter or "empty," there is not much cushion there (figs. 4.18 A & B).

Equine Podiatrist Dr. Ric Redden has also given us a general measurement we can use. As he explains, "The depth of the digital cushion can be estimated by placing your thumb in the shallow depression between the heel bulbs and placing the index finger of the same hand on the center of the frog. In light breed horses with strong, healthy heels, the distance between thumb and fingertip is in the range of 3–3½ inches. When this distance is well short of the normal range, one can expect to see evidence of soft tissue compromise radiographically."

You can also learn to feel how dense and strong the digital cushion is by placing your thumb on top of the heels and your fingers on the frog, and giving the area under your thumb a good squeeze (fig. 4.19). A weak digital cushion will feel

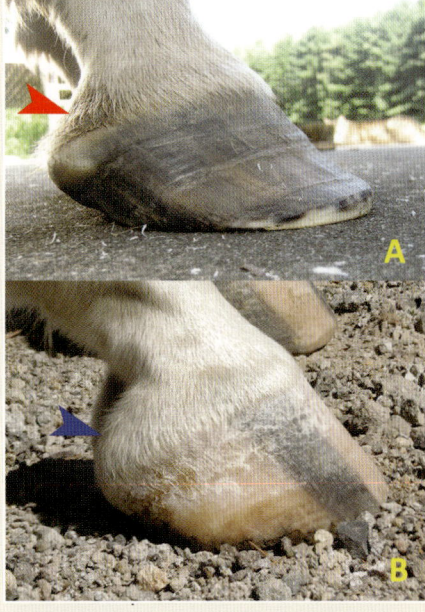

4.18 A & B The foot in Photo A has many problems, one of which is the flatness of the heel bulbs (red arrow)—a telltale sign of an underdeveloped digital cushion. The foot in Photo B shows the full, rounded heel-bulb shape (blue arrow) indicative of a healthy digital cushion.

- It absorbs concussion.

- It helps protect and support the navicular bone and the back of the coffin bone, and aids in the prevention of a negative palmar/plantar angle.

- It is the location of most of the proprioceptors in the foot, helping the horse to feel and respond to the ground.

- When it compresses during weight bearing, it helps to move blood through the blood vessels in the lateral cartilages.

This contributes to the perfusion of the foot, and also helps the development of the lateral cartilages.

Under conditions in line with what nature intended, the digital cushion changes quite a bit as the horse grows. When a foal is born, the digital cushion is mainly made up of adipose (fat) tissue,

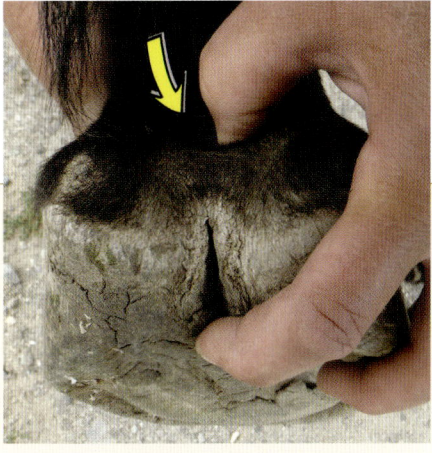

rather spongy, while a healthy one will feel quite firm.

To get an idea of what you are looking for, try squeezing the muscle of your thumb when you are making a fist, then squeezing it again with your hand relaxed (fig. 4.20). It will feel firm and elastic when you're making a fist, and softer and squishier when your hand is relaxed. A healthy digital cushion will feel more like the first version. You will likely have to feel the feet on a number of different horses to get a good sense of how the firmness varies.

If you believe that your horse's digital cushions are not as strong as they should be, don't despair, as it is never too late for these amazing structures to improve—at least to some degree. For this to happen, your horse will need plenty of movement, and you will

4.19 A squeeze with your thumb in the depression between your horse's heel bulbs will allow you to feel the digital cushion. It should have a bit of give, but should not feel soft and spongy.

need to work with a competent hoof-care professional to determine how to get your horse moving heel first, and how you can get the sole and frog to be active players in supporting the weight of your horse. Be aware that fixed frog pressure, such as that applied with heart bar shoes, is not the best solution for this issue, as the digital cushion requires both pressure and release with each step in order to develop properly.

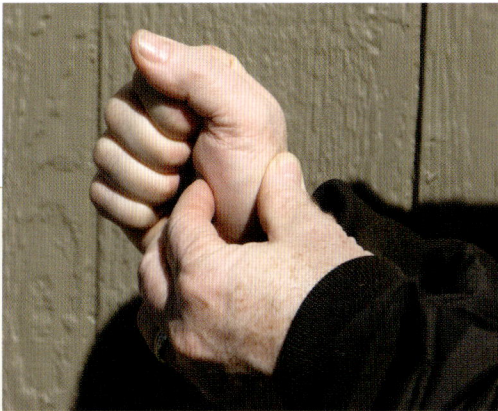

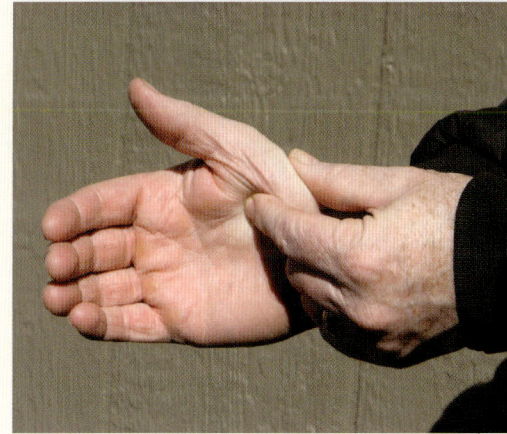

4.20 You can use your thumb muscle to get a sense of what a robust digital cushion should feel like.

which is quite soft and spongy. This spongy tissue provides just the right amount of anti-concussive protection for the light little foal. But, as the baby matures, movement over varied terrain stimulates the digital cushion to grow a dense network of collagen bundles and fibrocartilage, making it much firmer and helping it to support the youngster's increasingly heavy body.

However, in order for movement to have the effect nature intended, the horse also has to have a foot that functions as nature intended, which means that the frog, sole, and walls must all share in the weight bearing, and the foot must land heel first. Anything that promotes peripheral loading—meaning that the walls alone are bearing the horse's weight with the frog and sole lifted away from the ground—will inhibit the development of the digital cushion.

Unfortunately, domestic horses don't always get the movement and hoof care to develop firm, robust digital cushions. The result is that we can end up with fully grown, adult horses walking around on soft, underdeveloped digital cushions. Think of a Mack truck driving around on baby carriage tires, and you'll have an idea of why this is not a good thing. Underdeveloped digital cushions are commonly seen in horses that have been continually shod from an early age, horses that grew up in confined areas or on soft ground, and sometimes in barefoot horses with chronically overgrown walls.

Horses with poorly developed digital cushions have greater vulnerability to hoof and leg ailments that can result from increased concussive forces and diminished blood perfusion. The horse's attempts to compensate for the increased sensitivity and pain in the back part of the foot may also play a role in the development of disease and injury. You can get an idea of what difference a well versus a poorly developed digital cushion makes by putting a thin sandal on one of your feet, and a good running shoe on the other. Jog down a paved road for a few steps and feel the difference in the concussive forces that your bones, joints, and soft tissues have to contend with.

The Laminae (aka Stratum Lamellatum, Lamellae, or Lamina)

A note on terms: while out and about in the horse world, you will hear a number of different terms used to describe the specialized structures that connect the hoof wall to the inside of the foot. Here is a little chart of the ones you are most likely to come across:

Singular Noun	Plural Noun	Adjective
Lamina	Laminae	Laminar
Lamella	Lamellae	Lamellar

We have used the noun form "laminae" throughout this book, but when it comes to adjectives, we use both "laminar" and "lamellar," choosing one or the other based on what is most commonly used in each particular instance. The *laminae,* in very basic terms, are two sheets of tightly connected, intricately folded tissue that attach the inside surface of the hoof wall to the outside surface of the coffin

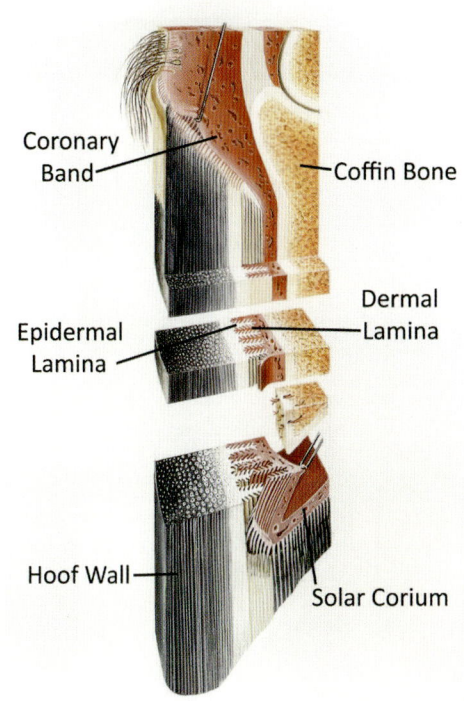

Coronary
Band

Coffin Bone

Epidermal
Lamina

Dermal
Lamina

Hoof Wall

Solar Corium

4.21 A The epidermal and dermal laminae (plural of lamina) form a tight connection that holds the coffin bone to the hoof capsule.

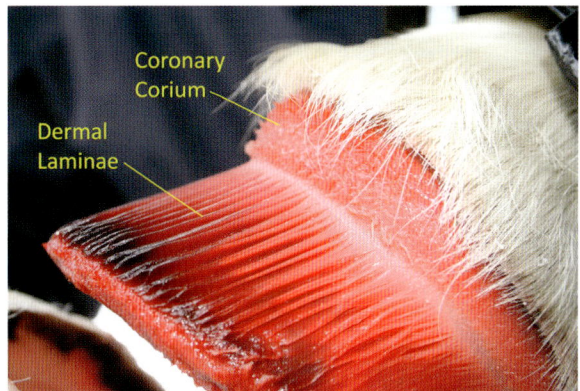

Coronary
Corium

Dermal
Laminae

4.21 B Here we can see the dermal laminae below the coronary corium. They tend to clump together when exposed like this, but if you look at their origin just below the coronary corium, you can see how fine they are and how many.

4.21 C This is a close-up of the inside of an actual hoof capsule. The fine, gill-like structures are the epidermal laminae.

bone. Their two main functions are to keep the coffin bone suspended within the hoof capsule, and to absorb shock. The sheet lining the hoof wall is called the *epidermal* or *insensitive* laminae (often called the "horny laminae," in lay terms), while the one lining the coffin bone is called the *dermal* or *sensitive* laminae (figs. 4.21 A–C). Together these act like super-strength equine hoof Velcro®. Ask your farrier or veterinarian if they have ever done hoof dissections in their studies, and they will confirm how extremely difficult it is to separate the laminae of a healthy foot.

Both the epidermal and dermal laminae have multiple folds of material that create a huge surface area for attachment—about 1.4 square yards packed into each foot. When viewed under a microscope, the folds form a bristling forest of inter-locking, fern-shaped structures, each one having a primary lamina with a fringe of secondary laminae branching off it. Each foot has 550–600 primary laminae, and each of these has 150–200 secondary laminae (fig. 4.22).

In a healthy foot, all of the laminae are neatly zipped into one another, and where they interface,

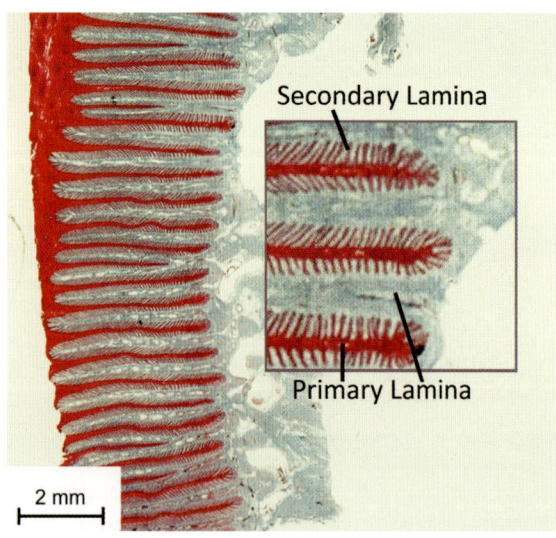

4.22 Although the primary and secondary laminae are individually small, their combined surface area is enormous, providing tremendous strength of attachment.

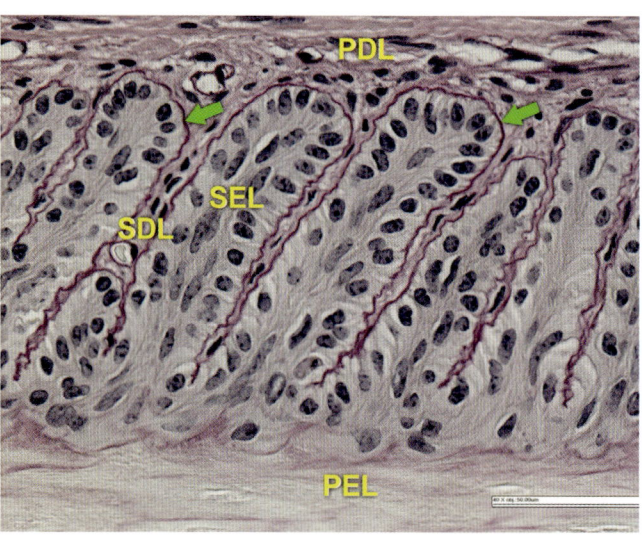

4.23 The green arrows in this image point to the basement membrane. PDL and PEL are the primary dermal and primary epidermal laminae, while SDL and SED are the secondary dermal and secondary epidermal laminae.

Delving Deeper:
MMPs and TIMPs

The hoof wall and its laminae grow down from the coronary band, which begs the question—how do these epidermal laminae, bonded as they are to the dermal ones on the coffin bone side, travel downward as they grow? We can thank Chris Pollitt, BVSc, PhD, and his team of researchers at the University of Queensland for the answer to this mystery.

Pollitt's work has shown that there are two classes of enzymes that create a constant, precisely controlled remodeling of the laminae, allowing them to migrate down the foot without separating. The first class, called *metalloproteinases* (MMPs), signal the basement membrane to "let go" just enough to allow the cells of epidermal laminae to slide down the tiniest bit. That process is then halted by the release of another type of enzyme called *tissue inhibitors of metalloproteinase* (TIMPs). The result is a perfectly timed dance of healthy, growing tissue that maintains its integrity to keep the coffin bone suspended and protected. According to Pollitt, laminitis results from something triggering the release of an overload of MMPs, causing the laminae to separate (see *Laminitis*, p. 163).

they are bonded by the basement membrane, an incredibly strong mesh of collagen and glycoprotein molecules the science types call an *extracellular matrix* (fig. 4.23). The amount of force that this membrane and the laminae deal with is truly amazing—a full ton with each running step on the forelegs of an average-sized horse.

Laminitis, in its many forms, causes damage to the basement membrane, loosening the bond between the laminae and causing separation of the epidermal and dermal laminae (see *Laminitis*, p. 163).

The Corium

The *corium* is a type of specialized tissue rich in blood vessels through which it supplies nutrients needed for growth. The corium has five main parts, each named for the structure associated with it (fig. 4.24). The five coria are lined with a layer of germinal cells from which the corresponding part of the hoof grows. All parts of the corium, except the lamellar (aka laminar) corium, are covered in fine, velvety, hair-like projections called *papillae*. Each tapered papilla fits tightly into a hole in the interior of the hoof capsule.

Starting at the top is the *perioplic corium,* a thin strip located in the groove above the juncture where the wall meets the coronary band. This part of the corium produces the periople and the stratum externum.

Next is the *coronary corium*, which is the main supplier of groceries for the hoof wall, and the place from which the majority of the hoof wall grows. Each one of the papillae of the coronary corium fits into a corresponding hole in the

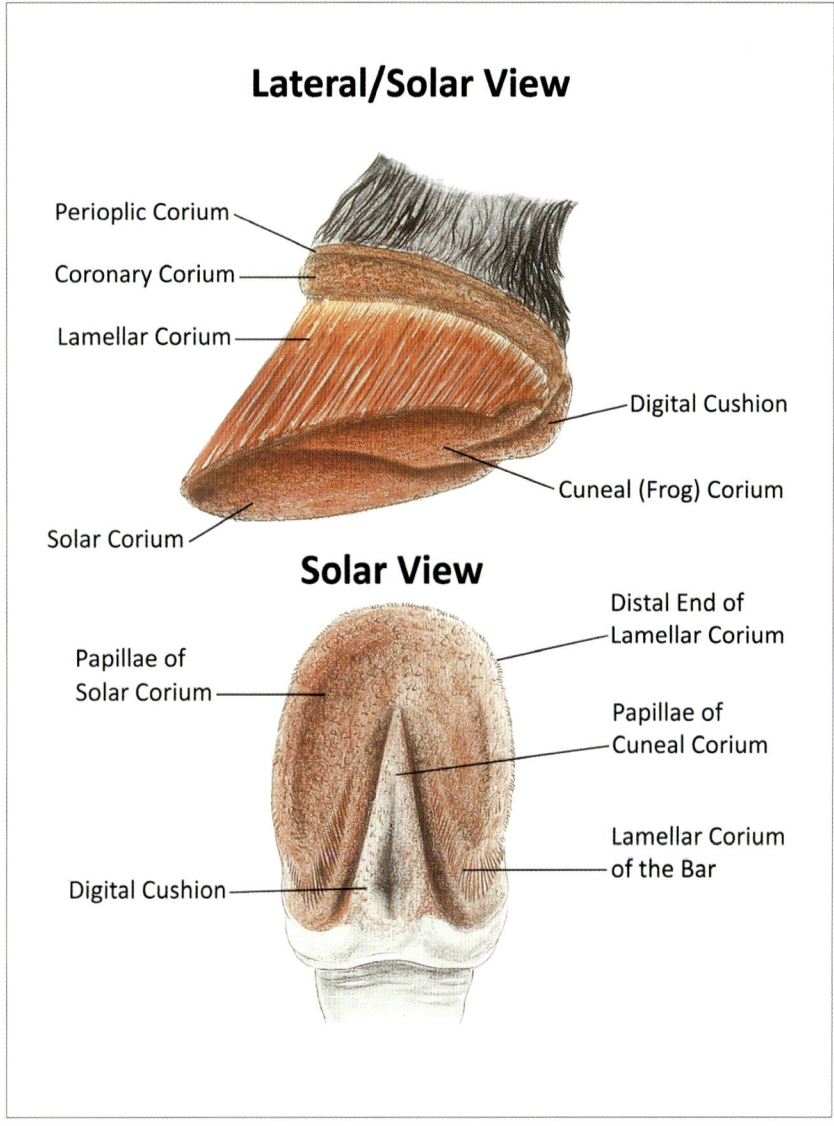

4.24 The five coria all carry nutrients to various parts of the hoof capsule, but the lamellar or laminar corium is also part of the interlocking laminae system that attaches the hoof capsule to the coffin bone.

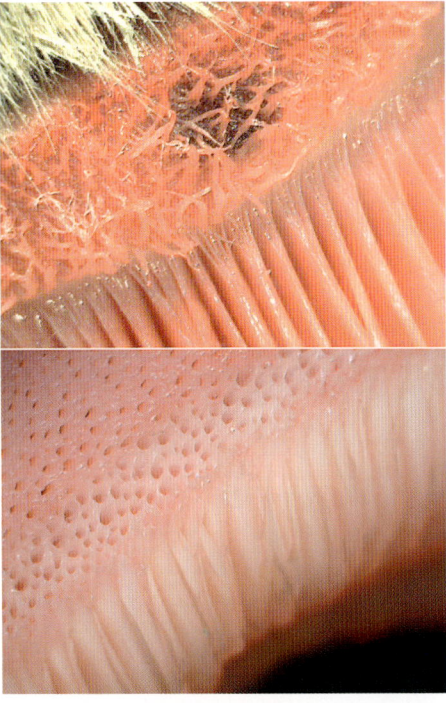

4.25 Each one of the papillae of the coronary corium (above) fits into an individual hole in the coronary groove (below).

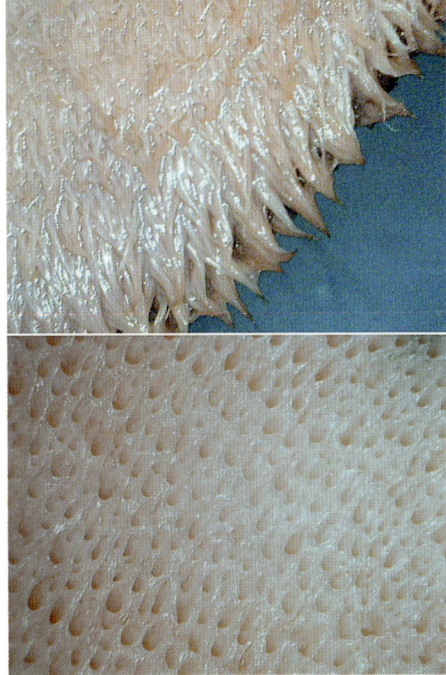

4.26 The papillae of the solar corium, like the other papillae of the foot, are tapered at the ends (above). Each papilla fits into a corresponding hole in the horny tissue of the sole (below).

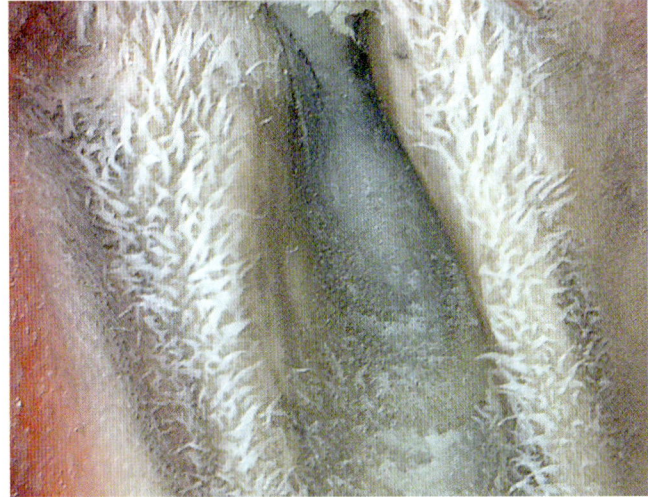

4.27 The velvety cuneal corium creates the elastic tissues of the frog.

coronary groove at the top of the hoof capsule, where it feeds and shapes one individual hoof tubule (fig. 4.25).

Moving on down, you find the *lamellar* or *laminar corium*, which attaches to the coffin bone and lies underneath the dermal laminae. This corium supplies the dermal laminae with nutrients, and it provides sustenance for the epidermal laminae via capillaries that pass through the basement membrane. The lamellar corium also produces some of the intertubular horn of the inner hoof wall.

Lining the inside of the bottom surface of the hoof is the *solar corium*. Like the coronary corium, it is covered with velvet-like papillae. These orient downward and insert into holes in the horny tissue of the sole, providing nutrients and growing the sole itself (fig. 4.26). Similarly, the papillae of the *cuneal (frog) corium* attach into the frog and are the source of its growth (fig. 4.27).

Section Two:
Recognizing Healthy and Unhealthy Feet

I f you made it through the previous section on anatomy (the hardest one, we promise!), you now have a helpful level of familiarity with the exterior and interior structures of the hoof. Unfortunately, knowledge of the interior structures doesn't make it any easier to *see* them, which, unless you are Superman, is impossible to do without expensive technology. The good news is that the external appearance of the hoof can usually give you a vast amount of valuable information about that hoof's state of health—inside and out. A foot that looks well-formed and robust on the outside has a good chance of being well-formed and robust on the inside, too. The key is learning how to recognize whether the foot looks healthy or not.

In order to do that, the first thing you need to understand is that when it comes to domestic horses, there is often a big divide between what is *common* and what is *healthy*. In fact, the horse industry has become so used to looking at unhealthy feet that many of us don't recognize problems when they are right in front of us. This section will compare healthy and unhealthy feet, pointing out the features you can look for to tell the difference. Not quite as good as X-ray vision, but a huge step in the right direction.

Size, Shape, and the Hoof Wall

Size Does Matter

If you ever get a chance to see Mustangs living out in the wild, you might notice that while the horses are usually on the small side, their feet are often proportionally large (fig. 5.1). This is because the pressures of natural selection, coupled with miles and miles of daily movement, result in large, sturdy feet ideally suited to the intense demands of a free-roaming life.

Domestic horses, on the other hand, are sometimes seen sporting dainty little feet better suited to animals half their size, a scenario that makes them more vulnerable to a whole slew of hoof and limb ailments, including laminitis and palmar heel pain (aka "navicular syndrome").

It all boils down to simple physics: in this case, pounds per square inch (PSI). The more PSI you have on a given area, the greater the load that area has to bear. It follows that if you distribute the same load over a larger area, the PSI goes down. Larger feet mean fewer pounds per square inch of load on the structures of the hoof (fig. 5.2).

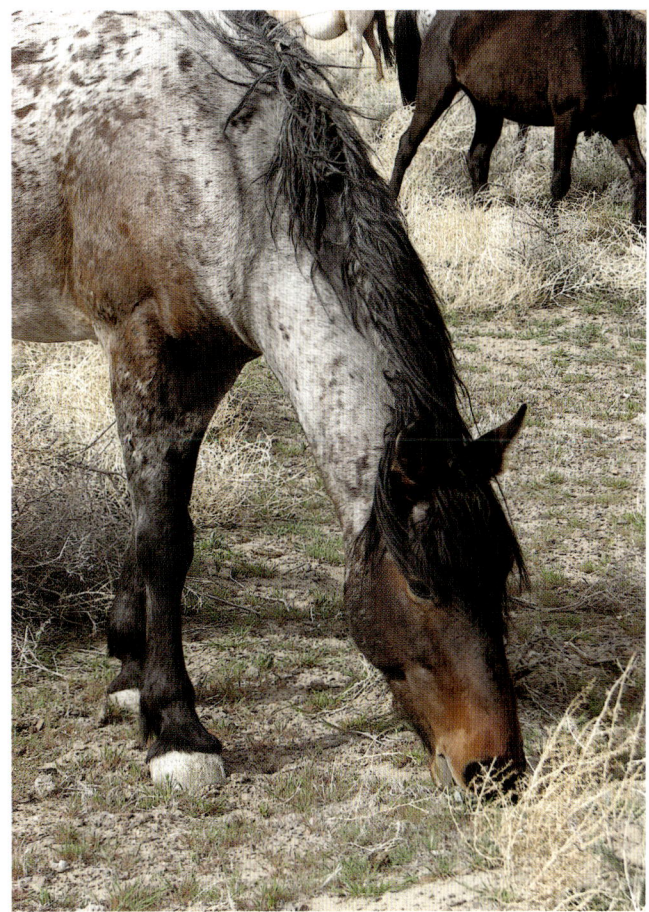

5.1 This wild Mustang stallion is only about 14 hands, but his feet are bigger than many domestic horses that would tower over him.

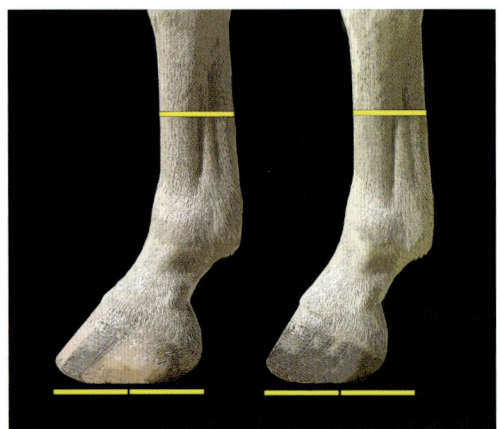

5.2 The image on the left shows a foot nearly twice the measurement of the leg. The image on the right is closer to one and a half. Assuming these horses are the same weight, the right foot would have to bear many more pounds per square inch.

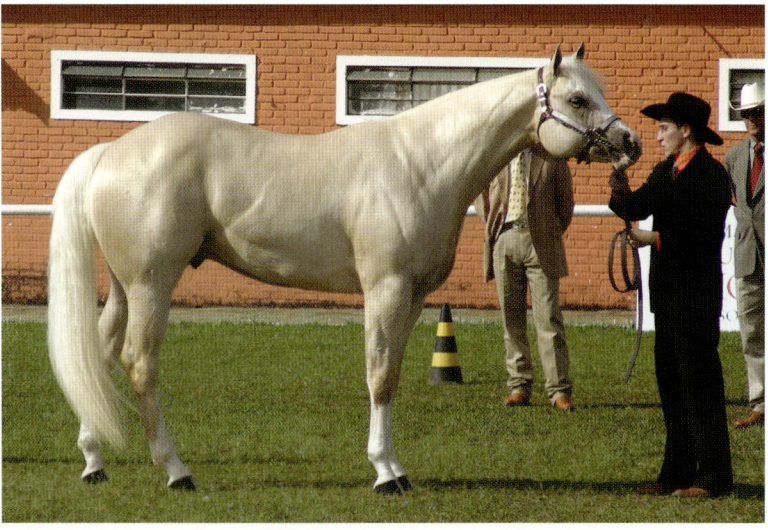

5.3 When the feet are small in proportion to the body, the hooves can have trouble handling the horse's body weight. This problem will be more pronounced when the horse is bred to be extra heavily muscled.

Of course, there are variables that can alter this equation, particularly when the hoof is peripherally loaded, meaning that the walls are the only structure holding up the weight of the horse. This is an unnatural situation, raising the PSI on the walls much more than they are designed to handle. Thus, a smaller foot that has the sole, frog, and walls each playing a part in weight bearing will have significantly lower PSI than a larger foot that is peripherally loaded. The best scenario is to have a healthy, large foot with all the right parts sharing the load, which gives you the lowest possible PSI.

So, if large feet are such a good thing, why is it that so many of our domestic horses have hooves that are smaller than ideal for their body? One reason has to do with breeding—that process by which man throws natural selection out the window and "improves" upon nature. One notorious

improvement in the horse world was the fashion among certain breeds to selectively breed their halter horses to have oodles of muscle and tiny hooves (fig. 5.3). The logic was that those wee hooves would make the muscles appear even bigger in proportion, the result being that we had thousands of horses that were simply too heavy for their own feet. Sadly, it was the horses that suffered the consequences of the hoof problems that inevitably resulted. Fortunately, many breeders eventually realized that this was a really bad idea, but the problem still exists, as it was bred into and continues to be perpetuated in a number of popular bloodlines.

Two other factors that can result in a horse having smaller feet than he should are soft terrain and lack of movement. Soft terrain, whether grass, sand, shavings, or some other kind of highly conformable surface, simply does not apply the type of pressure

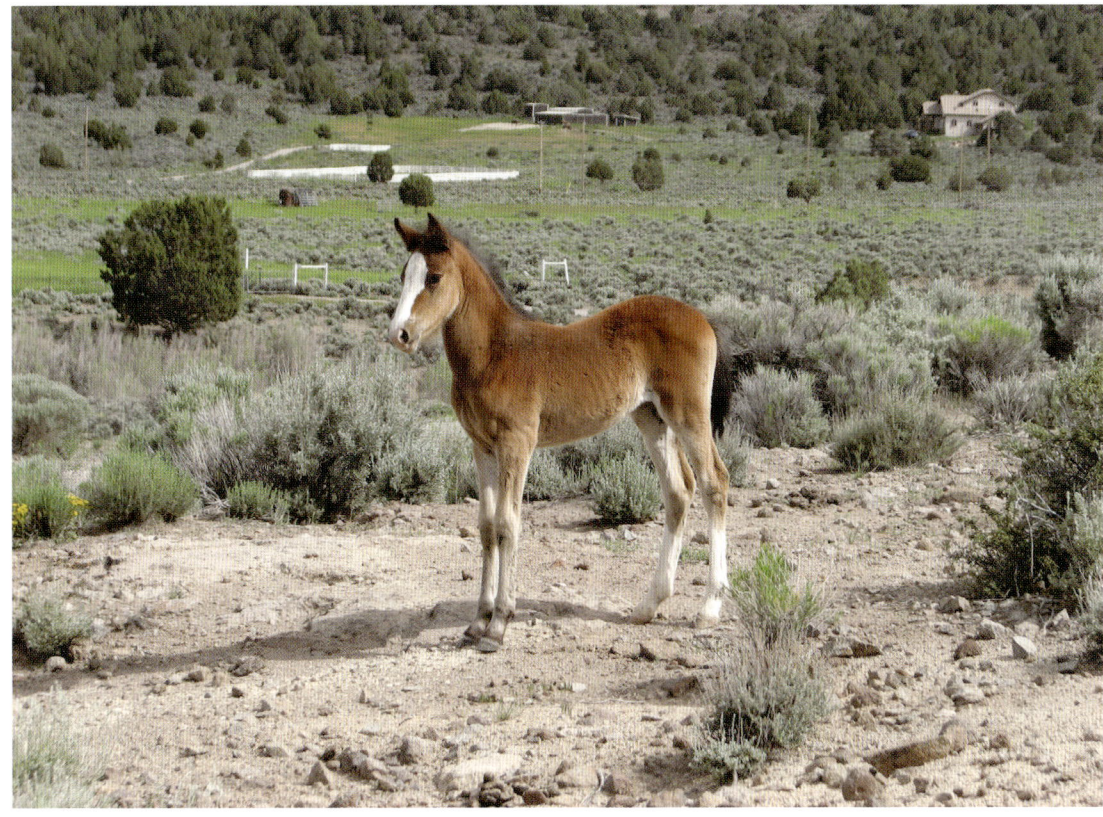

5.4 This foal has plenty of room to move on terrain that varies from soft, grassy patches to areas that are hard and rocky. While this may not be the "perfect pasture" we often visualize, it is a much better environment for healthy hoof development.

on the foot that encourages a developing hoof to spread and grow. In fact, perpetual exposure to soft footing may actually cause contraction of the hoof—the opposite of what you want to see.

Confining horses in small spaces has a similar effect: a lack of expansion due to too little of the pressure and release the hoof experiences during motion on varied terrain. As many of our domestic horses get the double whammy of being raised in confined spaces on soft footing, they are at a real disadvantage. Foals raised with plenty of room to roam over varied terrain have the best chance of developing big, strong, healthy feet (fig. 5.4).

Shoeing horses at a young age is also thought, by some, to have an effect on the ultimate size of the foot. The theory is that because the coffin bone and the entire hoof capsule should continue to increase in size until the horse is about five years old, shoeing before that time will "lock" the hoof into the size of the shoes being used.

In reality, since young horses are often shod at the time they begin training, it is difficult to know what effects on their feet are actually due to shoeing, as opposed to other stresses put on them by training. And, since we can't experiment by leaving one hoof shod and the other bare, there is no way

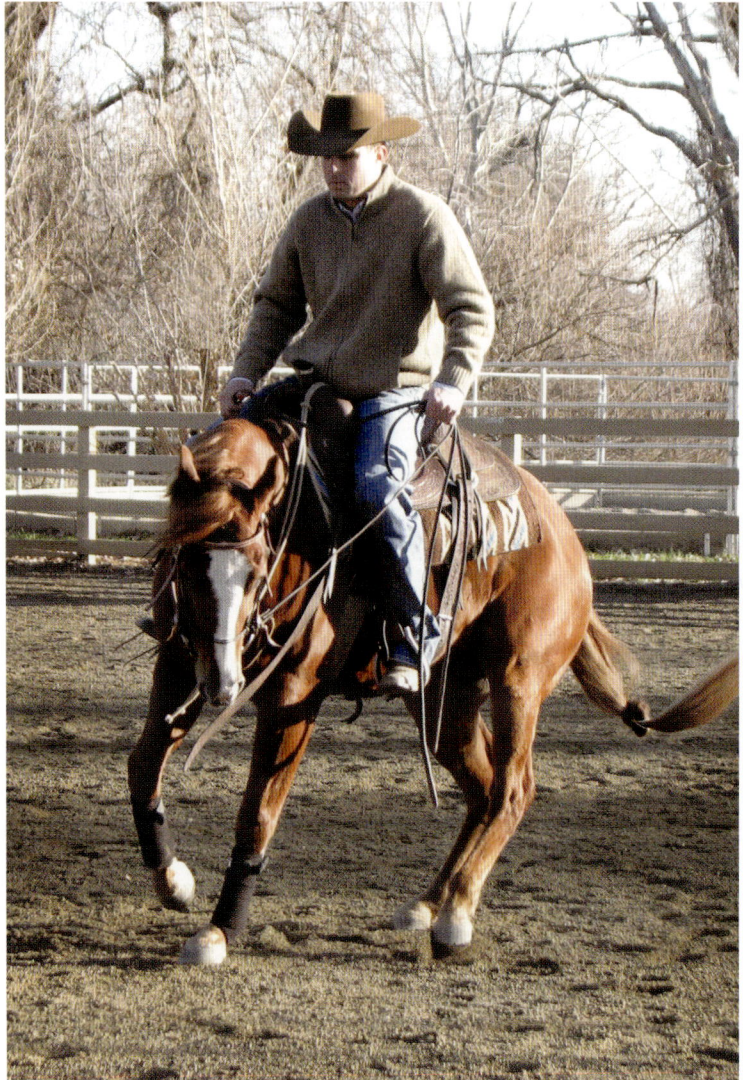

5.5 Great care must be taken when shoeing young horses, as early shoeing and the stresses of training may be detrimental to the developing foot. The bones and other structures of the equine foot, if allowed to develop naturally, will keep growing until about the age of five. This young horse's feet appear to be an appropriate size for his age and body size, indicating that measures are being taken to safeguard his hoof development.

to know what size a horse's feet would have been if left unshod longer.

What we do know for sure is that the feet of young horses often start to deteriorate once they are shod. Therefore, it is safe to say that shoeing a young horse should only be done if it cannot be avoided, as remaining barefoot does provide numerous advantages to the growing foot. If you are thinking about shoeing a youngster because he is entering training, you might want to try delaying shoeing to see how the horse does without the shoes. Many owners are surprised to find that the youngster didn't "need" shoes after all.

If you are having shoes put on a young horse, the farrier should keep in mind that the foot is not fully mature, and do whatever possible to encourage the foot to continue to grow and develop in a healthy manner (fig. 5.5). This includes making sure the shoes are large enough, having short intervals between shoeings, and periodically giving the feet time off to recover from the effects of shoeing, as most farrier textbooks recommend.

One last note on foot size: a foot that is flared can give the impression of being much larger than it would if the walls were well attached. So, when evaluating hoof size, be sure to check for flares (see *Flares*, p. 99).

Bottom line: When evaluating a hoof, you want it to be relatively large (though not splayed or flared) in proportion to the overall size of the horse.

Cone Shaped vs. Contracted

When a foal is born, his hoof walls are quite upright and the heels are close together, resembling a contracted hoof in many ways. But if the hoof develops correctly, it will gradually spread and take on a cone shape, meaning that the circumference of hoof is larger where it meets the ground than at the coronet (figs. 5.6 A & B). The walls should slope out from the coronet at pretty much the same angle on both sides, though it is extremely common and perfectly okay for the medial wall to stand slightly more upright than the lateral wall.

Contrast this to a contracted foot, which is shaped more like a soda can than a cone (fig. 5.7). In such feet, the footprint will be about the same circumference as the coronet, or in some cases, the hoof is actually smaller at the ground level than at the coronet.

Why does this shape matter? We learned earlier that arched or vaulted forms are enormously strong in terms of weight bearing, and the cone shape of the hoof contributes to the incredible strength of the hoof in the same way. However, it does something else that is extremely important: it allows the hoof to flex more easily upon impact. The flexing of the hoof not only dissipates energy but is also a critical part of what is known as "hoof mechanism," in which the expansion (upon loading) and contraction (upon lifting) of the hoof actually pumps blood and lymph (a fluid rich in infection-fighting white blood cells), through the feet and back up the legs. A contracted

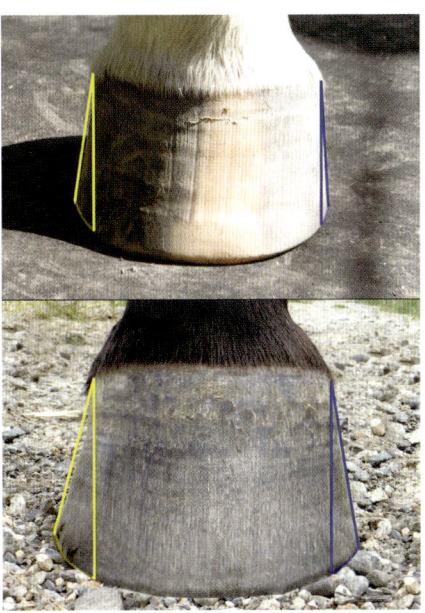

5.6 A The foal's foot in the upper photo will grow into the cone shape of the mature foot in the lower photo if nothing impedes its development. Notice that on each foot, the medial wall (right) is slightly more upright than the lateral wall (left).

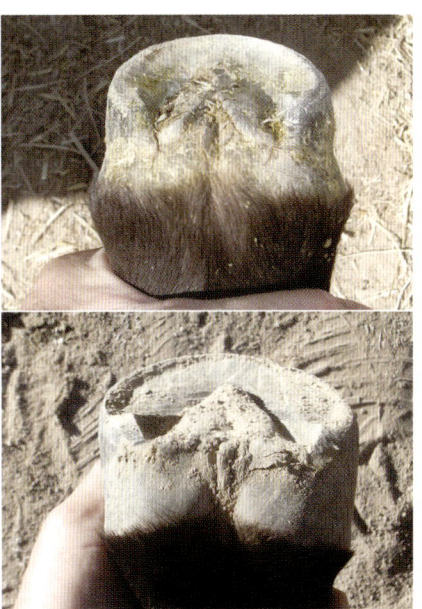

5.6 B The upper photo shows a normal foal's foot at three weeks, when it still has a narrow, "contracted" appearance. However, by five months (lower photo), the foot has opened up and developed quite a bit. This foal is fortunate to be afforded plenty of movement on firm terrain and regular hoof trimming, both of which are contributing to the healthy development of his feet.

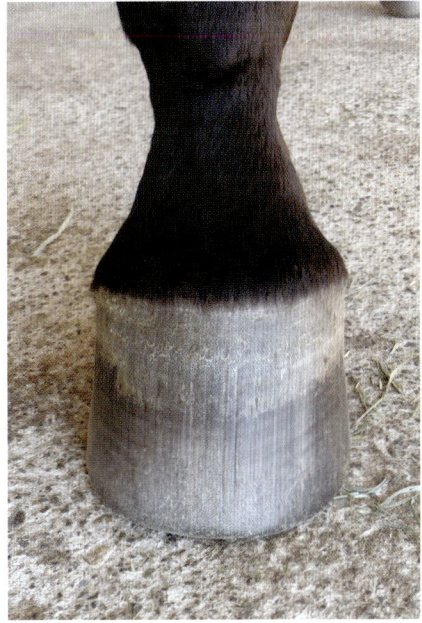

5.7 The contracted, "soda can" feet of this horse subject her to increased concussion and impaired circulation, both of which can cause a slew of problems.

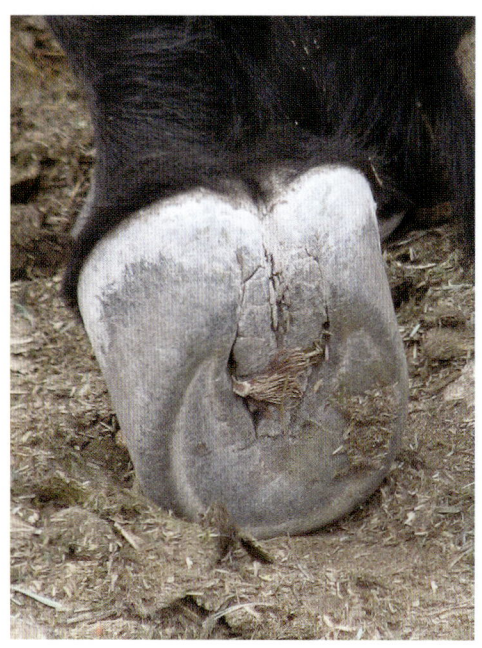

5.8 This wild Mustang's foot is quite contracted, with the circumference of the solar surface smaller than the coronet. As this horse grew up with plenty of movement on varied terrain and was never shod, the condition is likely congenital or developmental in origin.

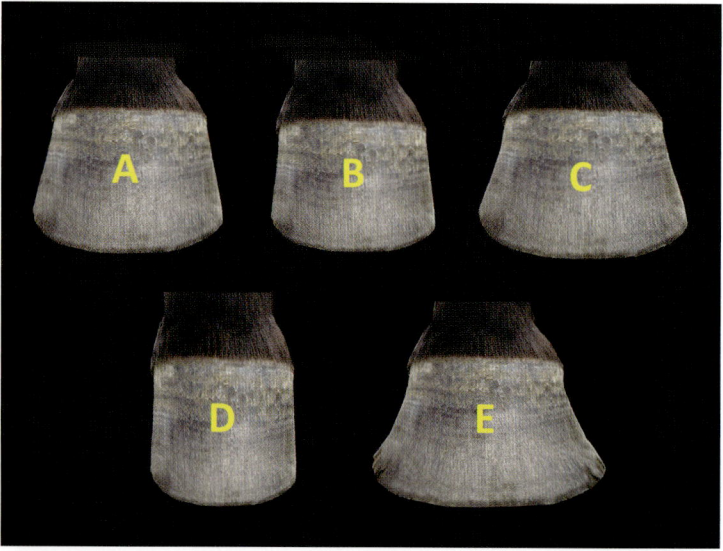

5.9 A normal, average, cone-shaped foot (A); within normal range for a young or small horse or a pony (B); within normal range for a large, heavy horse (C); contracted foot for a horse, though within the range of normal for a donkey (D); flared "pancake" foot likely to crack (E).

foot will have a harder time expanding upon impact and therefore cannot contribute to circulatory function in the way it was meant to. Impaired circulatory function in the foot can have devastating consequences, including poor growth and underdevelopment of the internal support structures.

The contracted foot is also unable to dampen concussive forces as well as its cone-shaped counterparts. The result is that more force travels up through the foot and the limb, increasing the likelihood of damage or injury over time. Contraction is most often noted and discussed as *contracted heels,* but when you've got an all-around upright, soda-can foot, this means the entire foot is contracted. That said, it is quite normal for the feet of donkeys and mules to be more upright than those of horses, and smaller, lighter equines such as foals and ponies

often have hooves that are less dramatically cone-shaped than their heavier brethren.

As a general rule, the more pounds coming down on the hoof, the more likely it is to spread out and become more obviously cone-shaped. This is why big, heavy horses often have more sloping hoof walls than you will see in the typical pony.

Horses can also have genetic factors that predispose them to having cylindrical hooves. One particular type of hoof distortion, called a *club foot,* is thought to be hereditary in many cases. A club foot can be extremely upright and contracted (see *Club Feet,* p. 85). Non-hereditary causes of contraction can include heel pain, poor shoeing practices, lack of movement, lack of exposure to firm footing, and developmental disorders (fig. 5.8).

If there is too much slope in the walls, sometimes

called a "pancake" foot, the wall connection is compromised, causing them to flare outward. When this happens, the foot can easily develop cracks, white line disease, and other problems. Cracked, pancake feet are commonly observed in draft horses, so much so that it is often thought that this is simply how draft horse feet are due to the weight their hooves have to bear. This is a fallacy. While the heaviness of draft horses can make it

more challenging to keep the walls from flaring, appropriate, physiologically correct trimming, done often enough, can make an enormous difference as it prevents the walls from bearing more of the load than they can handle (fig. 5.9).

Bottom Line: When viewed from the front, the hoof should be cone-shaped, with the angles of the medial and lateral walls close to the same.

Shoes and Contraction:
A Matter of Debate

There has been much discussion about whether or not shoeing a horse causes contracted hooves. Some argue that metal shoes inevitably cause some degree of contraction, as they do not allow the walls to grow wider as they grow longer. In other words, if you take two normal feet of exactly the same size and shape, shoe only one of them, then let them grow for some weeks, the bottom edge of the unshod hoof will typically have become wider as the foot gets taller, while the shod foot, being locked in by the shoe, will be the same width, despite being taller. This means that the angle from the coronet to the edge of the wall will have become steeper (more contracted) on the shod foot (fig. 5.10).

Although this seems logical enough, it is simply not a universal truth. If it were, every

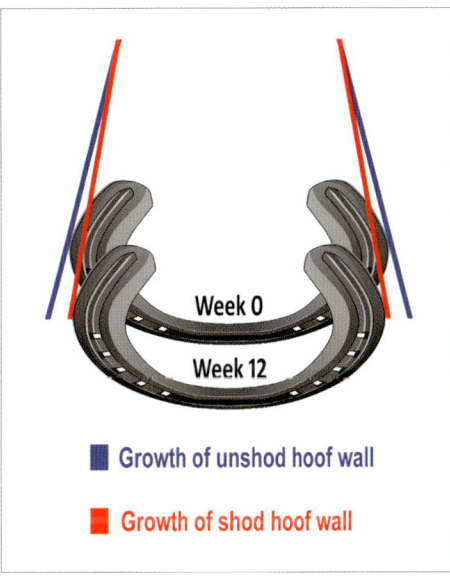

5.10 An unrestricted, healthy, cone-shaped foot will expand in circumference as it grows longer. A foot with rigid shoes, on the other hand, is locked in by the size of the shoe.

Week 0
Week 12

■ **Growth of unshod hoof wall**
■ **Growth of shod hoof wall**

shod horse would have contracted feet (they don't), and every shod horse's shoe size would decrease over time (also not the case). Nonetheless, poor shoeing practices can, and often do, cause contraction, so it is important to size shoes appropriately, and not to go too long between shoeings.

Straight and Narrow: The Hoof Tubules

Now, here is where things can get just a tad confusing: while walls that are straight and tubular are bad, walls with straight *tubules* are good! As you recall from the anatomy section, the hoof tubules are the tiny, keratin-based, straw-like structures that make up the majority of the hoof wall. They form a sort of grain, similar to what we see in a piece of wood. But, unlike wood grain, which can bend in various configurations and differ in the thickness between the lines, the grain of the hoof tubules should ideally be even and straight, following the angle of the hoof wall (fig. 5.11).

When a well-balanced hoof is viewed from the front, the lines made by the tubules will be parallel to each other and perpendicular to the ground. When seen from the side, the angle of the tubules at the heels should roughly match the angle of the tubules at the toe. If the angles are significantly different or there is any "bending" (deviation) from a straight line in any part of the foot, this indicates that all is not well (fig. 5.12).

There are quite a few different issues that can lead to bending of the tubules, including injury, unbalanced trimming/shoeing, poor movement due to conformational issues, club foot, or laminitis. Since there are so many possibilities, it is important to get the advice of a competent hoof-care professional or veterinarian to try to determine what is causing the tubules to bend. If you suspect that unbalanced trimming or poor shoeing may be the root of the problem, don't be afraid to seek an opinion from a professional other than the one you use. It is your right and duty as a horse owner to look out for your horse.

Bottom Line: Hoof tubules should be straight and even.

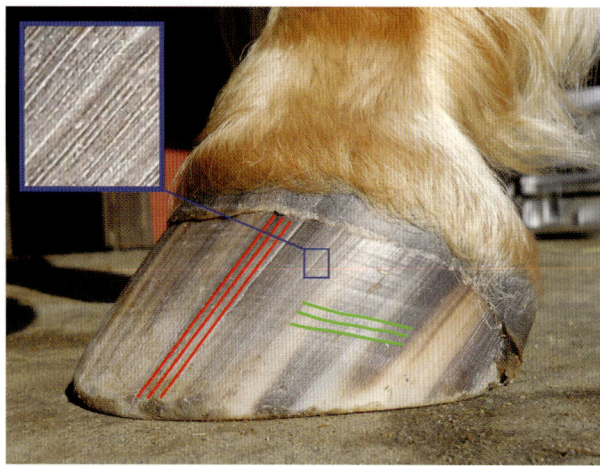

5.11 The stripes on this foot make it easier to see the hoof tubules, which run from the coronet down to the ground in the direction of the red lines. The blue inset shows what the tubules look like close up. Growth rings, which are not always visible, run side to side, in the direction of the green lines. The growth rings on this foot are slightly visible.

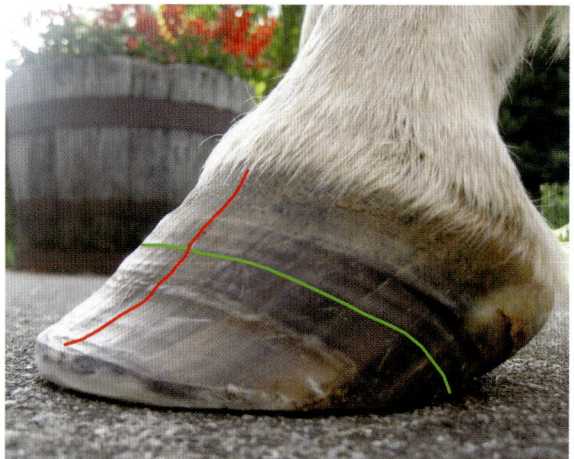

5.12 Notice the bend in the tubules, following the direction of the red line, on this unhealthy, distorted foot. You can also easily see the very pronounced growth rings, following the direction of the green line.

Wall Growth: A Variable Constant

The hoof wall, like your fingernails, is always growing. The average rate of growth for a typical adult hoof ranges from about ¼ inch to a bit less than ½ inch per month. It can take anywhere from 6-12 months for the hoof to grow from the coronet down to the ground at the toe on a foot of normal length, but typically only 4–5 months at the heels, as they are shorter. The actual growth rate, however, has normal fluctuations, and both the growth rate and the quality of the wall horn can be affected by many different factors, including:

• *Time of year:* Most horses see a slowing of growth in winter months, perhaps associated with metabolic changes meant to conserve energy in colder weather.

• *Age:* Foal feet grow much faster than adult feet, one of the reasons it is important to make sure youngsters get the hoof care they need.

• *Illness:* Stress or illness anywhere in the body can potentially affect hoof growth and horn quality. Hoof ailments like laminitis certainly change the rate of growth, strength, and shape of hoof, but even a simple fever can cause an abnormal ring in the hoof wall. Some problems can change the growth rate of the heels and toes relative to each other, so that one is growing much faster than the other.

• *Damage to the coronary corium:* As the center of growth for most of the hoof wall horn, the health of the coronary corium is essential for normal growth. Anything that damages it in any way can slow growth or cause a fault in the wall.

Hands-On Activity: Chart Your Horse's Hoof Growth

Using the chart provided on page 285, chart the rate of growth of your horse's feet. Doing this will allow you to see how much the growth rate changes at different times of year, as well as any other factors that might be affecting hoof growth.

• *Diet:* Hoof growth and quality can be affected by both nutritional deficiencies and nutritional excesses. Diets high in non-structural carbohydrates, for example, can weaken the hoof wall, as can diets deficient in key minerals like zinc and copper.

• *Exercise and terrain:* A horse that gets plenty of correct, heel-first landings on varied terrain is likely to grow hoof wall at a faster rate than a horse that is standing around in a stall, and its horn is also likely to be of better quality.

Growth Rings: Less Is More

In addition to the *vertical* lines made by the tubules, the equine hoof sometimes has visible, *horizontal* growth rings that run parallel to the ground. Very subtle growth rings without any distinct ridges may be due to changes in growth rates at different times of year, or they may reflect minor changes in the diet. This type of ring, as can be seen in figure 5.11, is no cause for worry.

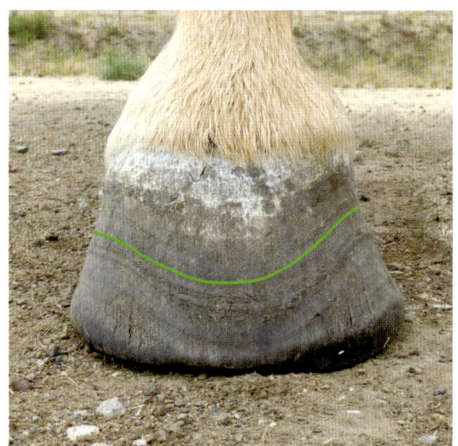 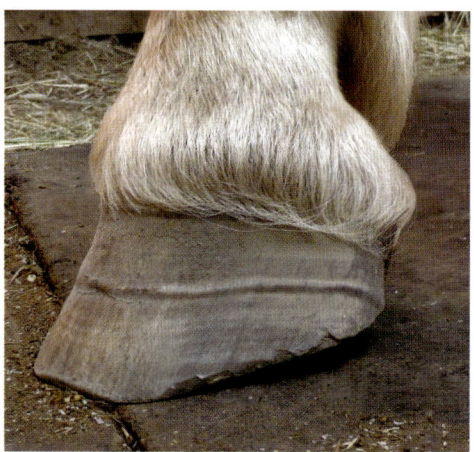 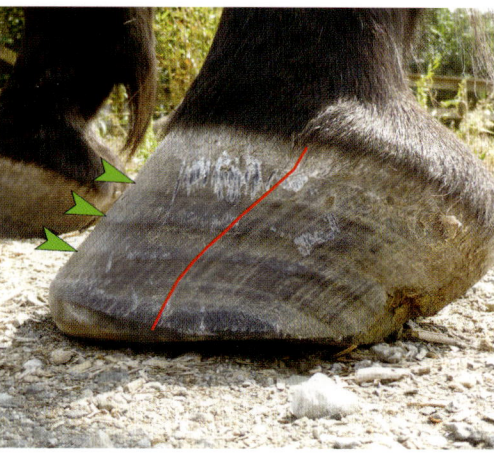

5.13 The curved growth rings on this hoof were caused by excessive pressure in the quarters. Notice that the curves rise up where pressure is high, and drop where pressure is lower.

5.14 The single, pronounced growth ring in this hoof was the result of an abscess that caused inflammation inside the foot. Though dramatic in appearance, it will simply grow out and disappear, likely without any lasting effects.

5.15 This foot has repeated, prominent growth rings (green arrows) indicative of an ongoing problem, and it also has bending in the tubules (following red line). If alarm bells are not ringing in the owner's head, they should be.

Rings that are more prominent indicate some kind of stressor at the time that part of the hoof wall was being produced. These stressors include illness; laminitis; a change of diet; a poor or overly rich diet; anxiety related to training, showing, travel, isolation, or separation from herd mates; and medications, vaccinations, or dewormers. All of these stressors can cause a degree of inflammation that may result in more pronounced ripples in the hoof wall. Noticeable curves in the growth rings also indicate a problem, generally some kind of imbalance in the hoof. Areas where rings are pushed higher indicate greater pressure, and lower areas indicate less pressure (fig. 5.13).

A single, pronounced growth ring, with the rest of the hoof wall being relatively smooth, indicates a specific event that caused a disruption in hoof wall growth and does not necessarily mean that there

is an ongoing problem with the horse. Some people, therefore, call them "event rings." While worth taking note of, a single ring is usually not cause for undue concern (fig. 5.14).

Multiple, pronounced rings are more of a worry, as they show you that something is going wrong in the horse's body on a continual basis (fig. 5.15). You often see this in cases of chronic laminitis. In some cases, the horse may not be so bad that he is exhibiting overt lameness, but he is, nonetheless, experiencing constant or repeated bouts of inflammation or those rings wouldn't be there.

When you see prominent growth rings on your horse, you need to get busy and figure out what is causing them. Most important is to take a close look at the horse's diet, as this is where the problem often lies. Excessive starches and sugars are frequently the culprit, so you might want to look at reducing or eliminating grain and other sources of "quick carbs" from your horse's diet (see *Feeding the Foot*, p. 238).

You also want to look for growth rings that are not parallel to each other, which most often appear as rings that are wider at the toe and compressed at the heel, or wider at the heel and compressed at the toe. If the rings are wider at the heels than at the toes, the horse could have laminitis, high heels, or a club foot. If the rings in the heel are narrower than the toe, the heel may be too far forward—a condition called underrun heels (see *Underrun Heels,* p. 78)—or bearing too much weight, or the toe might be too long. Any time you see rings that are not parallel, it is a good idea to call in your vet or farrier to assess hoof balance and check for other issues (fig. 5.16).

Bottom Line: Growth rings should be almost invisible and parallel to each other.

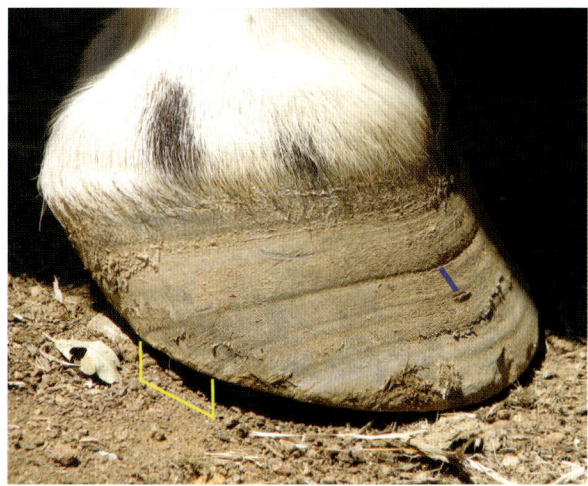

5.16 Although this pony was never overtly lame, the pronounced growth rings that are wider at the heels (yellow bracket) than at the toe (blue line) are the result of laminitis.

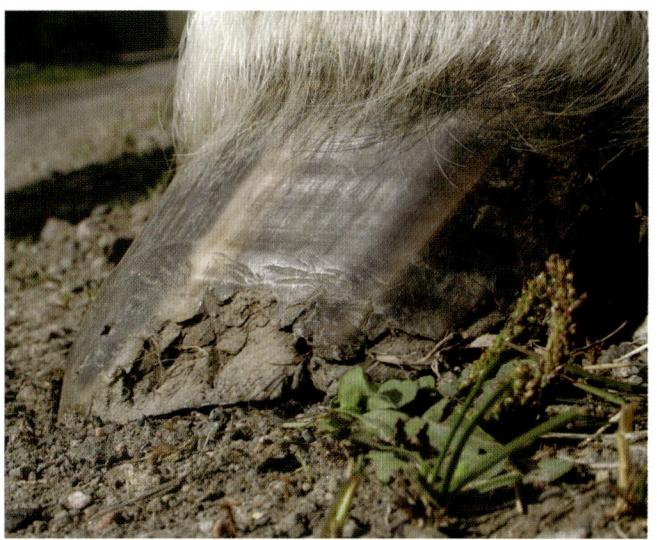

5.17 Thin, weak, or diseased walls tend to crumble or split, making it hard for a horse to hold a shoe.

Weak Walls

When a horse has hoof walls that tend to chip, flake, split, peel, or crumble if you breathe on them too hard, owners and farriers alike can feel like tearing their hair out (fig. 5.17). If the horse is shod, he may continually lose his shoes, costing the owner money and causing frustration due to lost riding time. The pulled shoes may also take substantial chunks of the weak wall with them, making it a real challenge to put the shoes back on. If the horse is barefoot, his feet may constantly chip, flake, and crack. And, whether they are shod or barefoot, horses with weak walls often have thin soles as well, which makes them tender-footed and puts them at increased risk of bruising, abscessing, and other sole-related problems.

Faced with this situation, most people quite logically think that the poor quality of their horse's hooves is the result of genetics, a nutritional issue, or both. Many people turn to hoof supplements, hoping to make up for some unknown deficit. However, while heredity and diet certainly play a part in creating such feet in some instances, there are frequently other factors in play.

One common problem is too much exposure to moisture, which breaks down the molecular bonds that give the hoof wall its integrity. Repeated bathing, morning dew on grass, wet weather, muddy ground, or anything else that soaks the foot can weaken the hoof wall and lead to chipping, splitting, peeling, or flaking. Water is more likely to cause a significant problem in feet that are already weakened by other issues (fig. 5.18). Further compounding the moisture issue is repeated bouts of very wet followed by very dry. For example, routine bathing of a horse after a workout and then turning him loose in a hot, dry sand paddock can exacerbate cracking problems brought on by excess hydration.

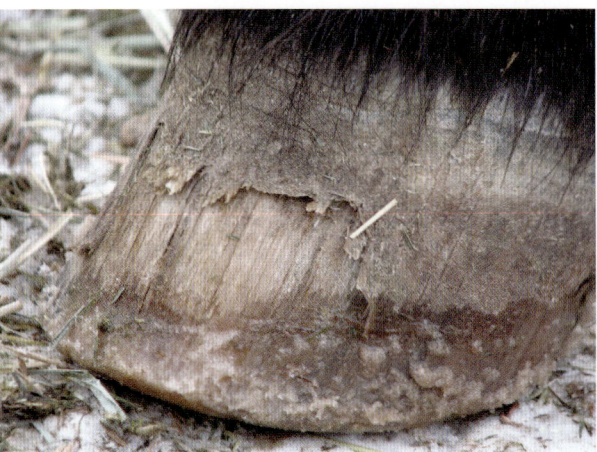

5.18 This horse's feet were affected by severe, prolonged malnutrition, but they looked relatively normal until wet weather set in, causing the already weakened keratin to break apart.

A more insidious issue that may very well be at the heart of many cases of chronic weak walls is compromised circulation within the foot. This starts to make sense when you remember that the hoof wall and sole both rely on nutrients supplied by the blood stream via the corium for growth. Damage the blood vessels and the groceries necessary to feed the growth of wall and sole horn are going to have a hard time reaching their destination. In order to have a chance of eliminating the weak wall/sole problem in such feet, you have to figure out what is causing the blood flow to be compromised in the first place. Fortunately, studying the foot will likely give you some answers.

Peripheral Loading

One frequently unrecognized problem to look for is peripheral loading. When the hoof wall, with or without shoes, is long enough to lift the frog, bars, and sole off the ground, the wall is put into the unnatural position of bearing the entire weight of the horse. This not only subjects the wall itself to tremendous stress, it also exposes the laminae, the lamellar corium, and the coronary corium to forces they are not designed to bear, which can damage their blood vessels and impede growth.

Correcting peripheral loading will often reverse this process, allowing a horse to grow much better and more strongly connected hoof walls. The best results tend to occur when the horse is allowed to remain barefoot, at least for a period of time. All farrier textbooks recommend giving hooves some time off from shoes, as doing so with a good trim will relieve any peripheral loading and improve circulation within the foot. It may seem ironic to leave a horse barefoot so that you can have an easier

Hands-On Activity:
Looking for Peripheral Loading

Peripheral loading is a serious and extremely common issue that may cause significant damage to the hoof over time. One way to check your horse's feet for peripheral loading is to take a look at the back of the foot when he is standing on level, firm ground. Keeping a safe distance, and with your horse tied or held so he can't back up on top of you, get down as low as you can and take a look at what parts are touching the ground. If it is only the heels, with a gap between the back of the frog and the ground, you likely have peripheral loading (figs. 5.19 A & B).

The "likely" part comes in because you also have to consider what type of footing the horse is moving and standing on day to day. Soft footing will allow the hoof to sink in farther than firm or hard footing, so if the horse is primarily housed and working on soft footing that is deep enough to allow the walls to sink in completely, the other structures on the bottom of the foot will share in weight bearing to some extent. If the horse spends any time resting, moving, or working on firmer footing, the wall is going to take the brunt of the horse's weight during those times.

Another way to look for peripheral loading is to examine your horse's footprints on various surfaces. The surface needs to be soft enough to create a footprint, or if it is smooth and hard, you can try wetting the horse's feet and seeing what the wet prints look like. The footprints of a peripherally loaded hoof will show nothing but a rim mark from the shoe or hoof wall, while the prints from a hoof that is not peripherally loaded will show that the frog made contact with the surface, at least toward the back of the foot (fig. 5.20). This experiment will not work on a horse with pads and packing material, as the pad will generally prevent the frog from making ground contact.

If you do suspect a peripheral-loading issue, talk to your hoof-care provider about changing your horse's trimming or shoeing to work toward getting the back of the foot more functionally involved in weight bearing.

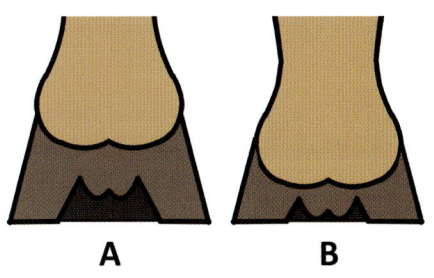

5.19 A & B A foot that is peripherally loaded has a gap between the frog and the ground (A). A foot that is not peripherally loaded will show the back of the frog making contact with the ground (B).

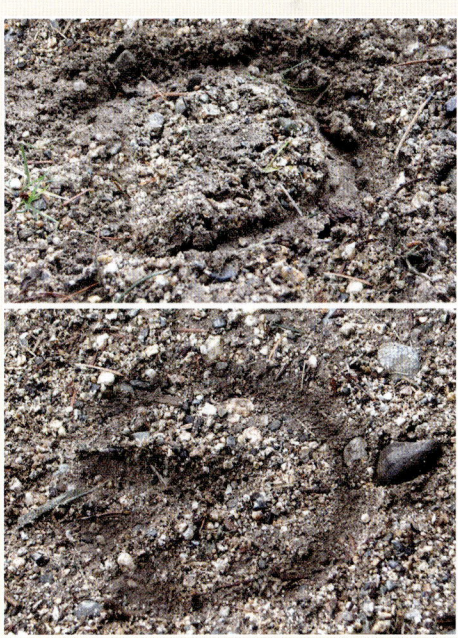

5.20 Two similar-sized horses walked across the same area of damp ground at the same time. The horse with peripherally loaded feet left only deep rim impressions (upper), while the other horse left shallower prints with clear impressions from his frogs (lower). Think of what this means in terms of weight distribution.

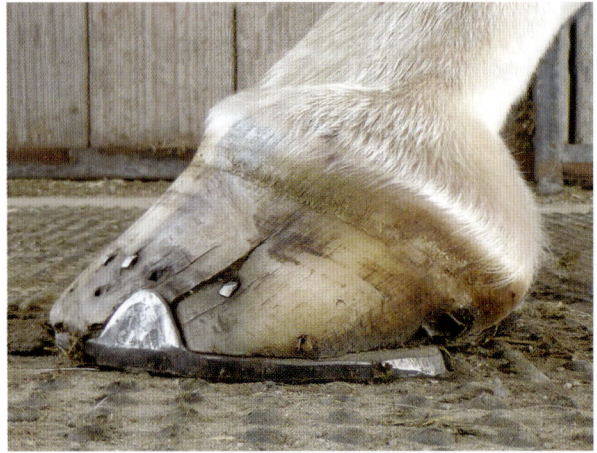

5.21 This horse's severely underrun heels leave little doubt that there are problems inside the foot as well. Is it any wonder that he can't grow a strong, healthy hoof wall? Notice that the worst cracks line up with the toe clips, which are applying additional pressure on an already weak wall.

time shoeing him, but it really does often work that way.

Other Factors

While peripheral loading is a common issue, there can be other factors such as hoof imbalance (underrun heels, for example), dietary issues, or underlying metabolic disorders that can lead to impaired circulation within the hoof. When any one or more of these problems are present, the horse owner may struggle with long-term wall and sole weaknesses (fig. 5.21). The bottom line is that if the "supply lines" are down, the foot can't get all the nutrients it needs for optimal growth, so no matter how great the diet is or what supplements get added in, the problem will remain. If you can address and rectify the underlying factors that are truly the root of the problem, improvement is far more likely.

Of course, it is never a bad idea to look at the diet of a horse with chronically weak walls to see if there actually is a deficiency or excess that could be creating or exacerbating weak wall issues. Many of the nutrients that contribute to good hoof health,

such as omega 3s, zinc, and copper, are pretty low in many hays and feeds. Most horses cope with these deficiencies without their walls falling apart, but it is worth thinking about if your horse is having problems. Excesses in the diet—particularly too much sugar or starch—are actually far more likely to be creating weaknesses in your horse's feet (see *Feeding the Foot*, p. 238).

When Chipping and Breaking Is a "Good" Thing

Sometimes, people with barefoot horses get alarmed when they start to see chips or little chunks missing around the bottom edge of the wall. Most of the time, a bare foot in this condition is simply ridding itself of excess hoof wall, a process referred to as "self-trimming" (fig. 5.22). Usually, all this means is that it is probably time for a trim, or that the hoof could use a little more beveling or rounding of the hoof wall when it is trimmed. Either way, minor chips or chunks are really just an aesthetic concern and do not necessarily indicate poor wall quality.

There are even cases where horses with badly overgrown feet will get some pretty big chips and chunk-outs as the foot attempts to self-trim, and even that can be a good thing. Long toes, for example, put stress on the laminae and can lead to strained tendons and ligaments, among other

White Line Disease

Sometimes, a weak, crumbly or cracking hoof wall is suffering from the fungal and/or bacterial infection known as *white line disease (WLD),* which is a common problem most often found in the toe and quarters. The term "white line disease" is somewhat misleading, as it is not actually the white line that

is affected. Instead, the invading organisms get up into the unpigmented, less dense inner zone of the stratum medium, where they eat away the wall material and cause weakening and separation within the hoof wall (fig. 5.24). If left unchecked, the infection can spread upward and fan out, eventually causing enough damage to destabilize the lamellar

problems, so if the foot can break off the excess toe horn, the whole limb will function better and be less prone to injury. Some feet can look pretty awful when they are trying to take care of themselves in this way, but if they are otherwise healthy, all they are likely to need is a good trim or two, and they will be just fine (figs. 5.23 A & B).

Of course, neglect that leads to excessively long feet is never a positive, but if you ever find yourself in a situation where you are considering taking on a horse and the only problem is that his feet look ragged, try to assess whether the foot is actually a healthy one trying to self-trim, or a foot that has real issues that won't disappear with simple trimming.

Another kind of chipping that isn't usually problematic often occurs after a horse's shoes have been removed and he is left barefoot. The nail holes weaken the hoof wall a bit, making it more vulnerable to breakage. When a horse's walls do break away around the nail holes while the hoof is growing out, this does not necessarily indicate weak walls or that the hoof is falling apart. It may just mean that the nail holes are growing out, and once they do, the hoof will be amply strong.

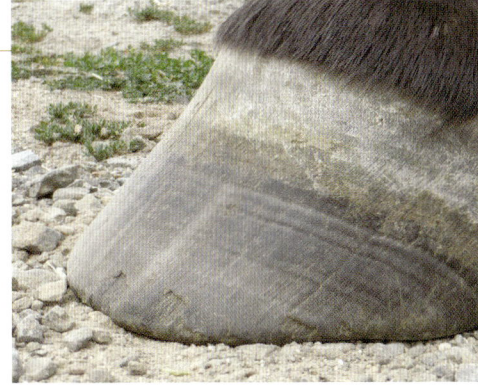

5.22 The small chips along the bottom of this hoof wall are just a bit of self-trimming at work and nothing to be concerned about.

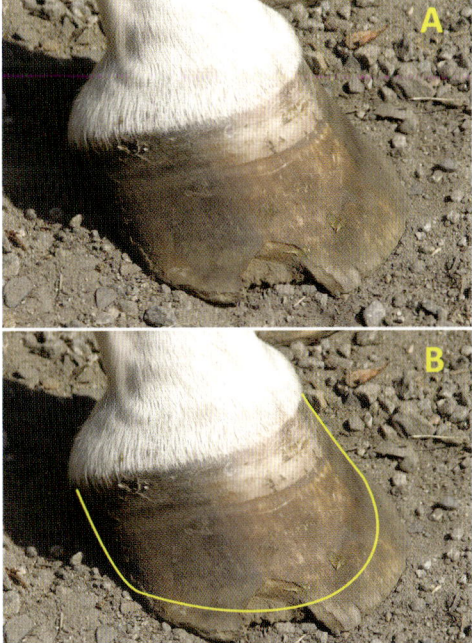

5.23 A & B Although this self-trimming wall isn't pretty, the foot is otherwise healthy and is simply trying to rid itself of all that overgrown toe (A). How can you tell the foot is healthy? Try imagining it with the excess growth taken away (B). If the remaining hoof has good balance, straight walls, and no other significant issues, chances are the foot is healthy and would look just fine in short order with proper care.

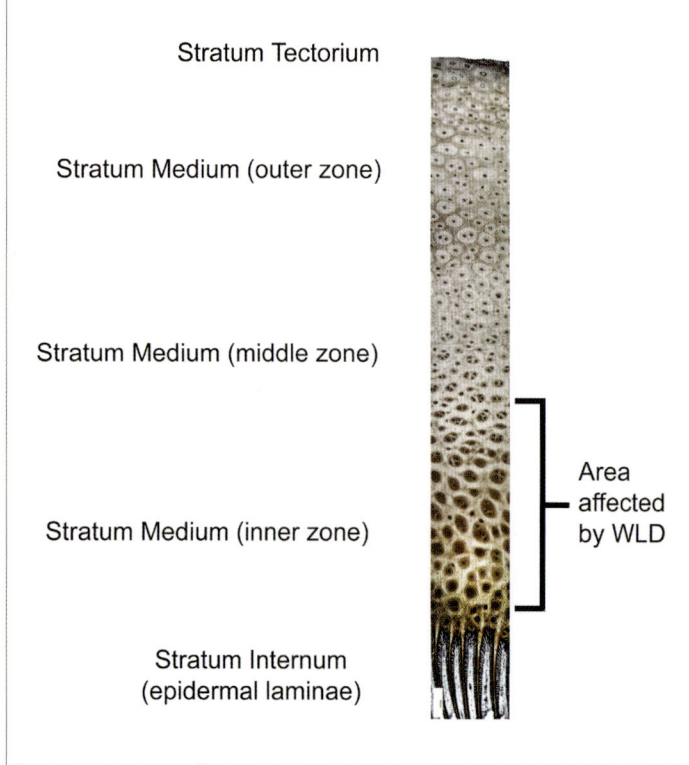

5.24 The area affected by white line disease (WLD) is the softer, less dense inner part of the hoof wall. This zone is more vulnerable to stretching and separating, which opens the door for opportunistic organisms.

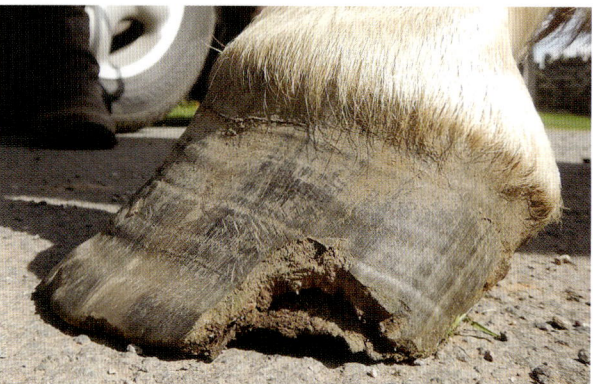

5.25 This hoof lost a large chunk of wall to WLD that went unnoticed.

connection and potentially cause displacement of the coffin bone.

White line disease is an opportunistic infection, meaning it needs the hoof wall to be already compromised in some manner before it can get a foot in the door. Usually, this involves some kind of separation or stretching of the hoof wall at the ground level, most often from laminitis or mechanical forces acting on an imbalanced or overgrown hoof. The separation created by these other issues allows the organisms to enter the tissues of the wall, and since they are anaerobic, they thrive in that closed environment. Once the infection takes hold, it will cause further separation as it spreads.

One of the problems with WLD is that it often goes unrecognized until the damage is extensive enough to cause lameness or serious wall degradation (fig. 5.25). By that time, the infection may have eaten away large portions of the inner hoof wall, and can be harder to deal with. The presence of WLD is often first signaled by a fissure, gap, or groove close to the sole/wall junction, which may be filled with soft, chalky material, black gunk, or dirt and debris from the environment (fig. 5.26). This opening—usually hidden under a shoe if the horse is shod—generally starts off small but gets wider, bigger, and deeper as more wall is damaged (fig. 5.27).

The problem is further compounded by the stuff that inevitably gets jammed up into the gap, effectively prying the already separated area open even more. Other signs may include wall cracks, walls that tend to chip or crumble away, walls that can't hold a shoe, and a hollow sound when the wall is tapped. Lameness is not usually

Labels on figure 5.24:
Stratum Tectorium
Stratum Medium (outer zone)
Stratum Medium (middle zone)
Stratum Medium (inner zone)
Stratum Internum (epidermal laminae)
Area affected by WLD

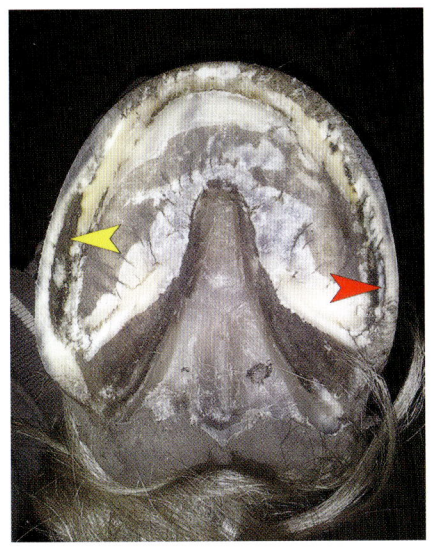

5.26 As the infected hoof wall separates, it forms fissures (red arrow), which eventually widen and may get packed with dirt and debris (yellow arrow).

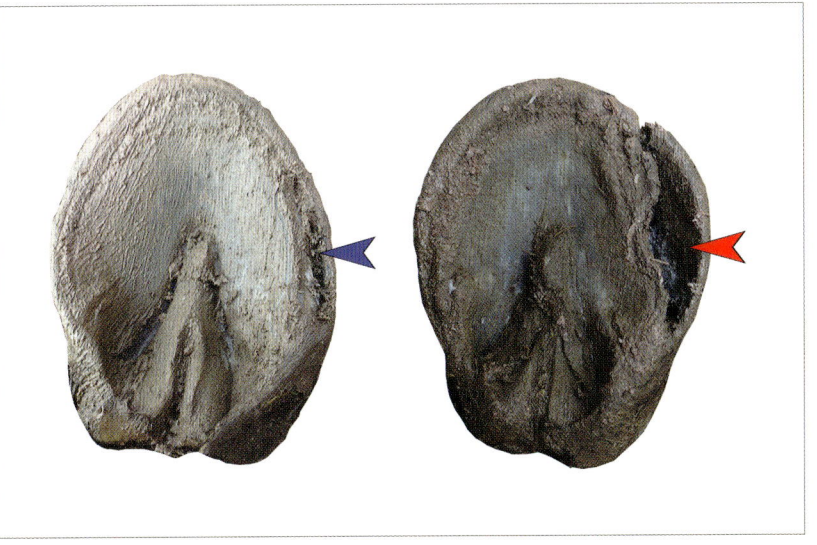

5.27 A small pocket of separation (left) can soon turn into a whopping one (right) if infection is allowed to spread. These are not the same feet, but without intervention, the one with the minor problem could easily end up like the more seriously damaged one.

present early on but can become severe as damage progresses.

As for how best to treat WLD, this is another one of those areas where opinions vary greatly. At one end of the spectrum are those who believe that you cannot get rid of WLD without resecting (cutting away) the separated portions of the wall, as they feel this is the only way to expose the anaerobic organisms and eradicate them (fig. 5.28). At the other end are those who argue that WLD is a secondary problem that will usually resolve on its own if you correct the underlying issues and maintain good hoof care. In between are the people who try to get rid of the infection with various soaks and topical treatments. Some report success with these treatments, but others try them to no avail, possibly because the active agents are unable to reach all of the infected areas.

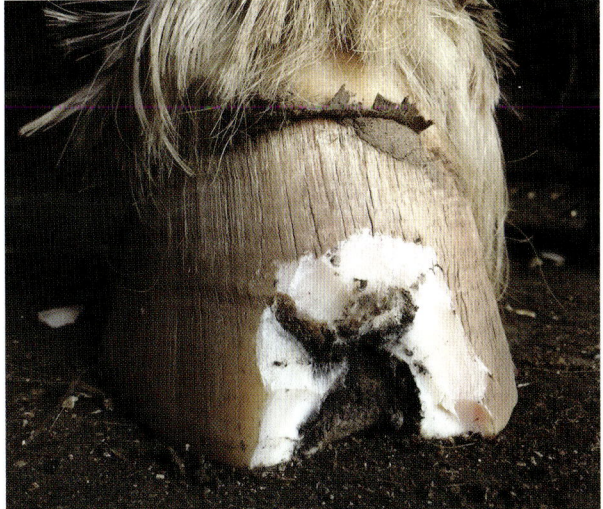

5.28 This hoof is undergoing a resection, in which the detached, diseased outer hoof wall is removed. The process exposes the anaerobic organisms to the air, which makes it impossible for them to survive. Though it looks awful now, the hoof wall will eventually grow down and be just fine if the underlying causative factors are dealt with.

Many experienced hoof-care providers will tell you that all of these approaches are valid, depending on the extent of the infection. When they do end up resecting significant portions of the hoof wall, some providers will want to put a shoe on to support the foot, while others may accomplish the same thing with hoof casting. Either way, great care must be taken if covering the opened area with any kind of packing or support material, as this can negate the whole purpose of exposing the anaerobic organisms to the air. Effective antibacterial/antifungal agents must be employed in these instances. If the resected area is left open, you want to be sure to keep it as dry and clean as possible.

Whatever treatment is employed, it is unlikely to succeed if the underlying issues that made the foot vulnerable to WLD are not addressed. To start with, look at the balance of the foot. If it has any issue causing the wall to distort or flare, this needs to be taken care of if at all possible. Often, this is simply a matter of better or more frequent trimming, though there are horses with permanent issues that cause them to load their feet unevenly no matter what you do, which can make dealing with WLD an ongoing battle. Still, keeping the foot as well-balanced and tight as it can be is your primary line of defense against WLD.

But, you can have the best trim in the world and still end up in a never-ending struggle with WLD if there are dietary issues causing continual or repeated bouts of subclinical laminitis (fig. 5.29). Usually, the problem is too many non-structural carbohydrates, which can be found in hay, grain, and grass. Getting serious about diet often ends up being the turning point in cases of stubborn WLD, so it is critically important that horse owners

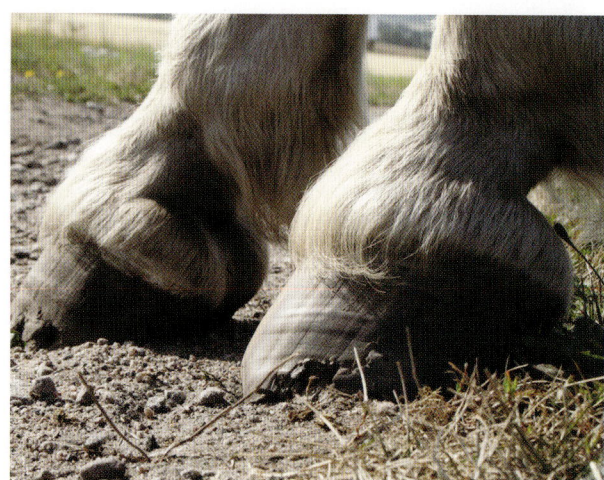

5.29 Both of these feet are so damaged by WLD that they can no longer hold a shoe. They are unlikely to get better if the horse continues on the same diet, which is the probable cause of the continual bouts of subclinical laminitis creating all those pronounced growth rings.

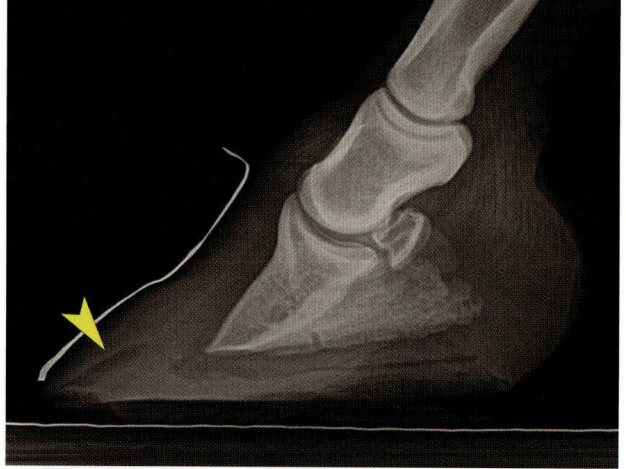

5.30 Because horn tissue damaged by WLD is less dense than healthy tissue, it shows up as a darker area on an X-ray, as pointed out here by the yellow arrow. (Note: the whitish line running along the front of the hoof wall is radiopaque material used to demarcate the hoof wall surface on the X-ray.)

understand the connection between what is going in a horse's mouth and what is going on in his feet.

You also need to recognize that advanced WLD can have consequences similar to laminitis in terms of displacement of the coffin bone, so if the infection is extensive, X-rays are a good idea to assess the extent of the damage to both the hoof wall and the internal structures. On an X-ray, WLD shows up as a darker area in the hoof wall, as the disrupted, infected tissue is less dense than the rest of the wall (fig. 5.30). Any internal damage is certainly going to make recovery more complicated, but with good treatment, horses can and often do recover from terrible bouts of WLD, even if the entire hoof wall has to be resected.

Get This Straight: The Coronet

Besides being the wellspring where much of the hoof wall originates, the coronet is important for another reason: it tells you a lot about the balance of the hoof and the position of the coffin bone within the hoof capsule.

From the Front

Since the hoof wall is anchored to the coffin bone, the angle of the coronet, when viewed from the front, generally reflects the coffin bone's orientation to the ground. Therefore, the coronet of a well-balanced hoof forms a straight line parallel to the ground when you are looking at the front of the hoof. The horse needs the bottom, front edge of the coffin bone to be parallel to the ground, as that orientation allows the horse's weight to be distributed evenly across the bottom of the coffin bone (fig. 5.31).

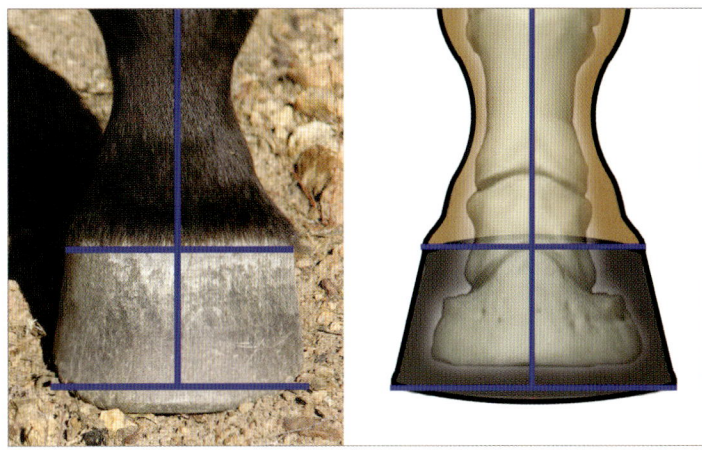

5.31 The foot on the left belongs to a horse with nicely balanced hooves, reflected by the almost perfectly straight coronet. If you were to X-ray this foot, you would see that the bones align much as they do in the illustration on the right.

5.32 The medial wall (left) of this hoof is significantly taller than the lateral wall, resulting in a tilted hairline. This means the coffin bone is tilted too, with the right side lower, thus bearing more weight.

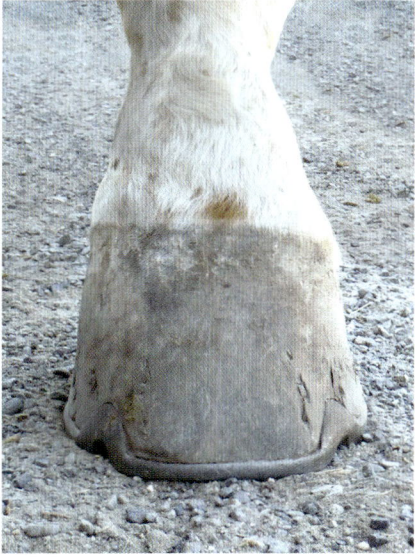

If the coronet is higher toward the inside or the outside of the hoof, you are looking at *mediolateral imbalance*. When that happens, the coffin bone will also be tilted relative to the ground. The result is uneven loading, with the side that is closer to the ground carrying more weight and becoming more vulnerable to breaking down (fig. 5.32). Unfortunately, that uneven loading carries on in the bones above the coffin bone, as they must all compensate for the crooked foundation they are stacked

5.33 This horse's feet became extremely unbalanced from long-term neglect. Her bones were forced to compensate, resulting in the crookedness seen here. Note that the space between the bones are wider on side A than side B. You can also see the formation of sidebone (C) from the excessive strain on that side of the limb. The good news: her bone alignment and hoof balance improved tremendously with good hoof care. While some believe that such changes can only be accomplished with shoes, this mare was never shod during her rehabilitation.

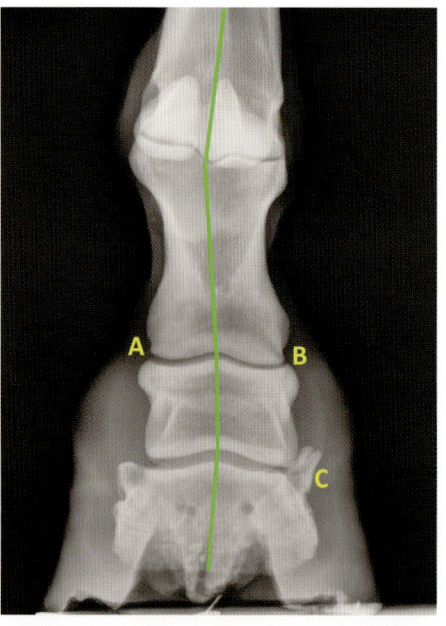

upon (fig. 5.33). Over time, this can lead to problems like arthritis of the joints, demineralization of one side of the coffin bone, and/or sidebone (ossification of the lateral cartilages), particularly on the side taking the additional pressure.

It is often possible to correct this kind of imbalance if the cause is something like bad trimming or a temporary injury. However, if a fully grown horse has a permanent conformational defect such as *carpus valgus* (knock knees) or *carpus varus* (bow legs), it is likely impossible to achieve a ground-parallel coronet band (and coffin bone) without placing harmful strain on the joints of the limb

5.34 This six-year-old grew up with *carpus valgus* that was never addressed. While it would be tempting to try to aggressively correct his resulting mediolateral imbalance and get those hairlines straighter, trying to drastically alter his hoof angles now would put strain on his joints and likely do more harm than good.

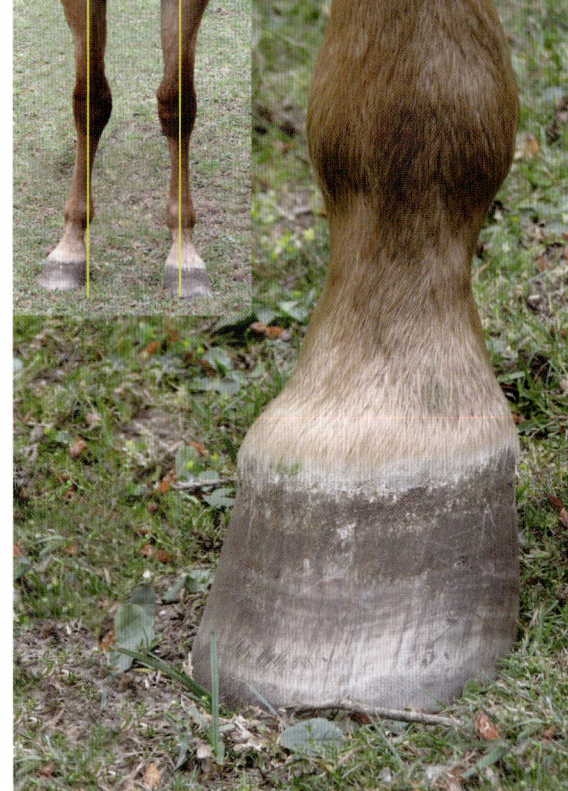

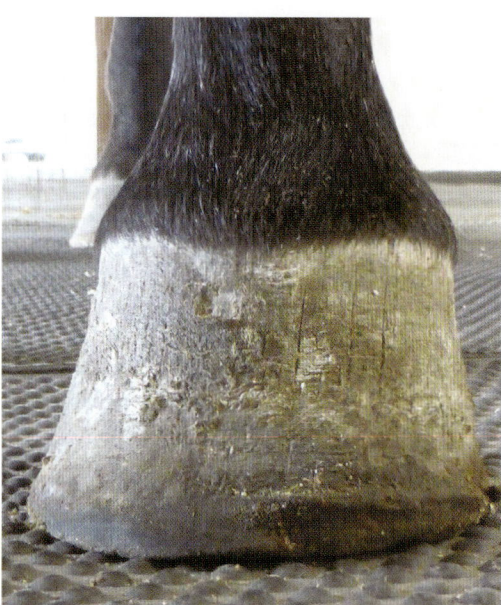

5.35 The dip in the center of this foot's coronet indicates that the coffin bone may have descended within the hoof capsule. X-rays would be a good idea to confirm this and see what other problems might be lurking, because distal descent (sinking of the coffin bone relative to the hoof capsule) can lead to a variety of issues.

(fig. 5.34). In such cases, you have to make the best of a less-than-ideal situation by trimming the foot regularly to minimize distortion. It is also worth investing in some X-rays to help your farrier see exactly what is going on in order to keep your horse as sound as possible.

Another abnormality we sometimes see is a dip in the center of the coronet. If you see this, there is a good chance that the horse has had an episode of laminitis or chronic peripheral loading that caused the coffin bone to "sink" within the hoof capsule, a process known as *distal descent.* In a healthy foot, the extensor process is suspended high up in the hoof capsule, keeping the coronet "full." You can actually feel this if you palpate the area. If the coffin bone sinks, it drags the extensor process down, leaving an empty space in the center of the coronet which you can both see and feel (fig. 5.35).

From the Side

With the hoof on the ground and viewed from the side, the coronet should be highest at the toe, sloping down toward the ground at the heels in a

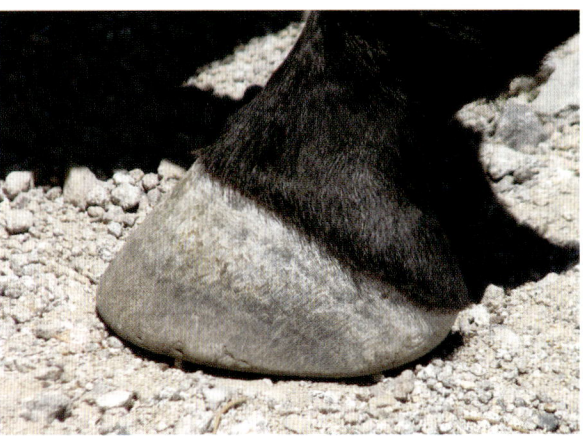

5.36 This horse's coronet forms a fairly straight line as it angles toward the ground, which is what you want to see.

fairly straight line (fig. 5.36). A slight upward arch is sometimes seen in healthy feet, but there should be no dramatic arch in this line, no "wave" up and down, nor should it be anywhere near close to parallel with the ground. If you see any of these features, you are probably looking at some sort of imbalance, with high heels and long quarters being two common issues that can cause these problems (figs. 5.37 A–C).

Club feet can also develop a very altered hairline, in part because their heels can get quite tall, and in some cases, the altered position of the coffin

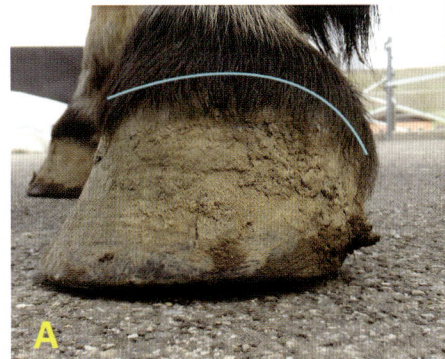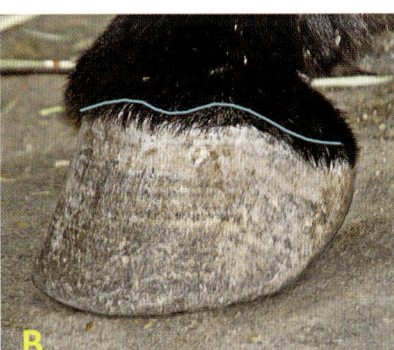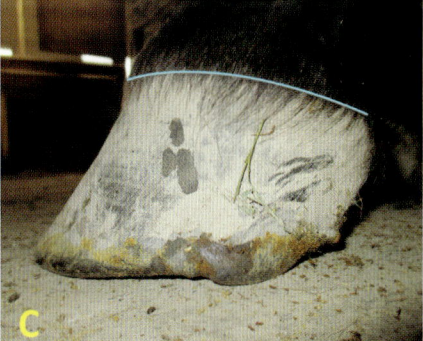

5.37 A–C You don't want a hairline that curves upward too much (A), waves up and down (B), or is too high in the back, making it close to parallel with the ground (C). Any part that is higher than it should be usually has too much pressure on it from an overly tall area of the wall.

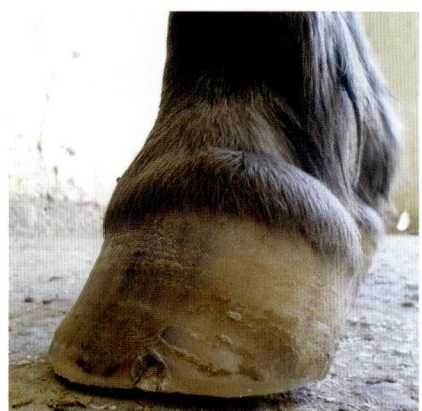

5.38 Club feet like this one can develop very arched hairlines if the heels are high and the front of the coronet is pulled downward by the position of the coffin bone.

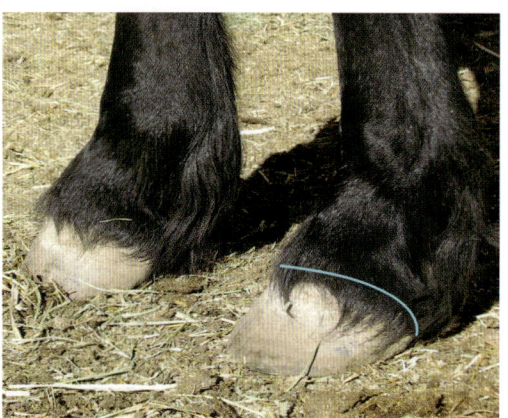

5.39 The long hair on this horse's feet makes it hard to see what is really going on with the hairline, but it looks as if she may have some minor bulging upward in the quarters.

bone can pull the front of the hairline downward, creating a very dramatic arch (fig. 5.38). Keep in mind that long hair around the coronet can obscure the true slope of the coronet, so you may have to do a little trimming job to get a good look if your horse has fuzzy feet (fig. 5.39).

As for the coronet angle, also called the *hairline angle*, it is important to note that there is no one hairline angle that suits all horses, and it is a mistake to try to force all horses into an angle that is unnatural for them. Doing so can make them sore or worse. That said, healthy hairline angles usually fall in the range of 20–30 degrees. When the hairline is less than 20 degrees, the heels are likely too high and the coffin bone is tilted too much onto the toe. When the hairline is greater than 30 degrees, there is a good chance that the back of the coffin bone is lower than the toe, putting excess pressure and strain on the back of the foot (fig. 5.40).

However, even if the horse's coronet angle is within the 20–30 degree range, that is no guarantee that the current angle is the best one for that horse. Some adjustments could still be in order, but you are less likely to have a serious problem than when the angle is outside of that range. If you do see angles that are overly steep or shallow, you definitely want to take a hard look at the horse's hoof form.

Bottom Line: The coronet should be straight and parallel to the ground when viewed from the front, and should form a basically straight line with a 20–30 degree angle when viewed from the side.

5.40 The top foot has a healthy hairline angle of about 20 degrees. The middle foot's angle, at 33 degrees, is concerning, but not surprising given its underrun heels. The bottom foot definitely has a problem, with high heels pushing the hairline angle down to 10 degrees.

Angles of the Hoof and Heel Assessment

Hoof Angle: Allowing for Natural Variation

In addition to the coronet angle, there are several other angles you want to look at when assessing the equine foot. The first is the angle the dorsal wall makes in relation to the ground, most often called the *hoof angle.* Veterinarians and hoof-care professionals used to be taught that the ideal angle for the hooves was 45–50 degrees for the front and 50–55 degrees for the hind. Some people took that even further, saying that all hooves should be exactly 45 degrees in front, and 55 degrees in back, and that we should strive to create these angles on all horses.

The problem with this idea is that it fails to take into account the fact that there is natural variation in how the bones of a horse's legs are put together. Forcing the feet to take on a certain angle that may be at odds with the angles of bones within and above them can wreak havoc with the function of the joints and related soft tissues, resulting in unnatural strain and potential injury, as well as degenerative changes over time.

Rather than aiming for a specific number, most hoof experts today believe that the angle of

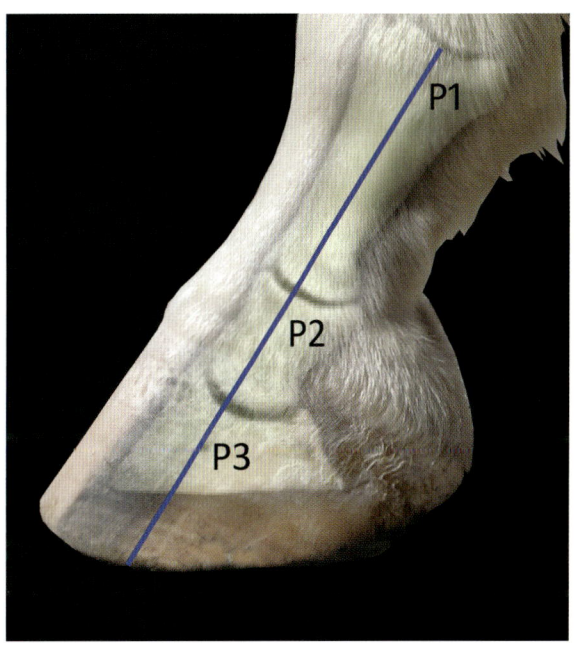

6.1 On a horse with a well-balanced foot, a line drawn through the middle of P1, P2, and P3 (the long pastern bone, short pastern bone, and the coffin bone) would be approximately parallel to the dorsal wall of the hoof.

the dorsal wall should be parallel to a line drawn through the coffin bone (P3), the short pastern bone (P2), and the long pastern bone (P1) (fig. 6.1). While we can't see the actual bones without an X-ray, we can see the angle of the long pastern bone, which is the part of the leg we call the pastern. A good rule

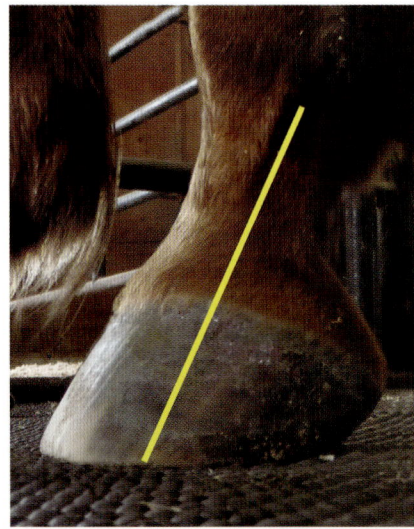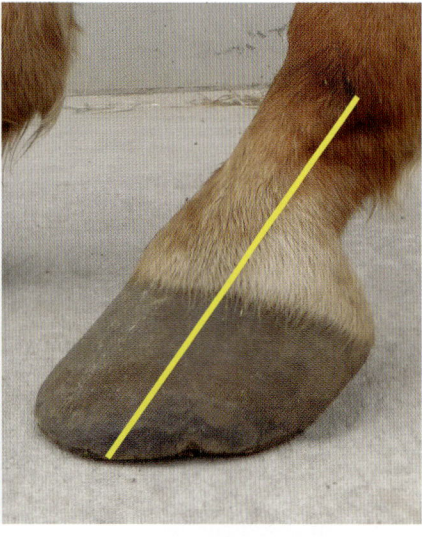

6.2 Even when the limbs don't have ideal pasterns, the angle of the dorsal wall should approximate the angle of the pastern. The horse on the left has short, upright pasterns, so his foot is appropriately a bit upright. The horse on the right has long, sloping pasterns, and his dorsal wall matches this angle, as it should.

of thumb is to look at the hoof-pastern axis, which is how the angle of the dorsal wall compares to the angle of the pastern bone. Ideally, these two will be parallel to one another. This means that a horse with more upright pasterns overall will have more upright hoof angles than a horse with more sloping pasterns, whose feet should echo that degree of slope (fig. 6.2). It also means that the hind feet will usually be slightly more upright than the front, as the hind pasterns of most horses are a bit more upright than the front.

"Broken" Axes

When the dorsal wall and the pastern don't line up, we say that the hoof-pastern axis is "broken." It can be broken back or it can be broken forward (figs. 6.3 A–C). Either way, if you spot a broken axis on your horse, it is definitely something you want to discuss with your hoof-care professional and possibly

your vet. In many instances, adjustments in trimming and/or shoeing can improve hoof-pastern alignment, such as a hoof with tall, overgrown heels causing a broken-forward axis, or a long toe and low heel causing a broken-back axis. However, there are cases where the misalignment of angles is permanent, such as a club foot on a mature horse, where it isn't going to be possible to achieve the ideal, and trying to force a "better" angle onto such a foot can potentially cause harm.

Broken Back Axis

When the axis is broken back, the hoof angle is lower than the pastern angle, which causes a number of problems for the foot (fig. 6.4). The coffin bone is likely to have a ground parallel or even negative palmar/plantar angle (p. 25), which puts excessive strain on the back of the coffin joint (the joint formed by P2, P3, and the navicular bone), as well as on the deep digital flexor tendon, since both of these are forced to extend more than is normal. As a result, the horse may develop inflammation in the DDFT or in the coffin joint itself, and

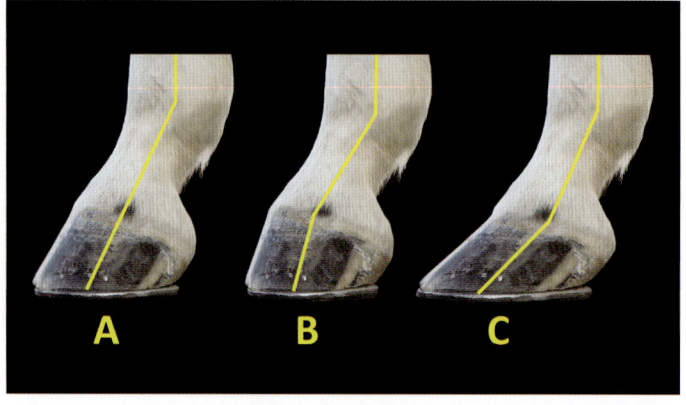

6.3 A–C A foot with a normal hoof-pastern axis (A); a broken-forward axis (B); a broken-back axis (C).

the navicular bursa can also suffer damage due to increased friction. These issues are often made even worse by long toe/low heel syndrome, which delays breakover and is frequently associated with broken back feet (see *Underrun Heels,* p. 78).

Another problem is that a broken-back axis shifts the focal point of weight bearing farther back in the foot, forcing the structures in the back of the foot to cope with abnormal compression and concussion. In such cases, blood flow to the back of the foot may be compromised, the digital cushion and the frog can deteriorate, and the foot may develop chronic heel pain, as well as visible marks of strain such as quarter cracks and cracks in the heels.

You may also see a prolapsed frog in a broken-back foot, where the frog is pushed downward due to abnormal pressures caused by the low palmar/plantar angle of the coffin bone inside the foot. As we've mentioned before, a prolapsed frog is not at all the same thing as a healthy foot with the frog making contact with the ground (p. 17). A foot with a prolapsed frog is very likely to be tender or downright painful in the back of the foot, whereas a healthy foot will not. Pain in the back of the foot, whether the frog has prolapsed or not, may cause the foot to start landing toe first, which in itself causes a problem and is now thought by some to be a factor in the development of palmar heel pain issues (see sidebar, p. 213).

However, when you come across a hoof with a broken-back angle and the back of the foot is already damaged, that is a chicken-and-egg situation, because while low hoof angles can cause deterioration in the back of the foot, it is also true that deterioration in the back of the foot, occurring for any reason, may lead to low hoof angles, as can

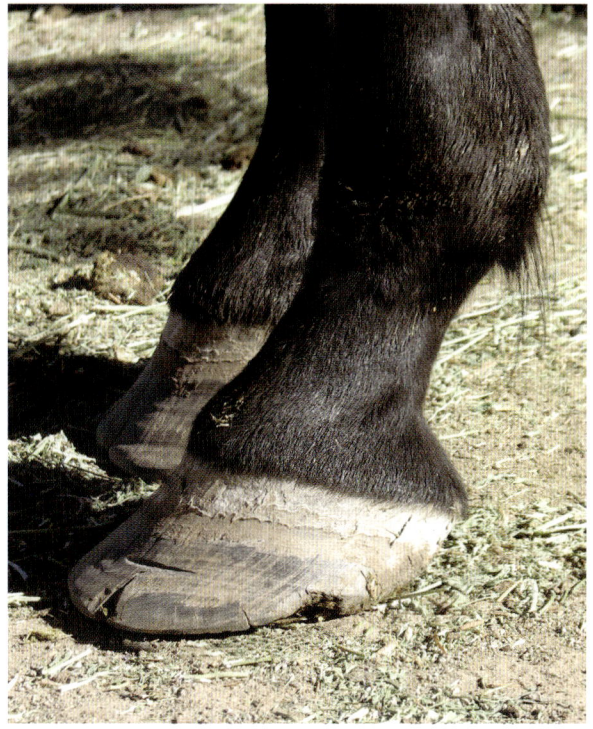

6.4 This horse's broken-back hoof-pastern axis is partially due to high/low syndrome, where one hoof is significantly more upright than the other, and partially due to the fact that he is well overdue for a trim.

laminitis. In the latter two scenarios, the low hoof angle is a symptom of the problem, and you must figure out and address the root of the problem to have the best chance of successful rehabilitation.

Whatever the cause, a broken-back axis needs to be addressed and corrected as much as the horse's conformation will allow. If the horse's axis is broken back simply due to overgrown, run-forward feet, there is a good chance that the problem can be corrected. However, as with any effort to change hoof angles, this one should be done gradually and under the guidance of a well-trained professional. Be aware that horses with long, sloping pasterns

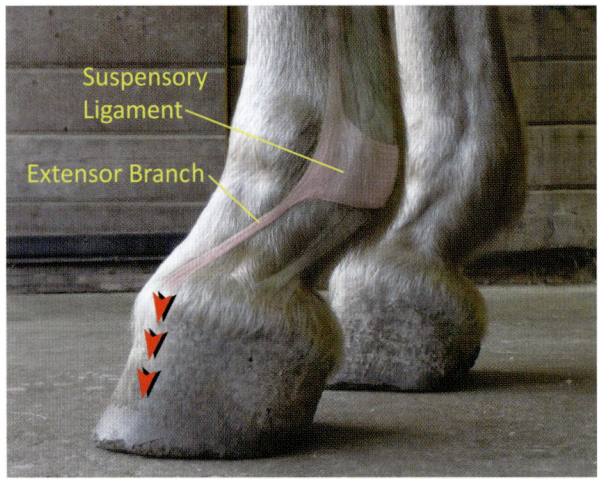

6.5 The continual downward pull on the extensor branches of the suspensory ligament is one of the abnormal stresses that come with a broken-forward axis, which in this case is the result of the horse's club feet.

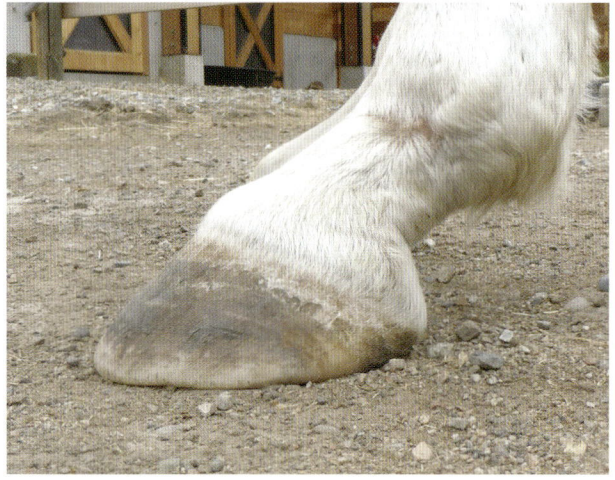

6.6 A When the suspensory ligament becomes slack due to degenerative suspensory ligament desmitis (DSLD), the fetlock and pastern drop, creating a broken-forward hoof-pastern axis, as well as a tendency to develop long toes and low heels, as this horse has done.

are more likely to develop a broken-back pastern axis, and can therefore be more of a management headache.

Broken-Forward Axis

A broken-forward hoof-pastern axis is also a problem that needs to be corrected to whatever degree is possible—but not forced if it is going to hurt the horse. Broken-forward conformation puts stress on the front of the coffin joint due to excessive flexion. It also puts strain on the suspensory ligament, as the ligament's extensor branches experience a constant downward pull (fig. 6.5).

Problems caused by this conformation include inflammation (desmitis) of the suspensory ligament, inflammation of the coffin joint, and damage to the coffin bone, particularly along the front edge (pedal osteitis). In some cases, load bearing is shifted forward, causing the horse's toes to tend to wear

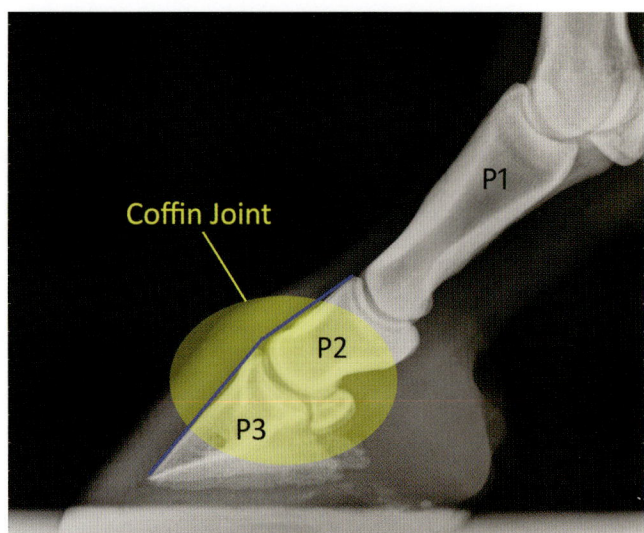

6.6 B An X-ray reveals that as this horse's pastern angles are dropping due to suspensory ligament deterioration, the coffin joint, made up of P2, P3, and the navicular bone, is taking on a broken-forward axis (blue line). However, when looking at such X-rays, do keep in mind that the coffin joint normally does have some mobility, so its axis can change to some degree depending on how the horse is standing.

down, while the heels will grow too high due to lack of pressure and wear. This can be exacerbated by changes in blood flow, where the coronary corium gets compressed and thus the toe wall has less blood flow than the heels, making toe growth slow relative to heel growth. Growth lines that are wider at the heels are common when this happens. The sole in the toe region may also become thin due to compression of the solar corium. Causes of a broken-forward axis include congenital or developmentally caused club feet (see *Club Feet,* p. 85), injury, as well as poor trimming or shoeing.

Degenerative Suspensory Ligament Desmitis

There is also a soft tissue condition called degenerative suspensory ligament desmitis (DSLD), now sometimes called equine systemic proteoglycan accumulation (ESPA), that can create a broken-forward axis, but this is quite a different situation. In these cases, it is not the hoof that has rotated downward in relation to the pastern, but rather the pastern that has dropped to a lower angle due to degeneration of the suspensory ligament (figs. 6.6 A & B). Horses with this condition will have a tendency

Hands-On Activity:
Evaluate Your Horse's Hoof-Pastern Axis

Evaluating your horse's hoof-pastern axis can give you important information about his trim and conformation, and possibly help you to head off problems that could result if something is amiss.

To get a correct read on your horse's hoof-pastern axis, make sure the horse is standing on firm, level ground. It is also extremely important that the horse is standing square, which means all four feet are placed so that the cannon bones are perpendicular to the ground and the feet are weighted evenly. This allows you to see the true relation of the pastern angle to the hoof. If the horse is not standing square, his joints will flex to some degree, giving you an inaccurate reading of the hoof-pastern axis (fig. 6.7).

Once your horse is standing square (it may be helpful to have someone helping to keep him that way), move to the side, crouch down at a low angle, and take a look at how the front of the hoof wall lines up with the middle of the pastern. You might want to take a photo and draw some lines on it for easier assessment. If you see a broken-back or broken-forward angle, discuss it with your hoof-care provider and/or vet at the next opportunity.

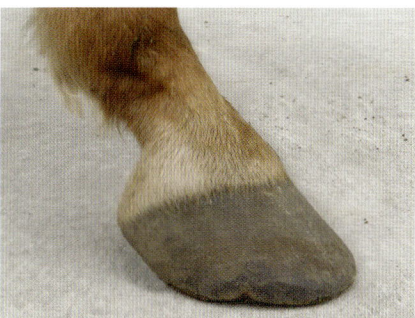
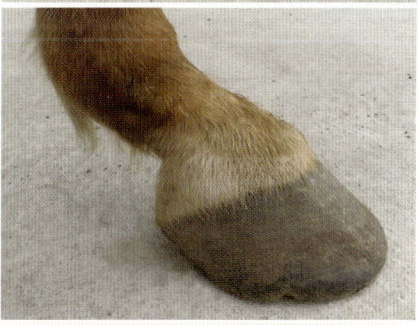

6.7 This is the same foot, but the hoof-pastern axis looks very different in the two photos. In the top picture, the horse was standing square with all four feet weighted evenly. In the bottom photo, he was weighting this foot much more heavily than the others, making it look like he has a broken-forward axis.

to develop long toes and low heel angles, as weight bearing is shifted backward. Because of this shift, damage inside the foot is in some ways more similar to what you see with a broken-back angle, even though the foot looks broken forward.

Heel Angles

The angle of the heels should match or come close to matching the angle of the dorsal wall, assuming the dorsal wall is not distorted in some way. If the wall is distorted, the heel angle may match it, but both could be unhealthy (fig. 6.8). When the angles don't match, the issue is almost always that the heels have a lower angle than the dorsal wall. Whether the angles of the toe and heel match

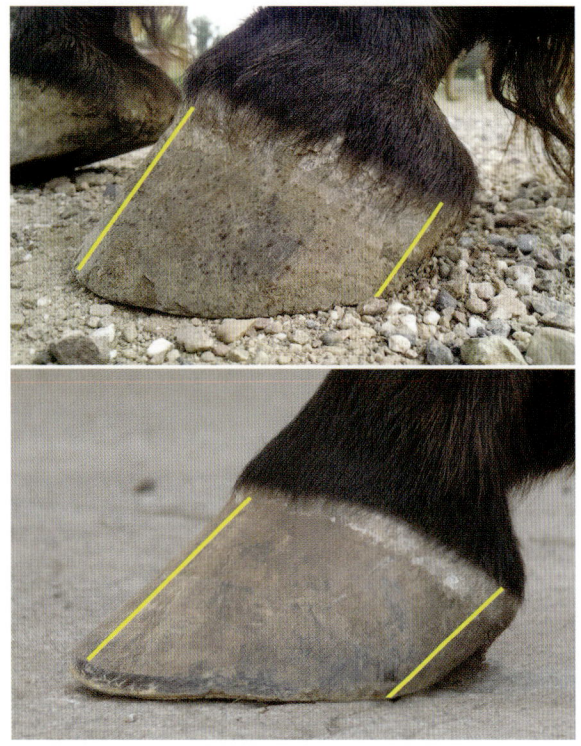

6.8 While both of these horses have heel angles that are very similar to their toe angles, the bottom foot's toe and heel angles are rather low. Although you can't see much of the pastern angle in this photo, it does not match the angle of this long, low toe or the heel that is starting to become underrun. This foot is a good example of why "matching" doesn't always mean "healthy" when it comes to toe and heel angles.

or not, if the heels are farther forward than they should be, we call them *underrun,* or sometimes, *underslung.* One of the main problems with under-run heels is that they don't support the bony column of the leg properly. We'll talk more about that in a minute, but first, let's look at the different ways you can examine the heels for overall health.

Assessing the Heels

Heel Height

The heels of the horse can be assessed in a number of ways. One is the height of them, as viewed from the side. While there is no one perfect heel height that is right for all horses, healthy heel height allows the coffin bone to maintain a slightly positive palmar/plantar angle, meaning a few degrees raised in the back (see fig. 4.7, p. 25). On most horses, this will equate to a heel height of around 1 inch to 1½

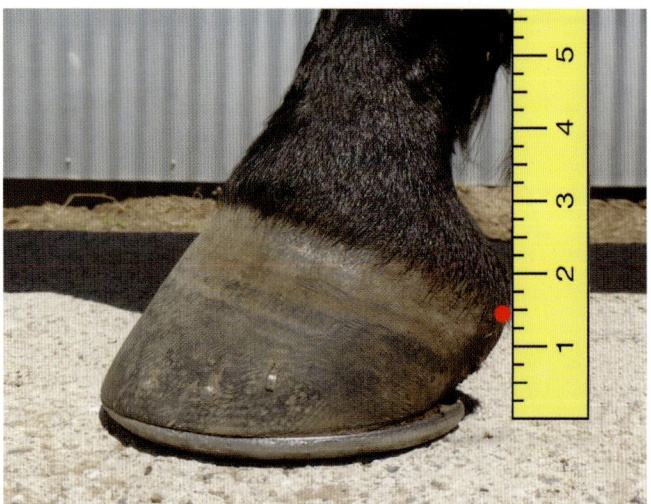

6.9 Domestic horses with healthy feet tend to have a heel height of about 1 inch to 1½ inches, as you see here. If your horse is shod and you are taking this measurement, be sure to factor in the height of the shoe.

inches measured from the hair line to the ground when barefoot, or the top of the shoe when shod (fig. 6.9). However, there are certainly horses out there with heels a bit higher or lower that do just fine, so if your horse doesn't quite fit into that range but is perfectly sound, it is likely nothing to fret about.

Too High

More important than measurement is whether or not the heels are the right height to align the coffin bone in a correct orientation with the ground. When the heels are too high (fig. 6.10 A), they can create a broken-forward hoof-pastern axis, tip the coffin bone forward, place excessive pressure on the solar margin of the bone and on the toe wall, and put strain on the front of the coffin joint and the ligaments that attach to the front of the coffin bone. All of this can lead to inflammation and tearing of the laminae, separation and white line disease, thinning of the sole in the toe region, ligament damage, arthritis, and other problems. Another issue with high heels is that they can lift the frog off the ground, rendering all of the shock-absorbing mechanisms in the back of the foot useless.

Too Low

When the heels are too low, they may cause a broken-back hoof-pastern axis, which tips the coffin

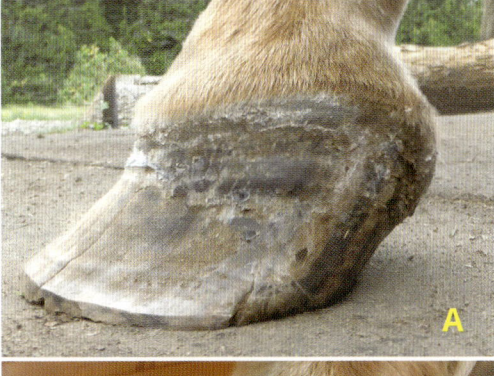
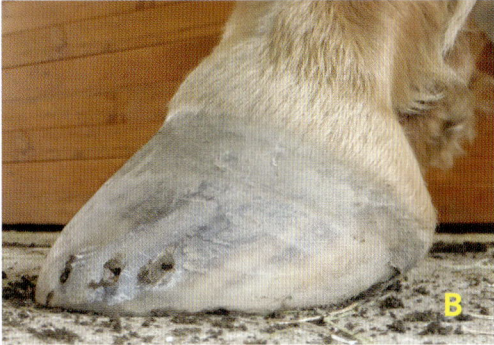

6.10 A & B You don't need an X-ray to know that the coffin bone of the foot in the upper photo is lifted up far too high in the back. As for the lower photo, the "bullnose" profile of this hind foot indicates that the coffin bone has a negative plantar angle, a consequence of the foot's too low, underrun heels.

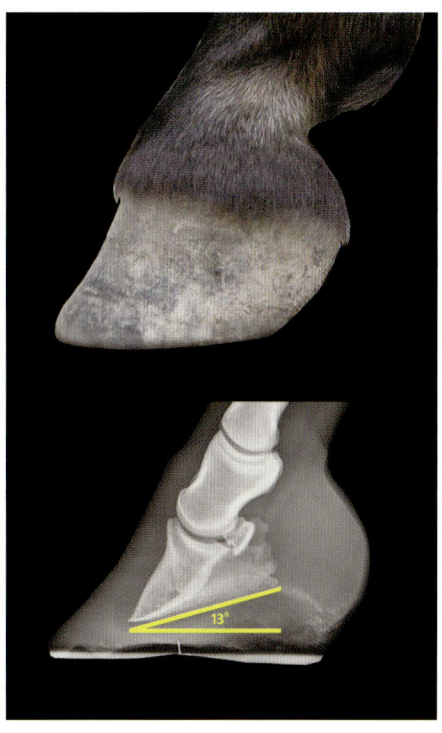

6.11 This horse had serious lameness issues, in part because her heels were allowed to get extremely high. The X-ray (below) of her foot (above) shows the 13-degree palmar angle of the coffin bone. A healthy angle is approximately 2–5 degrees. (Note: The foot is shown at a slightly more forward-facing angle than the X-ray.)

bone backward, straining the various structures in the back of the foot and compressing the solar corium. Sometimes, when the heels are too low, the dorsal wall will take on a convex profile, called a "bullnose," which results from the front of the coffin bone pushing up against the inside of the wall (fig. 6.10 B).

But whether the walls are too low or too high, it will affect the biomechanics of the entire foot and leg, which can lead to strain, imbalance, and possible injury (fig. 6.11). It is, therefore, very important

6.12 While heel height is measured from the hairline to the ground (blue line), heel length is measured from the hairline to the back of the heel buttress (yellow).

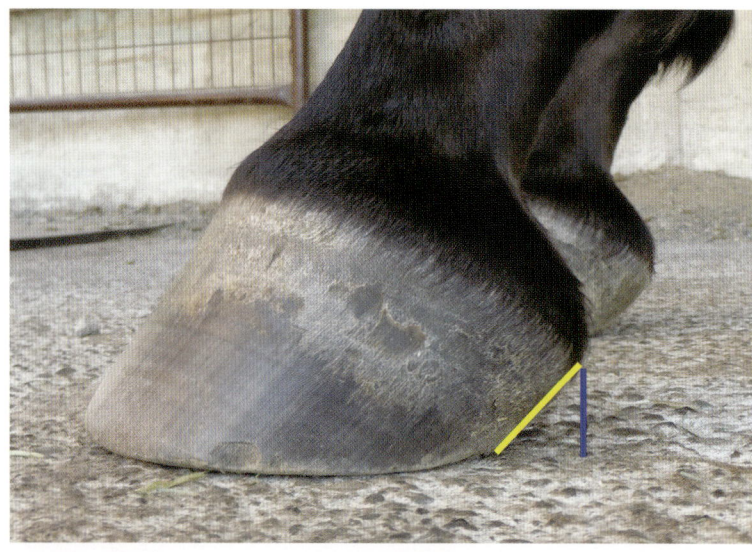

6.13 All four of these horses have long heels. The top left heel is long and high, as is the top right. The bottom left heel is a reasonable height, but is too long, nonetheless. The bottom right is long and is starting to get too low, putting it in danger of crushing.

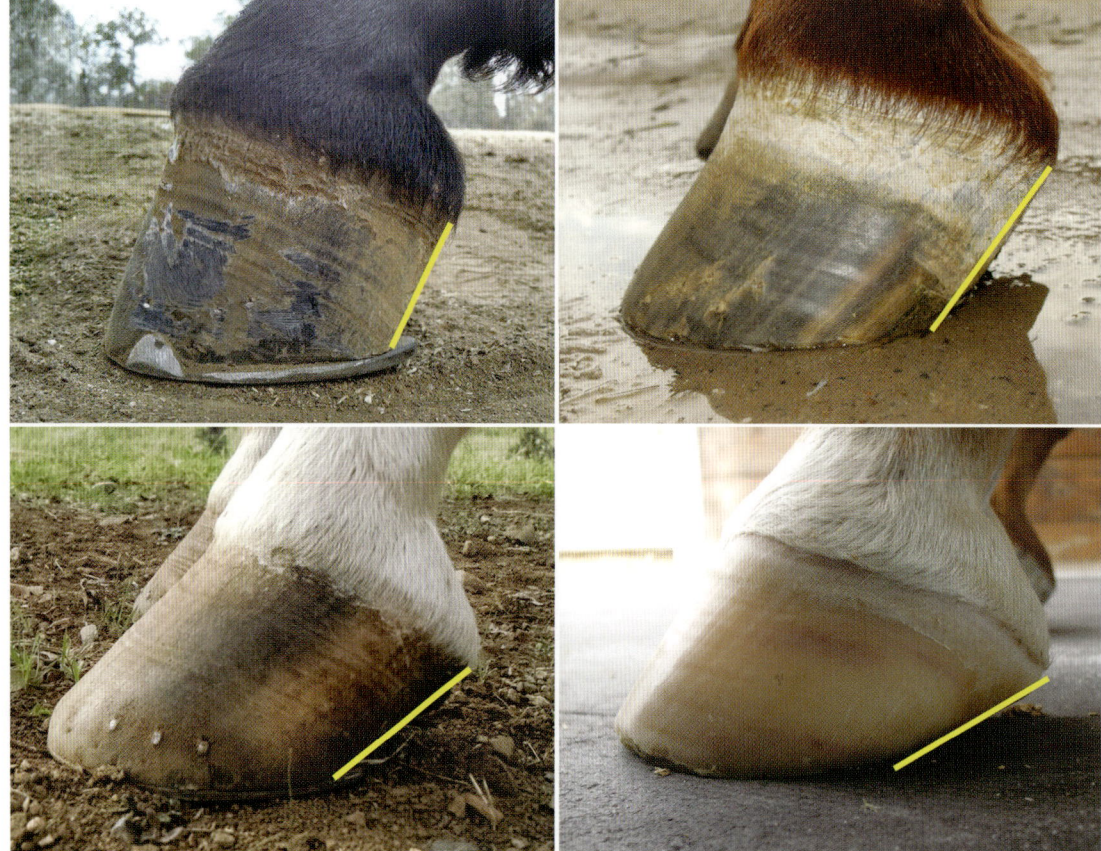

to make sure that your hoof-care provider is keeping your horse's heels at the right height for his conformation.

Heel Length

The second aspect of heel health to look at is the length of the heels, which is not the same thing as the height. While height is measured from the hairline to the ground in a perpendicular line, length is measured along the slope of the heel itself, from the hairline to the point where the back of the heel buttress touches the ground (fig. 6.12). Healthy heels will be fairly short. It is important to recognize that heels can be long and high, what we might call a "stacked" heel, but they can also be long and low (underrun), thus farther forward than they should be (fig. 6.13). Long, low heels are at risk of failing and collapsing altogether, at which point they are called "crushed heels" (fig. 6.14).

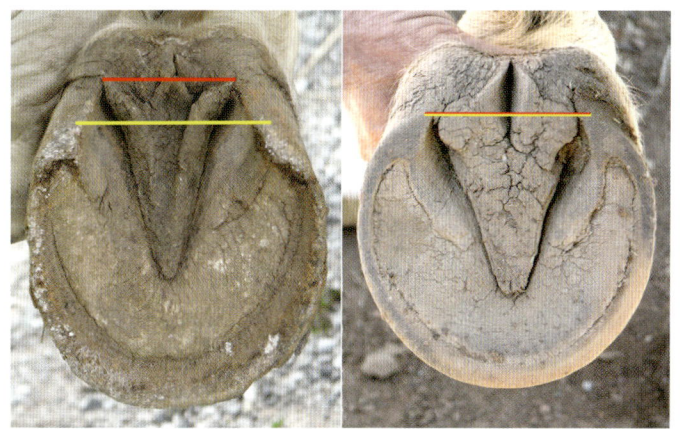

6.15 These two photos show the same foot. On the left, the heels—measured at the yellow line, which marks the farthest-back point at which the heel buttresses touch the ground—are quite run forward, well ahead of the widest part of the frog marked by the red line. Only a few months later, a change in diet, 24/7 turnout on firm footing, and the implementation of physiologically correct trimming have changed the entire foot, including getting the heels back in line with the widest part of the frog. Note that the yellow and red lines are now in the same place.

Heel Placement

Next, you want to look at the bottom of the foot (solar view) to see where the heels are in relation to the frog. Healthy heels are far back on the foot, with the heel buttresses ending in line with the widest part of the frog (fig. 6.15). Underrun heels end farther forward than the widest part of the frog. In this position, the heels cannot provide optimum support for the bony column of the leg, as they will be ahead of the focal point of weight bearing. This puts significant strain on the tendons and ligaments of the limb, particularly up the back of the leg, and the navicular bone and bursa can be affected as well. It also puts additional pressure on the heels, which are already weakened if they have run forward.

Viewed from the side, the back point of the heel buttresses in heels that are in the correct position

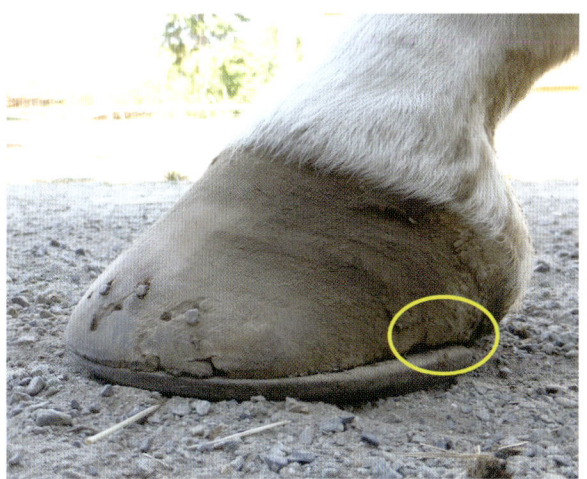

6.14 Long, low heels are subjected to tremendous strain. The farther forward they migrate, the more force is exerted on them, and the more likely they are to become crushed, as you see here. Notice that there is no angle at all to this heel—it is completely flattened.

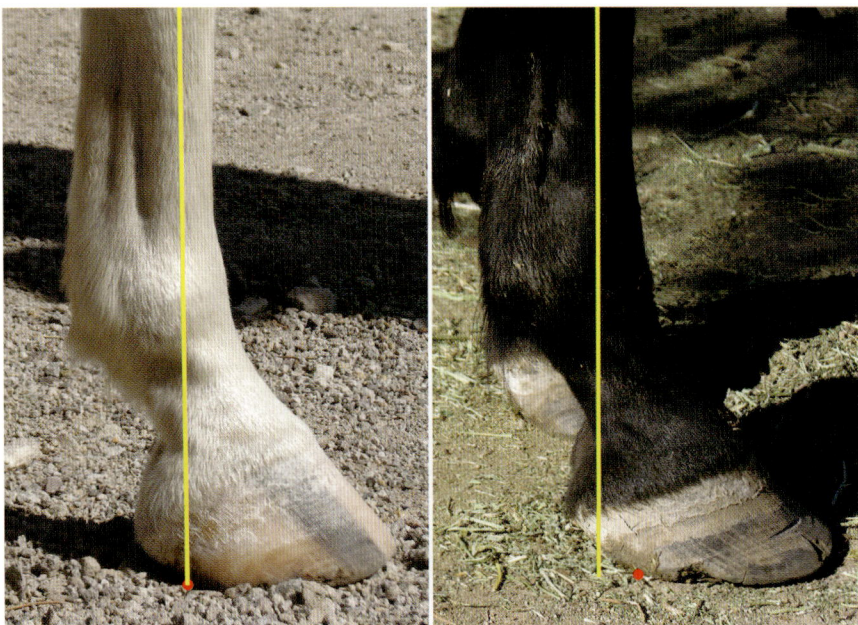

6.16 The back of the heels should align with the middle of the cannon bone in order to provide optimal support. The leg on the left has good alignment, but the right one's heels are too far forward (see red dot), placing them ahead of the focal point of weight bearing (bottom of yellow line).

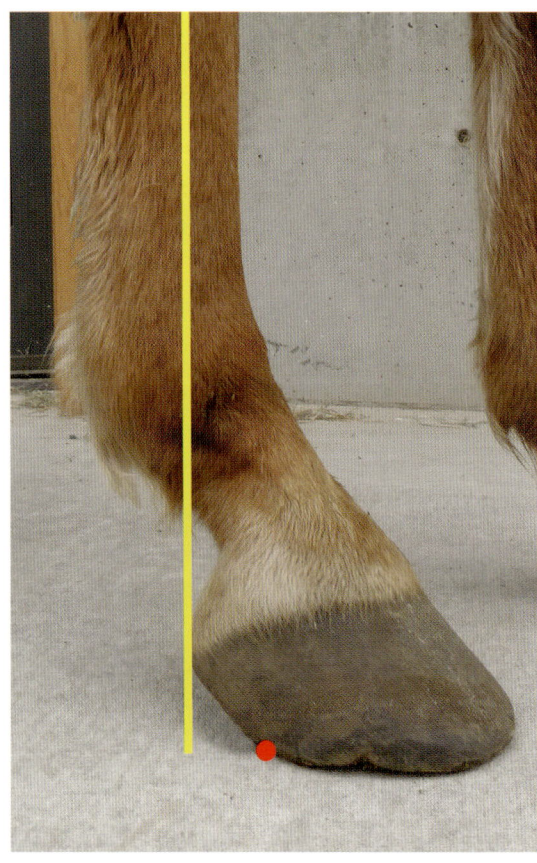

6.17 A horse with long, sloping pasterns like this one will often have his heels well ahead of the cannon bone (see red dot), even when the heels are aligned well with the frog.

line up with the center of the cannon bone, providing maximum support for the limb, while the point of the heel buttresses of underrun heels will be ahead of that point (fig. 6.16). Horses with long, sloping pasterns may also have heels that are ahead of the center of the cannon bone, even when their heels are in line with the widest part of the frog (fig. 6.17). This is one of the reasons why this conformation can cause lameness issues.

Heel Width

The next assessment—the width of the heels—is also easiest to assess from the bottom of the foot. Healthy heels are far apart, quite wide in relation to the total width of the foot. This allows plenty of space for a robust frog to grow and creates a good base of support for the limb (fig. 6.18). A strong frog works together with good heels to form a large "landing zone" for the foot, providing a tremendous amount of shock-absorbing capacity. Contracted heels (see p. 75) result in a narrow frog and compromised shock absorption, among other problems.

Heel Bulbs

The final aspect of heel health to look at is the symmetry and width of the heel bulbs, which requires a from-the-rear view. In terms of symmetry, what you want to see is that the heel bulbs are even in size, shape, and height. If one is noticeably different or higher than the other, there is some kind of imbalance in the foot or limb.

One problem to look for is *sheared heels,* which happens when the hoof is bearing more weight on one side of the hoof than the other, causing the over-weighted heel to remodel into a different shape with an upward displacement (fig. 6.19). The wall on the over-weighted side will also tend to be more upright than the other side, and if not well managed, it may even start to roll under in some cases.

Incorrect trimming/shoeing that leaves one heel longer or taller than the other has long been thought to be the most frequent cause of sheared heels, but some experts now believe that conformational defects such as an offset coffin bone or toeing-out may be more likely to lead to this problem (fig. 6.20). Pain issues that cause the horse to load his feet unevenly are another way that sheared heels can occur. For example, horses with osteoarthritis in the lower part of the hock joint ("bone spavin"), will often have remodeling of the medial heel, as well as the upright medial wall and flared lateral wall that tend to accompany sheared heels.

6.19 A conformational issue causes this horse to bear more weight on one side of this foot (right), which has led to shearing of the heels.

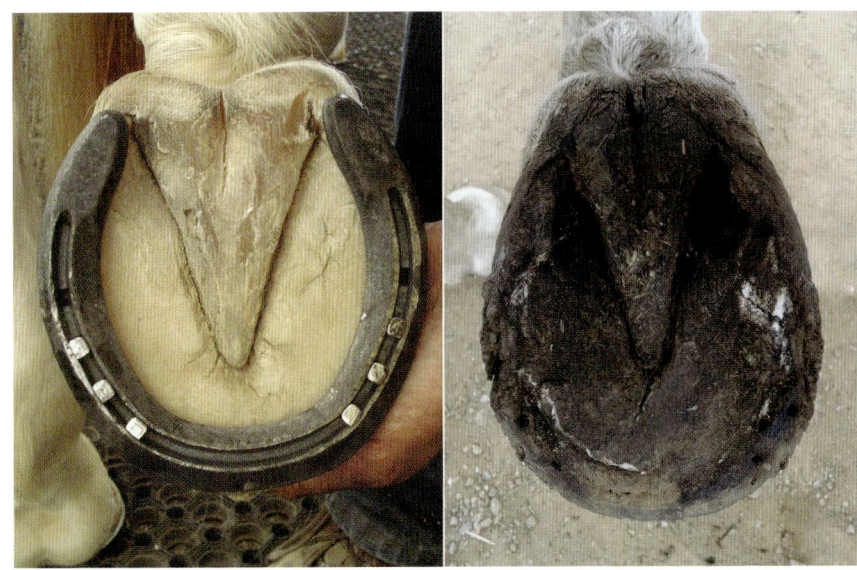

6.18 The broad, supportive heels and picture-perfect frog on the left are markers of a healthy caudal (back part) foot. Though it is hard to see from this angle, the back of the frog has been allowed to grow so that it makes contact with the ground, contributing significantly to the overall health of this shod foot. The contracted heels and pinched frog on the right cannot provide nearly the same support or shock-absorbing capacity as those on the left.

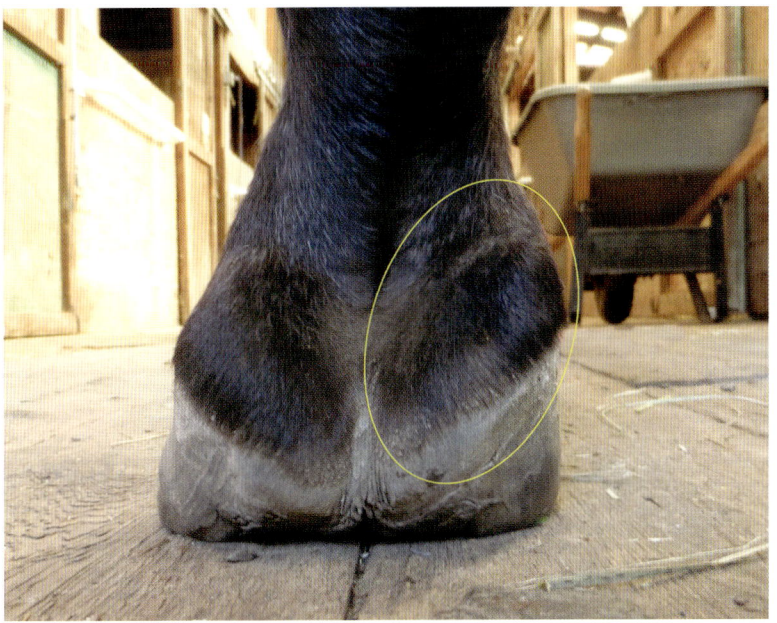

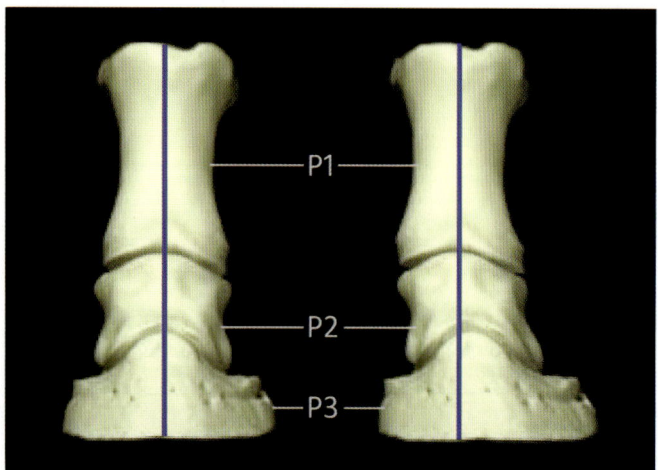

6.20 Normally, the coffin bone (P3) lines up directly underneath P2 and P1 (left). In an offset foot (right), the coffin bone is off to one side, usually shifted laterally. This causes more loading on the medial side of the foot, which may make the inside heel shear upward.

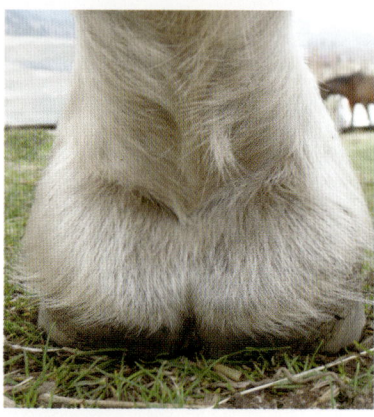

6.21 Healthy heel bulbs are wide-set, of even shape and height, and have no distinct cleft or fissure running up between them.

As for width, the heel bulbs should be wide-set, like the heels themselves, without any distinct cleft between them (fig. 6.21). If you see a "plumber's crack" between them, that means the heels are contracted and squishing the bulbs together (see p. 75). While the cleft between the bulbs may start out as just a fold, it will very often develop into an actual fissure due to deep infection of the frog (thrush), which commonly takes hold when the back of the foot is contracted (fig. 6.22).

Another hallmark of contracted heels is a V-shaped heel hairline that results when the bulbs are pushed together. A healthy foot will have a heel hairline that is fairly straight and parallel to the ground (fig. 6.23).

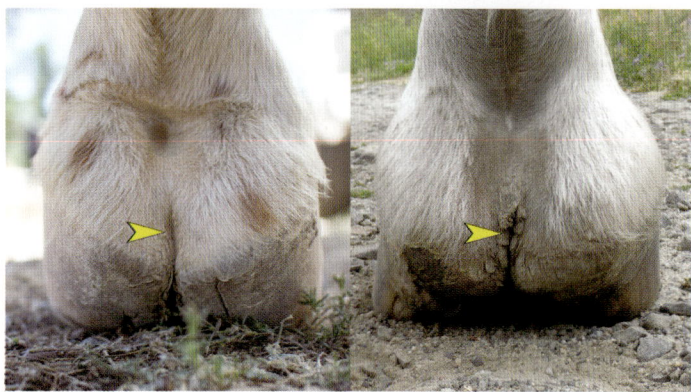

6.22 Both feet have contracted heels. The "plumber's crack" on the left is still just a fold, but as thrush is already present in this foot, it would not be surprising to see that fold turn into an actual fissure, as we see on the right.

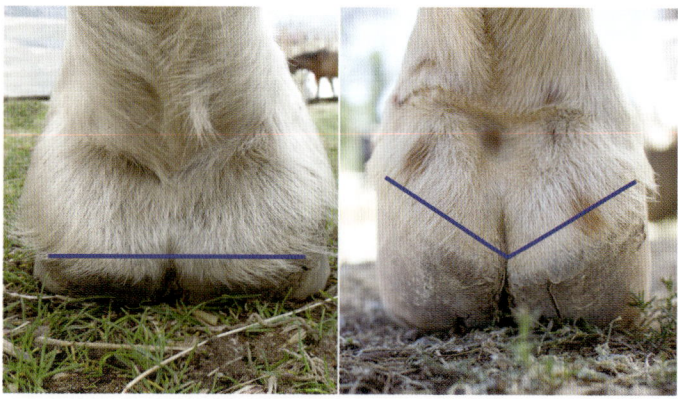

6.23 The V-shaped heel hairline of the foot on the right is typical of what you see when the heels are contracted. The straight hairline on the left is what you want to see from this angle.

Contracted Heels

Contracted heels are such a rampant problem that many people don't even recognize them as an abnormality. Heels can end up contracted for a number of reasons, with the most common being toes that have been allowed to grow too long. When the toes get long, leverage forces on the front of the foot are increased, which have the effect of "pulling" the whole foot forward. As mass shifts to the front of the foot, the heels migrate forward and pinch together (fig. 6.24).

Another major cause of contraction is pain in the back of the foot, as discomfort in this area will often cause a horse to land toe first in an attempt to protect the sore caudal area. This unnatural landing pattern leads to contraction, in part because it is the pressure and release of weight bearing that produces strong, wide heels. If the back of the hoof goes without the stimulation of weight bearing for any length of time, the internal structures can weaken, which then causes further contraction.

Other causes of contraction may include using shoes that are too small, going too long between shoeing or trimming, an injury causing a horse to favor a foot for an extended period, or spending too much time on soft footing. Soft footing does not encourage the hoof to spread, and some believe it may even put inward pressure on the walls.

So, why are contracted heels and overall "soda-can" feet (see fig. 5.7, p. 45) so bad? We already mentioned the possible atrophy of the internal structures, which are necessary for the support and correct functioning of the foot. If the contraction originated in heel discomfort, your horse can also end up in a vicious circle of pain: the heel pain leads

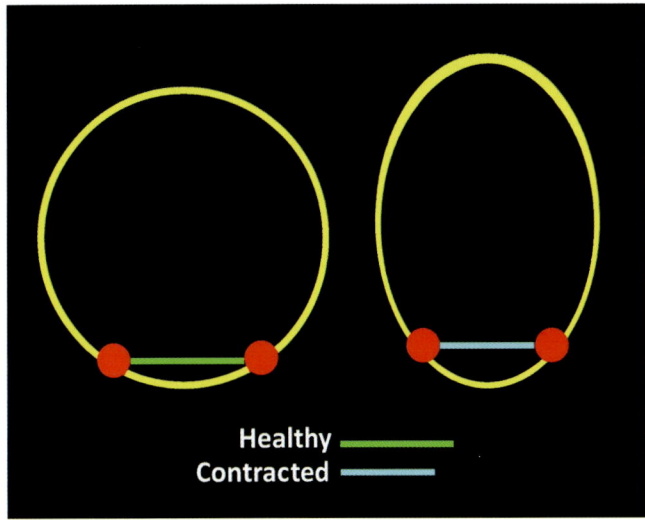

6.24 In this diagram, the round shape on the left represents a normal hoof, and the shape on the right is a contracted hoof. The red dots denote the heels. Notice that when the round shape is pulled forward into a contracted shape, the space between the heels (green and blue lines) gets smaller, and the heels also move forward.

to favoring the heels, which leads to contraction; then the contraction itself squeezes the foot, creating additional pain and causing the horse to favor the heels even more. Back in the olden days, they used to call this condition "hoof-bound," which was aptly descriptive.

Another problem with contraction is that it really messes with the health of the frog. First off, the blood supply to the frog corium can be compromised, both by the walls squeezing inward and by the horse favoring the back of the foot. The frog cannot grow optimally under such conditions, so it tends to become thinner, meaning it has less depth than it should. The result is less material to protect the sensitive inner structures and absorb concussion, so bruising is more likely, and more energy gets transferred up into the foot and limb.

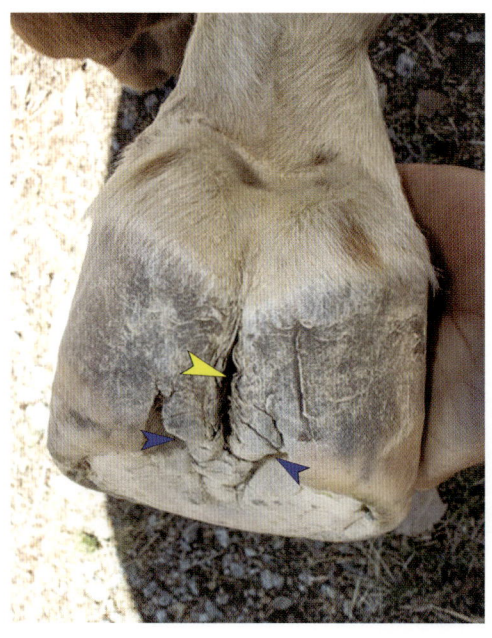

6.25 Contraction of the heels has caused the frog on this foot to become narrow, thin, and dysfunctional. Notice the deep, tight central sulcus (yellow arrow) and closeness of the collateral grooves (blue arrows). All of this has resulted in chronic thrush deep within the central sulcus, a common problem in horses with this type of hoof-capsule distortion.

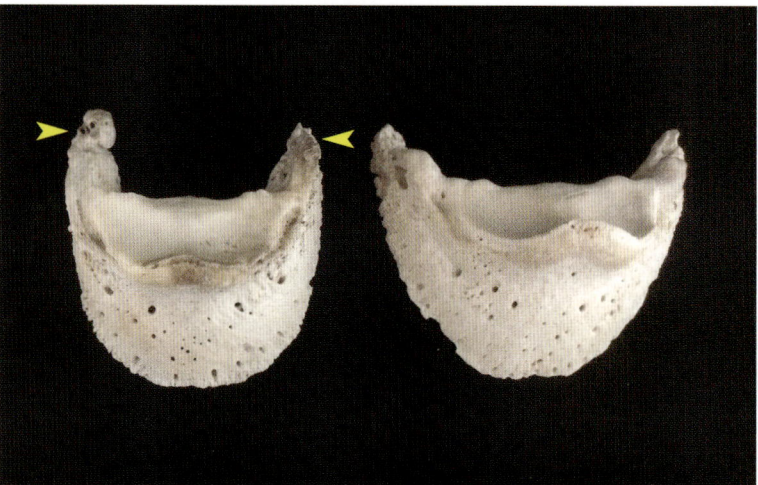

6.26 While the coffin bone on the right is a normal shape, the one on the left demonstrates what can happen in cases of long-term contraction. The bone has narrowed to the point that the sides are nearly parallel, and the lateral cartilages (yellow arrows) have begun to hook inward and ossify.

The walls shifting inward also cause the frog, the collateral grooves, and the central sulcus to get narrower, which has two important consequences: the "landing pad" area of the foot is smaller (as well as thinner), and the narrower grooves and sulcus create an inviting home for dirt and muck (fig. 6.25). Since the overall health of the frog is already diminished, it is very easy to end up with thrush, a potentially serious infection of the frog caused mainly by the anaerobic bacterium *Spherophorus necrophorum* (see *Thrush*, p. 115).

The good news is that contraction is often reversible when the cause or causes of the contraction are eliminated, and steps are taken to encourage the spreading of the hoof. In particular, the hoof needs plenty of movement on varied terrain—including some firm ground—to decontract. Unfortunately, there are instances where a contracted foot is not

going to improve. Long-term contraction, from whatever cause, can remodel the coffin bone to the point where it will reflect the narrowed shape of the hoof capsule, and it can also reshape the lateral cartilages so that they hook in toward each other in the rear. The lateral cartilages can then ossify (turn to bone—a condition known as *sidebone*), making those hooks more or less permanent (fig. 6.26).

Only X-rays can detect these kinds of changes for certain, so if your hoof-care provider is having an impossible time decontracting your horse's feet, it might be worth investing in them, as this will give you a realistic expectation of what can be accomplished.

Hands-On Activity:
Develop Your Eye for Contraction

There is normal variation in the shape of horse's feet, with some being very round and some naturally less round. While this can make learning to spot contraction a bit tricky, it is still a skill worth acquiring. We've talked about a few different ways to look for contraction, but here is another one that we call "thinking outside the box" (fig. 6.27):

Step 1: Have someone hold up each of your horse's four feet, and take a picture of the solar view of each foot. It may be helpful to use a marker and write "LF" on the sole of the left front, "RF" on the right front, and so on, to help keep your pictures straight.

Step 2: Print out your pictures.

Step 3: Draw a box that goes from the inside edge of the back of the heels, then straight down to the toe, as shown in figure 6.27.

Step 4: Draw a line from the edge of the box to the widest part of the foot on the left side of the box (blue lines in figure 6.27). Repeat on the right (green lines in figure 6.27).

Step 5: Using a ruler, measure the lines you have just drawn outside the box, and draw lines of those lengths inside the box, giving them space to overlap.

Step 6: What you want to see is that the width of the box is equal to or wider than the parts outside the box put together. That means that if your lines overlap, you are likely dealing with some contraction.

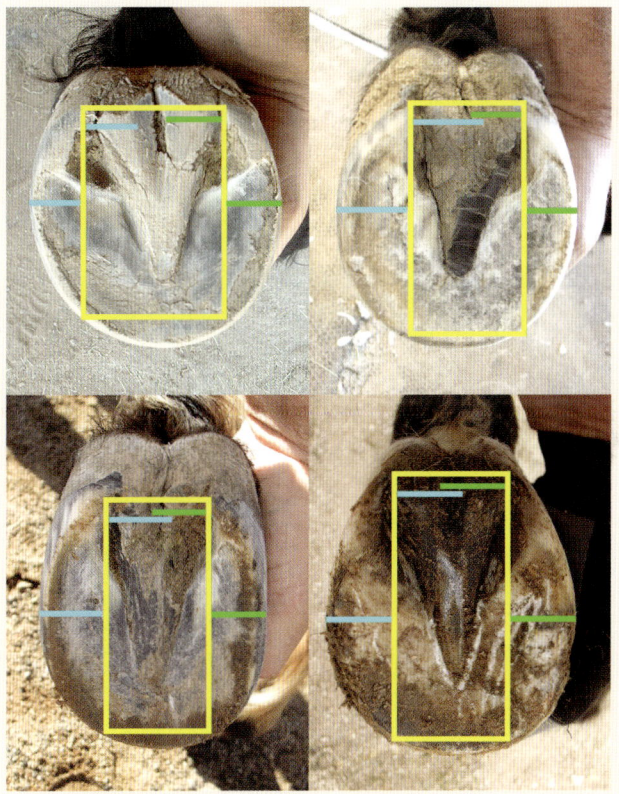

6.27 The yellow box in each photo is drawn from the inside edge of the back of the heels to the toe. On a healthy foot, the width of this box is greater than the widths of the parts to the left and right of the box (blue and green lines) added together. The top left foot has no contraction, but the other three all do.

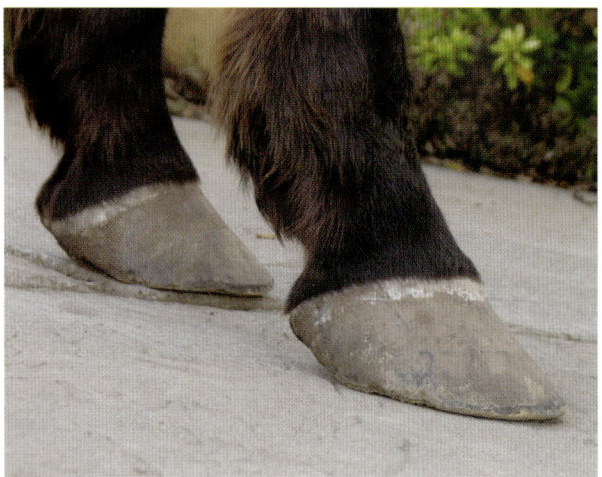

6.28 This is a classic case of long-toe/low-heel syndrome brought on by sheer neglect—what some people call "LOFD" (lack-of-farrier disease).

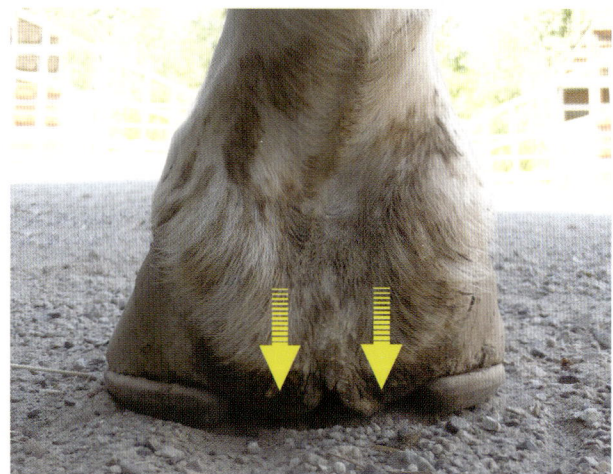

6.29 When the heels collapse, the inside of the foot is affected as well as the outside. Pressure from compression of all the internal structures in the back of the foot can push the frog outward, causing it to prolapse, as you see here. This should not be confused with a frog that has deliberately been allowed to grow down to the ground on a foot that is shod using physiologically correct trimming principles (see p. 250 and fig. 14.23, p. 251).

Underrun Heels

Now, let's get back to *underrun heels*, the problem where the heels have migrated farther forward than they should be. When a horse has underrun heels, you are probably going to see that he has long, low toes as well. This kind of dorsopalmar/dorsoplantar imbalance, which is referred to as *long-toe/low-heel syndrome* (fig. 6.28), is present in an alarmingly high percentage of domestic horses, and can wreak havoc in a number of ways:

• The entire foot is off-center in relation to the bony column of the leg, shifting the focus of weight bearing farther back than it should be.

• Blood flow in the back of the foot becomes compromised, leading to further atrophy of the digital cushion, lateral cartilages, and frog, thus reducing the shock-absorbing capacity of the back of the foot.

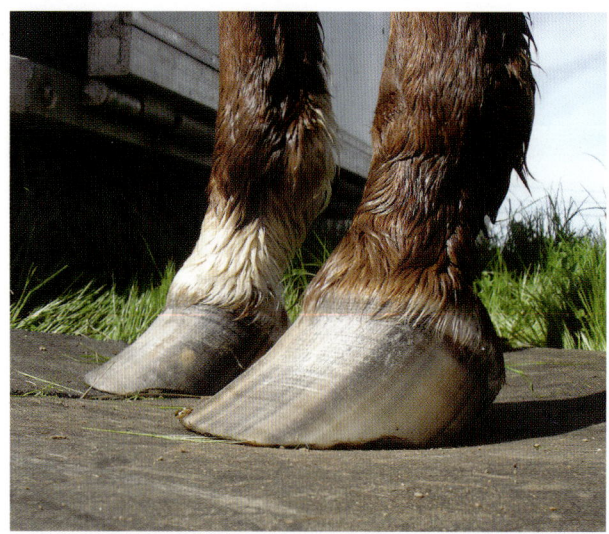

6.30 The more toe the foot has out in front of it, the greater the leverage is working to pull the laminae apart, and the more delay there is in breakover. This horse's toes are enormously long, affecting his movement and his overall hoof and limb health.

• Long, low heels are weak and can actually collapse. When this happens, the frog may become prolapsed, meaning it is bulging outward due to unhealthy pressure from within (fig. 6.29).

• The long toe delays breakover, meaning that it forces the foot to remain on the ground past the point where it should be rolling over itself and lifting off. This places strain on the tendons and ligaments running up the back of the foot and the limb, most notably the deep digital flexor tendon, which, in turn, puts excessive pressure on the navicular bone and nearby structures (see *Understanding Breakover*, p. 95).

• Long toes create leverage that puts strain on the laminae. The longer the toes, the greater the leverage (fig. 6.30). This can cause the laminae to fail, leading to separation of the hoof wall, white line disease, and other problems.

• Long-toe/low-heel often creates a broken-back hoof-pastern axis, which, as you've already learned, puts stress on the back of the coffin joint as well as the soft tissues.

• Heels tend to become contracted when the foot is pulled forward by a long toe.

All of the issues listed can become self-perpetuating, causing pain that makes the horse favor the back of the foot, weakening the heels and internal structures even more (from lack of use), and putting more pressure on the toe, which levers it farther forward. Ultimately, pain and damage resulting from the stresses of long-toe/low-heel conformation can lead to serious lameness, so it is critical to work with your hoof-care provider to correct this problem to the greatest degree possible.

Of course, prevention is light years better than cure, and in many cases, long-toe/low-heel syndrome can be nipped in the bud. Keeping up with trimming/shoeing is of huge importance, as going too long between trims is a common cause of dorsopalmar/dorsoplantar imbalance. Also be aware that horses with long, sloping pasterns are more prone to having feet that want to run forward. So, if you have a horse with any tendency toward developing long toes and low heels, you want to make sure to have his feet trimmed regularly and frequently. A 3–4 week cycle will help much more than a 6–8 week one. If your horse is barefoot, you might ask your trimmer to teach you how to rasp the toes between trims, which will help maintain your horse's feet in optimal condition and allow you to extend the time between professional trims.

One note of caution: When talking about a horse with long-toe/low-heel syndrome, it is often said that the heels are not only too far forward, but also too low. In some cases, this is certainly true, and the goal would then be to move the heel back and cultivate more heel height. However, when looking at such a horse, it is important to remember the difference between heel *height* and heel *length*. The underrun heel might actually have good height, but simply be too long. In this instance, you don't want to raise the heel, you just need to move it backward (fig. 6.31). Also keep in mind that what many believe to be good heel height is actually taller than is healthy, so don't get talked into "standing the horse up" (raising the heels) if it isn't necessary.

When working to improve feet with long-toe/low-heel syndrome, the primary focus generally should be on bringing the toe back because it may not be possible to do much with the heels at first.

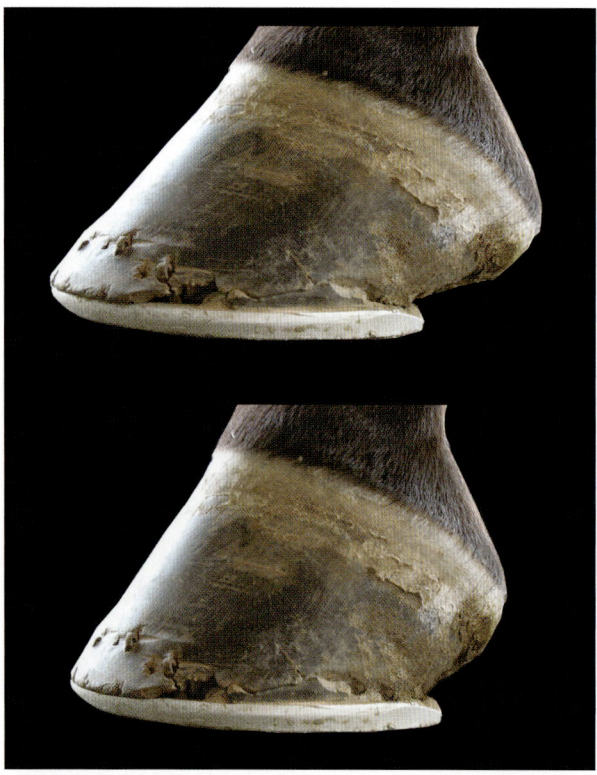

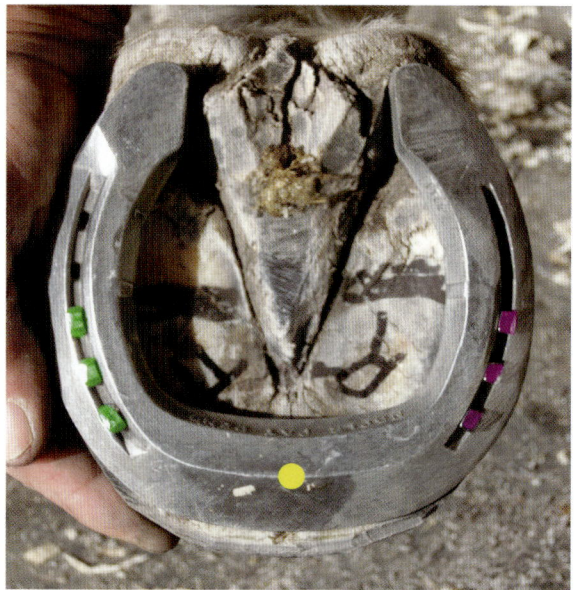

6.31 This horse (above) doesn't need his heels raised, he just needs them to be farther back than they are currently, and he needs his toes backed up as well. The digitally altered version (below) shows what this might look like, although the weak, crumbling walls would likely be improved as well by getting his dorsopalmar balance more in order (see figs. 1.6 & 1.7, p. 8).

6.32 This Natural Balance® shoe is set back a little behind the toe, and it also has a strong bevel built in, both of which help move the point of breakover (yellow dot) back. While this point of breakover may appear to be "too far back" if you are gauging it from the edge of the toe, it is actually correct in relation to the coffin bone and will help the foot attain better balance.

While it might seem reasonable to try to move the heel back immediately, removing material from a heel that is already too low is counterproductive and may cause the foot to continue to run forward. Raising the heels up with wedges to "support" them and change the angles might also seem logical, but many experts now believe this practice to be counterproductive, as it actually adds pressure to an area already damaged by excessive pressure.

In many cases, bringing the toe back as aggressively as is safely possible, while only minimally addressing the heels, will improve the biomechanics enough to start the foot moving in the right direction, encouraging the heels to grow faster and at a more normal angle. Once there is actually a bit of heel to work with, it is possible to start making effective changes through careful trimming. Moving the point of breakover farther back (closer to where it should be in relation to the coffin bone) by setting shoes back or using a shoe like the Natural Balance® shoe can also be very helpful for shod horses (fig. 6.32).

Balance and Symmetry

Nature loves symmetry. Symmetry indicates balance, and balance encourages good biomechanics. Developing an eye for symmetry and balance is definitely helpful in identifying hoof problems, though healthy hooves often show some minor asymmetries that are quite normal.

Normal Asymmetries

Medial vs. Lateral

If you draw a line down the middle of the sole from back to front, then compare the two halves, you want to see that the medial and lateral halves match fairly closely. But, even in a well conformed, good moving, and properly balanced horse, you will often find that the lateral half of the hoof is a smidge wider than the medial half (fig. 7.1). Similarly, peer closely at the medial and lateral walls when the horse is standing on a level surface, and you will probably see that the medial wall is slightly more upright than the lateral one.

Both of these minor asymmetries happen because the inside half of the foot is designed to bear a little more of the weight of the horse than the outside half does, while the outside half plays

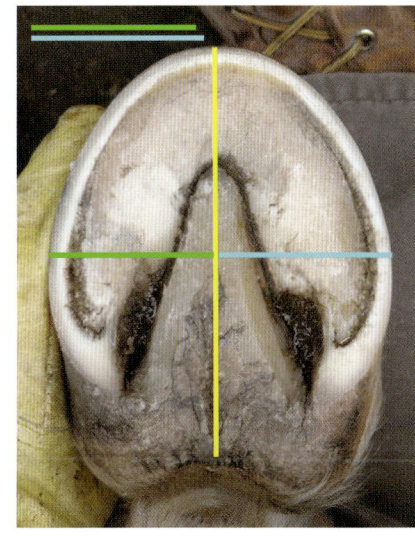

7.1 This hind foot has very good mediolateral symmetry, but even so, the lateral side (blue line), is slightly wider than the medial side (green line). This is perfectly normal.

a larger role in stabilizing the foot. The slightly steeper angle of the medial wall allows it to deal with the greater forces it encounters, but it also makes the inside half of the foot a little narrower than the outside half.

Front vs. Hind Feet

Another place where it is normal to see asymmetry is when you are comparing the shape of the front feet to the shape of the hind. Viewed from the bottom, healthy front hooves will usually be fairly round while the hind will be more oval-shaped or

7.2 The front feet on most horses are rounder (left) than the hind (right), which can be oval shaped, like this one, or sometimes a little more triangular.

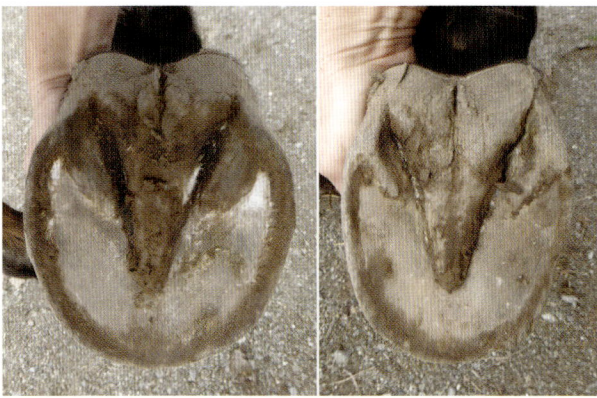

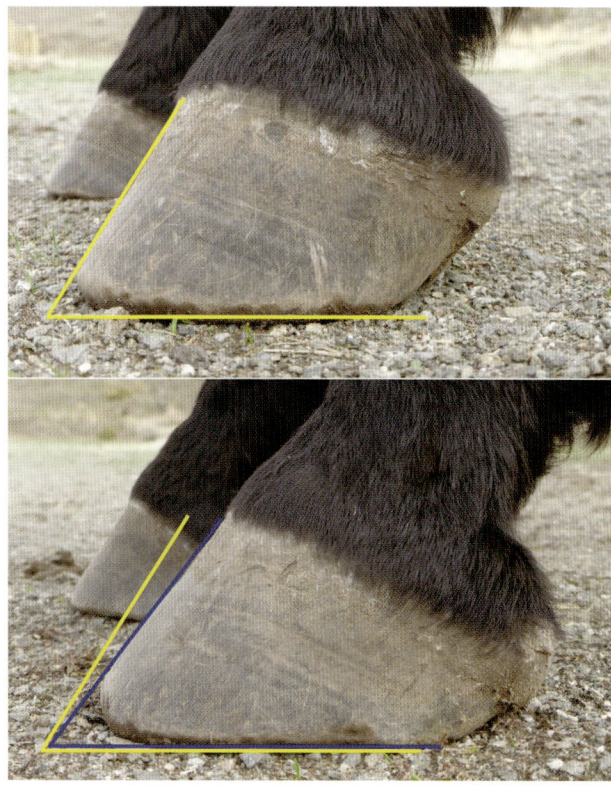

7.3 As is typical, the hind feet of this horse (above) have slightly steeper angles (yellow lines) than the front feet (blue lines) below.

a bit more pointed at the toe (fig. 7.2). Viewed from the side, the dorsal wall (front surface) and heel angles of the front will commonly be slightly shallower than those of the hind (fig. 7.3). The front feet are also typically larger than the hind, often a full size when it comes to shoes or hoof boots.

The fact that the hind feet are more upright might seem surprising given that we just said steeper walls reflect greater load-bearing capacity, and you've probably heard that horses bear more of their weight on the front limbs. But, while it is true that a *standing* horse carries more of his weight on his front feet, a *moving* horse shifts his weight back, where the hind feet to do the heavy work of pushing and carrying. The hind feet, therefore, need to be up to the task of more intense loading than what the front feet experience, which is reflected in the angles of the pasterns and hoof walls.

Left vs. Right Asymmetries: High/Low Syndrome

In a perfect world, the shape, size, and angles of your horse's left front foot would be identical to those of the right front foot, and the hind feet would also match one another. In the *real* world, the pairs

should still be quite similar, but slight differences are always present, especially in the front. However, minor differences do not make a horse's feet "mismatched," it merely makes them a realistic reflection of the fact that no animal as large and complex as a horse can exhibit perfect symmetry.

Horses can have any number of variances that will make one foot a little different than the other, but the most commonly encountered is that one front foot will be slightly more upright than the other. This difference is often due to the fact that horses, like people, tend to have a dominant side.

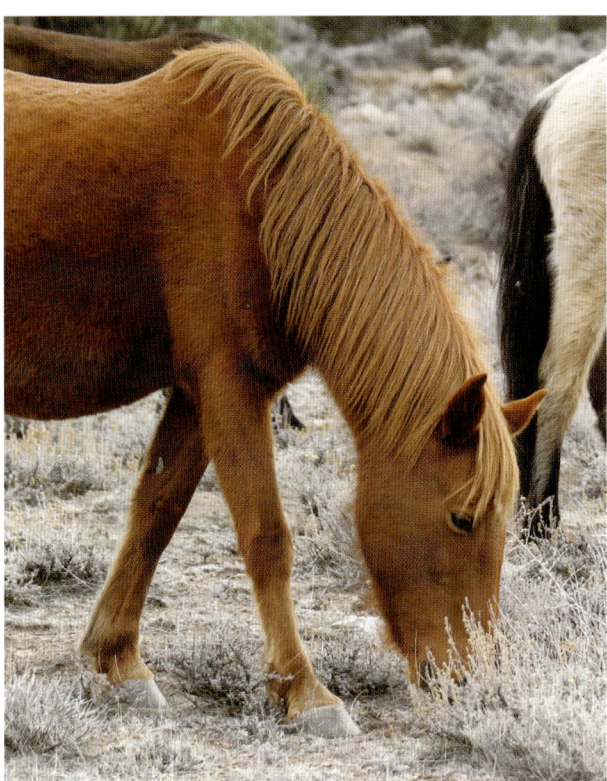

7.4 This mare prefers to have her right foot forward when she grazes, and if you look closely, you can see that it has a slightly lower angle than her left. Such differences are very common in horses with distinct "handedness."

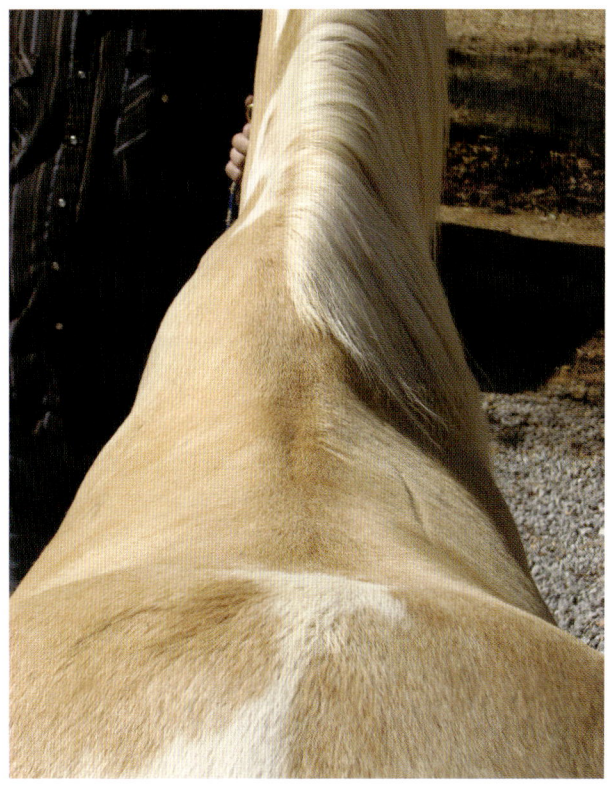

7.5 Even with the heavy mane on the right, you can see that there is more muscle mass on the left shoulder of this horse. Such uneven muscling is an extremely common finding in horses and usually correlates with a slightly lower angled foot on the more muscular side.

Left to their own devices, most horses prefer one canter lead over the other, and most will also habitually graze with a particular front foot forward more often than the other.

Over time, these preferences can change the shape of the feet, with the "forward" foot developing a lower angle, as it is bearing more weight toward the heel, and the "back" one becoming more upright (fig. 7.4), as it is bearing more weight toward the toe. The low-heeled foot is typically the more dominant side, which affects not only the feet, but the entire body. This is often noticeable as heavier muscling in the dominant shoulder, which is easiest to see when you stand above and behind your horse. A majority of horses are left-side dominant (fig. 7.5).

In most cases, if the difference between the angles of your horse's front feet is hard to notice unless you are really looking for it, it is probably not worth worrying about, though you may want to check it now and again to make sure it is not getting worse. A safe bet is that if the difference is less than 5 degrees, it is likely not causing issues for the horse, although most horses are more supple on their dominant (low foot) side. Riders can often feel this in their horse, as the horse will be easier to bend toward the low-footed side and will probably prefer to canter in that direction, as well. If your horse is like this, it would likely be beneficial to his overall balance and musculoskeletal health to work on strengthening and suppling the weaker side, though this may not have any noticeable effect on his feet.

If you are seeing a marked difference in the angles of your horse's hooves, you could be looking at *high/low syndrome*, an issue where one foot is significantly more upright than the other, and the lower-angled foot is usually larger than its partner (fig. 7.6). High/low syndrome can be hereditary (such as a club foot), acquired through a postural habit like the classic foal grazing stance, injury related, a

result of unbalanced riding and training, a saddle-fit issue, or a byproduct of any number of aches, pains, subluxations, dental issues, or other problems you may never discover.

High/low syndrome is another one of those chicken-and-egg scenarios in which you have to unravel the problem of, "Which came first?" On the one hand, a difference in the feet can cause other parts of the body to compensate for the imbalance, creating a cascade of problems such as muscle pain and stiffness, twisting of the vertebrae in the neck and spine, uneven muscle development in the shoulders and back, saddle-fit issues, and much more. On the other hand, various problems in other parts of the body can cause postural changes that affect the feet, and may be the cause of the high/low feet. Either way, careful and thorough assessment is in order.

Addressing the feet of a horse with high/low syndrome can also be a challenge. The first step is determining which foot is the primary one you want to change. To do this, you need to figure out if the low foot is closer to normal in terms of the hoof-pastern axis, in which case, the task will be to try to lower the angle of the more upright one. If the more upright one has healthier angles, the focus will be on trying to get the low-angle foot to stand more upright.

When you are working on high/low feet, it is important to recognize that high/low syndrome cannot always be "cured," and will thus require ongoing management. A lot depends on how long the high/low syndrome has been going on and how early it started, which will determine whether or not the two front coffin bones are entirely different shapes and sizes. If they are significantly different,

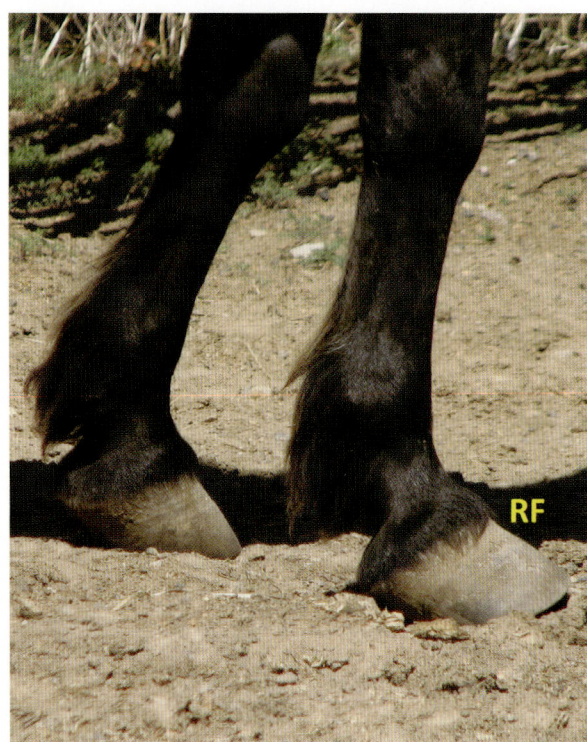

7.6 This wild horse sustained a serious injury to its left hind leg, which caused him to favor that leg for many months. As a result, the hind feet grew very unevenly, but the *front* feet, pictured here, also developed severe high/low syndrome. This occurred because the right front (RF) was forced to compensate for the injured left hind, bearing far more weight than normal. It was quite literally flattened by the strain.

RF

the chances of making the two feet match are about the same as winning the lottery. However, if the bones are the same size and shape, chances of regaining symmetry are significantly better, as long as the causative body imbalances are taken care of. Bodywork, stretching, and exercising to minimize muscular imbalances are all helpful in giving your horse's high/low feet the best chance to improve.

You must also keep in mind that while changes in trimming can sometimes minimize the differences in high/low feet, you have to be sure this creates a positive functional change, and not just an aesthetic one, as it is very possible to force a foot to look more like we think it should, but actually make it functionally worse. This is especially true with club feet.

Club Feet

Some cases of high/low feet involve a *club foot*, which is an upright foot caused by a shortening of the tendon and muscle of the deep digital flexor unit. The excessive pull on the DDFT turns the coffin bone downward, loading shifts to the toe area, and the hoof changes shape in response. The classic club foot is upright and contracted, and there may be a "fullness" in the coronet area due to the forward displacement of the extensor process of the coffin bone and the second phalanx just above it. The hoof wall will often show rippling and dishing in the front, and wider growth rings in the heels. However, club feet can vary quite a bit in appearance, and what they look like depends in part on the severity of the problem, and to a degree on the quality and timing of the hoof care they receive.

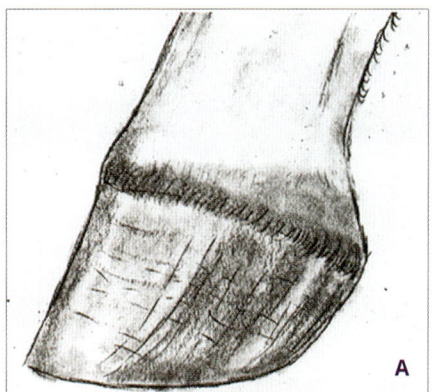
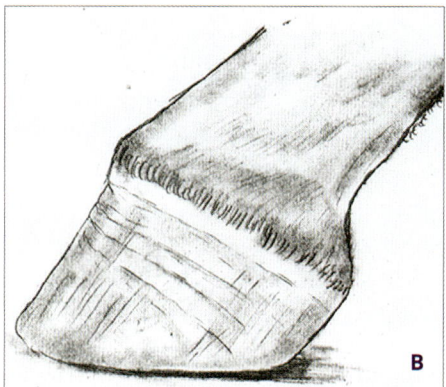
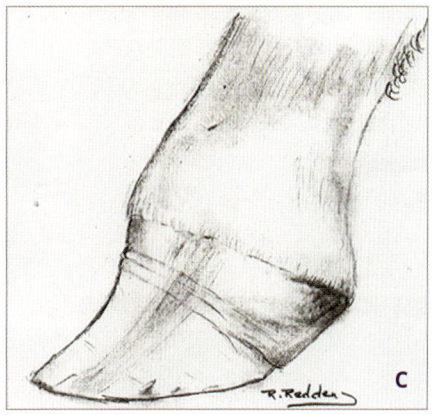
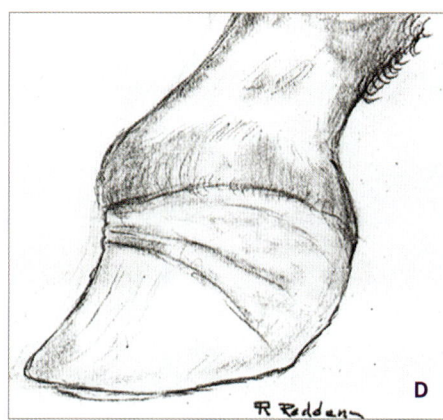

7.7 A–D Dr. Redden's Club Foot Classification.
Grade 1 (A): The hoof angle is 3–5 degrees greater than the opposing foot and a characteristic fullness is present at the coronary band due to subluxation (misalignment or partial dislocation) of P2 (short pastern bone) and P3 (coffin bone).
Grade 2 (B): The hoof angle is 5–8 degrees greater than the opposing foot with growth rings wider at the heel than at the toe. Heel will not touch the ground when trimmed to normal length.
Grade 3 (C): The anterior hoof wall is dished and growth rings at the heel are twice as wide as on the toe. Radiographically, P3 exhibits demineralization and lipping along the front of the bottom edge.
Grade 4 (D): The anterior hoof wall is heavily dished and the angle is 80 degrees or more. The coronary band is as high at the heel as at the toe, and the sole is below the ground surface of the wall. Radiographically, P3 is rounded due to extensive demineralization, and rotation may be present.

Club feet are graded on a scale of 1–4, with "1" being a mild case that may be hardly noticeable and "4" being severe (figs. 7.7 A–D). Higher grade cases may have limitations in terms of their ability to perform and to remain sound, but the majority of horses with lower grade club feet are able to lead quite normal lives with appropriate hoof care, and owners of grade 1 horses may not even realize that their horse has a club foot at all. Some horses with club feet have even been successful in high-level competition.

If your horse has a mild club foot that does not appear to be getting worse, it is something to be aware of and keep an eye on, but it is not a reason to panic. A competent hoof-care provider will know how to manage such a foot—most often by simply keeping the feet balanced and not worrying about trying to make them "match." Caring for a horse with a significant club foot (grade 2 or higher) is more challenging because such a horse is at higher risk for a variety of problems. The altered biomechanics of a club hoof can not only affect that foot, but also the limb, the other feet, and the rest of the body, which must compensate for the changes. As with feet that are mismatched for any reason, massage, chiropractic work, regular dental care, expert saddle fitting, and skilled riding exercises can be very helpful in keeping a club-footed horse sound and performing at his best.

Many of the problems that can be brought on by a club foot stem from the fact that the tightness of the DDFT is continually pulling the coffin bone around on its articular axis, causing the foot to want to land toe first. This puts an abnormal amount of pressure on the toe area while taking weight off the heel. Depending on the severity of the condition, the dorsal wall may ripple and dish in response to the increased loading, an issue that can be further compounded if the extensor process is pressing into the coronary corium, which can compromise blood flow and inhibit growth of the dorsal wall. When this happens, the heels still have an adequate blood supply and therefore grow at a faster rate than the toe.

But the possibilities for problems don't end there. If the club foot is putting excessive pressure on the toe, this can lead to inflammation of the laminae, white line separation and subsequent white line disease, and also make the front of the foot more vulnerable to cracks, bruising, and abscessing. Abnormal loading of the joints may cause osteoarthritis, and over time, the tip of the coffin bone can become deformed, demineralized, and may even fracture (fig. 7.8). And, if the coffin bone is displaced enough for that to happen, you can be sure there is some compression of the solar corium, which affects circulation and sole growth in the toe area.

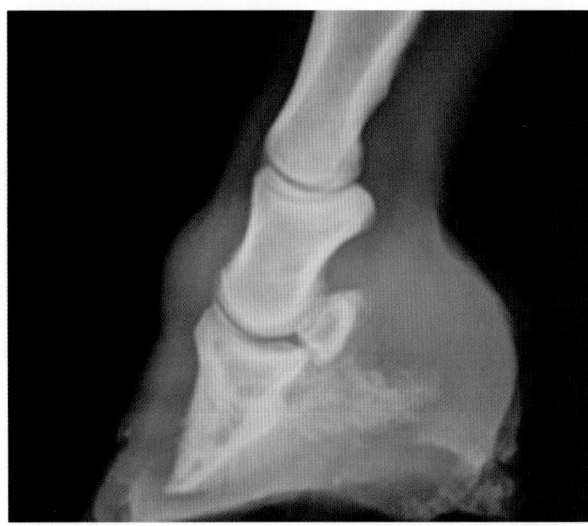

7.8 In addition to affecting what a hoof looks like on the outside, a club foot can cause profound changes inside the foot as well. The coffin bone of this grade 4 club foot already shows abnormalities, and this is only likely to get worse over time. Says Dr. Redden, "In grade 4 feet, the bone remodels quickly and shows signs of extensive bone resorption and remodeling, often appearing as a rounded off, very misshapen surface, indicating a large area of apex has been resorbed."

Recognizing Low-Grade Club Feet in Foals

Foal feet have a different shape than what we are used to looking at in adult horses, tending to be more upright and relatively tubular, as they have not spread out yet from years of weight bearing. Because of this, it can be difficult to recognize a low-grade club foot in a foal. If you know what to look for, however, the differences, subtle though they can be, will be easier to spot. Trying to note differences in the dorsal wall angles can be tough, as even a 5-degree disparity is hard to see without whipping out a protractor and taking actual measurements—not always the easiest thing to do with a bouncing baby horse.

However, there will also be differences in the heel angles, and sometimes, these are more obvious. The next clue you might be able to discern is that the feet will bear weight differently. The club foot will tend to weight the toe more than the heel, and the heel may even lift a bit off the ground. The opposite foot will load flat or with more weight on the heel (fig. 7.9).

Learning to see subtle differences in your foal's feet might just help you spot a problem early, which is the best way to keep any hoof issues from becoming life-long problems for the horse. Try to observe your foal's hooves on a regular basis, as they can change quite quickly when the foal goes through growth spurts. If you think you see something that could be a concern, don't hesitate to call your vet. Better to have the doc come out and tell you it is nothing, than miss what could be your best chance to help the foal.

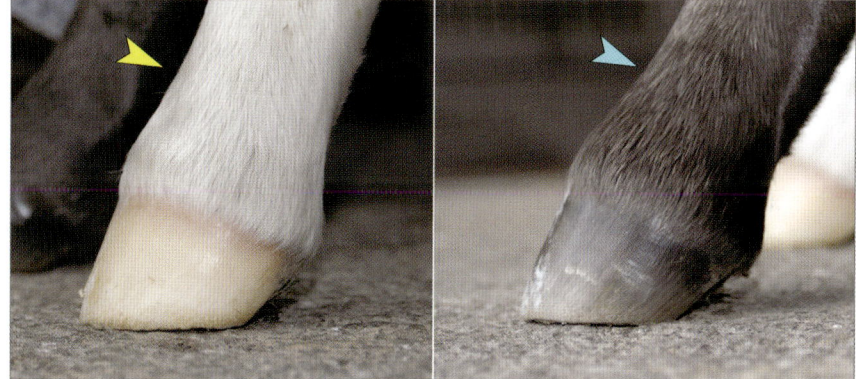

7.9 These are the two front feet of a young foal. Subtle clues show you that the white foot is a Grade 1 club. The minor difference in the dorsal-wall angle is hard to see, but the difference in the heel angle is more apparent. You can also see that the white foot is lifting up slightly in back, while the black foot is rooted in the heels. Lastly, the dorsal wall of the white hoof lines up very directly under the lower front of the pastern, giving that part of the pastern a "full" appearance (yellow arrow). This is due to the coffin bone rotating and the coffin joint pressing forward. The lower front of the black pastern, in comparison, has a little more of a "dish" to it (blue arrow).

This is why the sole in the toe region of horses with club feet is often painfully thin.

More issues can crop up in the back of the foot, as the heels typically contract in a club foot, causing the frog to recede and rendering the foot even less able to dissipate concussion. This, in turn, puts a greater amount of pressure on the already stressed toe and coffin bone, creating the potential for a really vicious circle of dysfunction. Then there is the navicular bone, which can also be affected by the increased pull of the DDFT. It is not unusual to see changes in the navicular bone quite early in horses with club feet.

In addition, the altered function of a significant club foot will almost always cause changes in other feet as well. Typically, the foot opposite the club, as well as the one behind it, will have a tendency to develop long toes and low heels, which bring their own set of problems to those feet. Frequently, the "low" feet will start having issues before any are noted in the club foot.

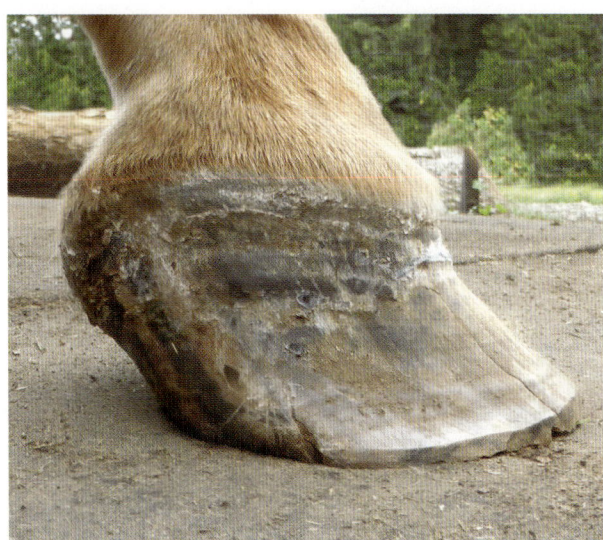

7.10 This foot has experienced the triple whammy of starting out as a club foot, then getting laminitis, and having poor hoof care for a long time. While the current hoof-care provider has been able to keep the horse more or less comfortable, the internal damage is too extensive for this foot to ever function properly or regain a normal appearance.

Because there are so many possible effects from a club foot, good management is absolutely critical. If recognized early enough—when a foal is born or very young—a club foot can often be corrected to the point where it will have little to no effect on the horse's long-term potential to remain sound. Early treatment involves corrective hoof care, sometimes in combination with surgery to relieve tension on the DDFT, all aimed at enabling the foot to load and grow more normally.

In an adult horse, the degree to which a club foot can be managed depends on a number of factors, including how bad it is, what caused it, and how long it has been that way. In long-standing cases, or any case where significant damage to the bones and soft tissue has already occurred, the potential for improvement may be limited, but an expert will be able to manage the foot to get it functioning as best it can and minimize problems (fig. 7.10). The Equine Lameness Prevention Organization (ELPO), co-founded by Gene Ovnicek, has specific guidelines that can help hoof-care professionals manage club feet and mismatched feet optimally.

Some adult horses may also be good candidates for a surgical procedure often used on foals, in which the inferior check ligament of the DDFT is cut, thereby lessening the tension that is causing the club foot. There is also another surgery called a deep digital flexor tenotomy (see p. 203), which is performed higher up the leg and may be a solution for grade 4 cases and grade 3s that have been unresponsive to other treatments.

Unfortunately, it is very easy to make a club foot worse with what might seem like the most logical thing to do—lowering the heels. While lowering the heels might indeed be called for, it has to be done with extreme care and with full understanding of the physiology and biomechanics of the structures involved. Far too often, well-meaning hoof-care providers will lower the heels too much, too soon, or without taking other critical measures, the result being that they cause the deep digital flexor apparatus to tighten more in response to the increased tension placed on it by the "missing" heel, and the foot may get tipped farther forward as a result. Club feet that have had too much heel removed (and sometimes even a little is too much) can end up with the heels literally hanging in the air (fig. 7.11). This is likely to make the horse sore, and could potentially cause serious harm.

In order to have any chance of truly improving a club foot, the key is easing the tension on the DDFT, which can often be at least partially accomplished by moving the point of breakover back. This may appear counterintuitive for a foot that already wants to "knuckle over," but if you don't help the foot get some slack into the DDFT, it will continue to pull itself in the wrong direction. The idea of facilitating breakover makes more sense when you realize that easing the pull *on* the DDFT is really the only way to ease the pull *of* the DDFT.

An apparent lack of understanding of this very important piece of the puzzle has led some hoof-care providers to try to correct a club foot by lowering the heels and then either leaving the toe long, or sometimes putting on a shoe that extends the toe beyond the front wall. While this may be a reasonable plan in certain cases involving young foals or immediately after check ligament surgery, it is counterproductive for an adult horse, unless it is a post-surgical measure to help realign the bones of the foot.

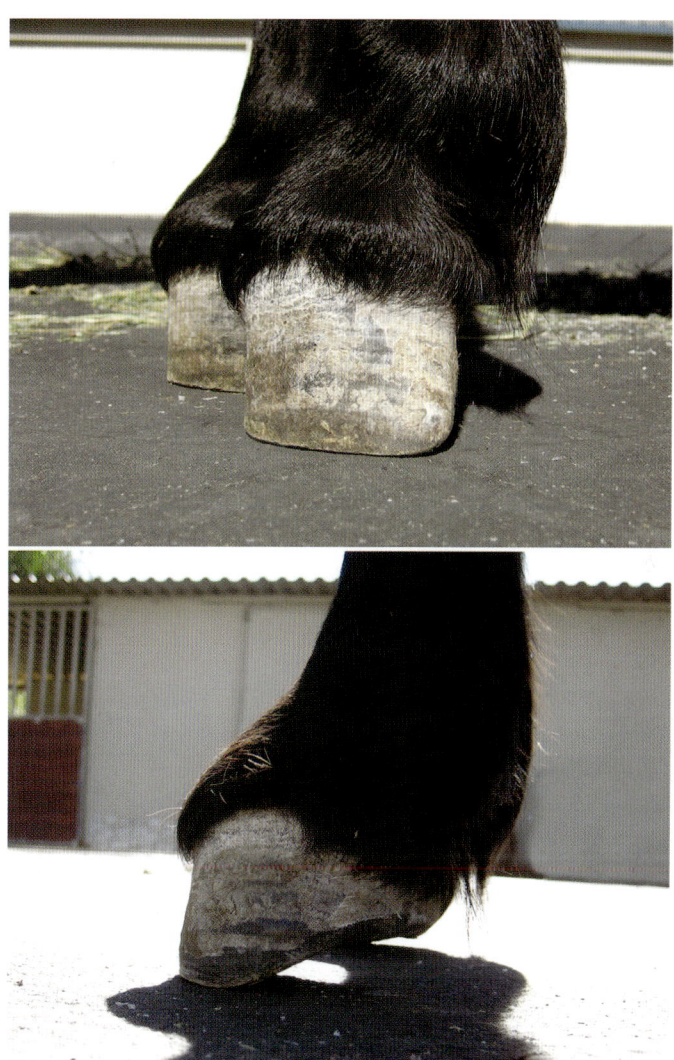

7.11 This miniature mare had severe club feet, as you can see in the upper photo. Though it went against his better judgment, the farrier followed the owner's request to remove a large amount of heel in one trim. The result (lower photo) was that the feet were left standing "en pointe" like a ballerina, with the heels up in the air. Her heels did sink down over time, and she did not appear to suffer any trauma. However, in a larger, heavier horse, the enormous strain such drastic trimming would cause could lead to severe injury.

7.12 The toe-extension shoe used on this foal was glued on and was very difficult to remove. It was then left on far too long, causing the foot to become contracted, as you can see by the narrow, deep central sulcus (red arrow) and close-together heels (yellow bracket). The foot's dorsopalmar balance was also affected, causing there to be more ground-contact surface in front of the widest part of the foot (green line) than behind it. This would be more obvious if the photo showed the foot straight from the bottom, rather than foreshortened.

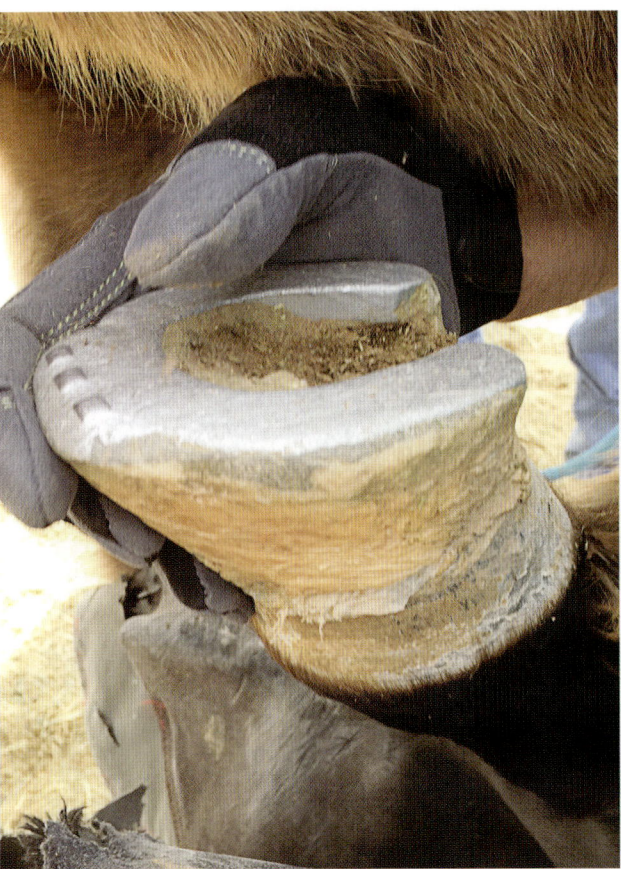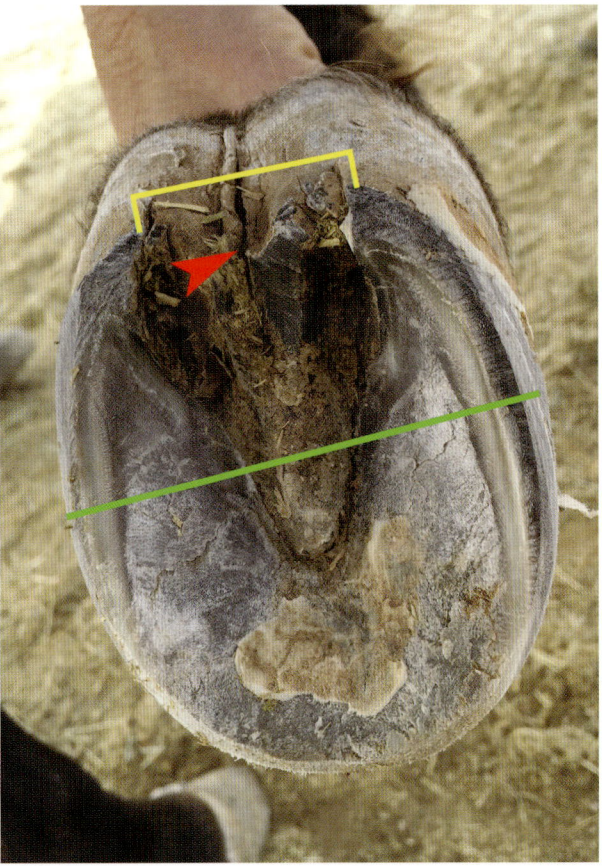

A toe (or shoe extension) that puts the point of breakover too far ahead of the tip of the coffin bone increases leverage on the already stressed laminae, and if you combine this with extra DDFT tension from lowering the heels, you will greatly increase the chances of the coffin bone tearing away from the hoof wall and rotating inside the hoof capsule. Even when used in foals, toe-extension shoes must be employed with great care, as they can cause other problems if left on for too long (fig. 7.12).

As for how club feet get to be that way in the first place, there are several possibilities. Some cases likely have a genetic component, as certain blood lines seem to produce more individuals with club feet than is typical. Most club feet start very early in the horse's life, either as a congenital limb deformity already present at birth, or as an apparently acquired limb deformity that develops as a result of the foal's tendons and bones growing out of sync. However, it is possible that some of the supposedly acquired cases already had the problem brewing when they were born, and it simply went unrecognized or was not manifesting observable signs at that time.

Many experts now believe there may also be a nutritional factor in some cases of club feet, citing overfeeding of nutrients and excessive caloric intake as the root problem (fig. 7.13). The thinking is that the too-rich diet causes developmental orthopedic disorders (DOD), and the pain from these problems leads to abnormal loading of one or more limbs, which then gets the club-foot ball rolling. Adult horses can also develop a club foot as a result of pain or injury that causes alterations in the loading patterns on their feet.

However they get started, club feet are best managed by competent, experienced hoof-care providers who understand when and how changes should be made, and when to leave well enough alone. The horse also needs an owner that pays attention, looking for any changes in the feet or the way the horse is going, and who is not afraid to ask questions or even seek out a different hoof-care provider if the foot is deteriorating. There are certainly cases where even the best professionals will not be able to alleviate the problems of a horse with a club foot, but if your horse takes a turn for the worse when changes are attempted, it may be that the methods being used do not suit your horse's needs.

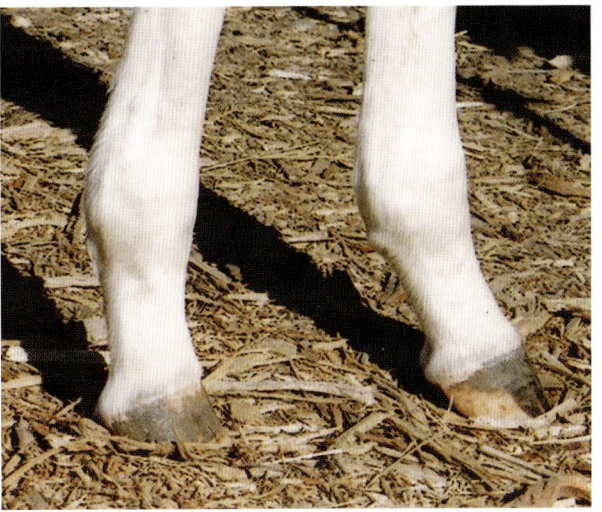

7.13 This foal was raised with free access to a big tub containing a mineral supplement that used molasses as a binder. He was frequently observed at the mineral tub, licking away, clearly enamored of the molasses. He soon developed a grade 1 club on his left front, seen here (foot extended forward). Was this due to excessive mineral intake? No one can say for sure, but such products should be used with caution.

Mediolateral Imbalance (aka Medial-Lateral Imbalance)

Another important type of asymmetry you want to keep an eye out for is *mediolateral imbalance*, which as mentioned earlier, is the term used to describe anything beyond minor asymmetry in the two halves of an individual foot. Mediolateral imbalance will be noticeable from one or more angles (fig. 7.14):

7.14 When looking for mediolateral imbalance, you want to observe the front, bottom, and back of the foot. Usually, if you see the imbalance from one angle, it will also be visible in one or more of the other aspects. This foot, on a horse with very toed-out conformation, shows mediolateral imbalance any way you look at it. In each photo, compare side A to side B, and notice how different they are. On a healthy foot, the two sides might have slight asymmetries, but nothing this drastic.

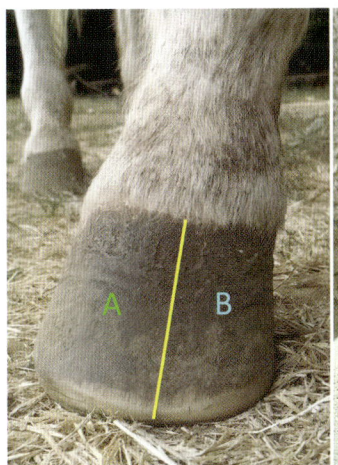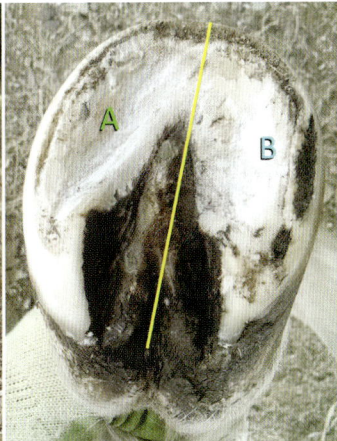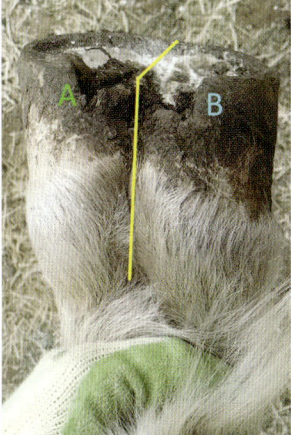

Dr. Ric Redden on

Treating the Club Foot

"The key to treating the club foot is best referred to as management, as the genetic code regulates the firing mechanism on the muscle and we are left to minimize the ill effects with two basic treatment concepts:

1) Attempt to improve the overall shape of the foot by removing the excessive heel growth and dish. This traditional concept offers temporary cosmetic appeal but invariably increases the tension on the musculo/tendon unit and associated components. Resisting the same force that caused the hoof distortion can be counterproductive.

2) We can reduce the tension that the muscle is exerting on the tendon, bone, and associated components, thereby enhancing the blood supply to compromised growth centers and ultimately improving the cosmetic appearance as well as soundness.

"The tension-reducing concept has advantages and fewer ill side effects, as it aids growth of the sole and the toe horn tubules, and can prevent hoof and bone distortion. Early detection of the effects of the increased suspension, and timely, efficient treatment can greatly enhance the overall appearance and soundness of the foot. Without appropriate management, the month-old foal with a slightly higher hoof angle may progress quickly to a grade 2 or 3, or it may remain a low grade

that will become more noticeable as the opposite foot develops a lower profile. The same applies to older horses.

"If you address the problem early, it may be that maintaining the foot with appropriate trimming is all that is necessary to reduce the slight suspension increase and prevent the foot from progressing to a higher grade. A foot that remains a grade 1 club throughout the life of the horse can be easily maintained as long as it is trimmed and/or shod in a fashion that does not drastically reduce palmar/plantar angle and thereby increase tension on the DDFT. Dropping the palmar/plantar angle of the club foot with every trim to match the opposite foot invariably increases tension on all structures and will slowly remodel the face of P3, the lamellar zone, sole depth, and articular surface.

"Good management of any club foot demands that you stay alert to the response and adjust treatment accordingly. If it becomes apparent that trimming alone or standard shoeing is allowing the foot to progress to a higher grade, therapeutic shoeing or surgery may be necessary. Whatever methods are used, it is very important that the elected treatment prevents excessive bone remodeling and horn growth center damage.

"In addition, it is extremely important to pay attention to any changes in the lower profile feet. The grade 1 and low grade 2 club feet are considered strong, healthy feet by most horsemen's standards, and rightly so, as they have an exceptionally strong heel and, as a rule, adequate mass (fig. 7.15). However, it is the opposite foot and the hind foot behind the apparently stronger club foot that confirm the club syndrome, and it is these lower profile feet that pose a threat to soundness

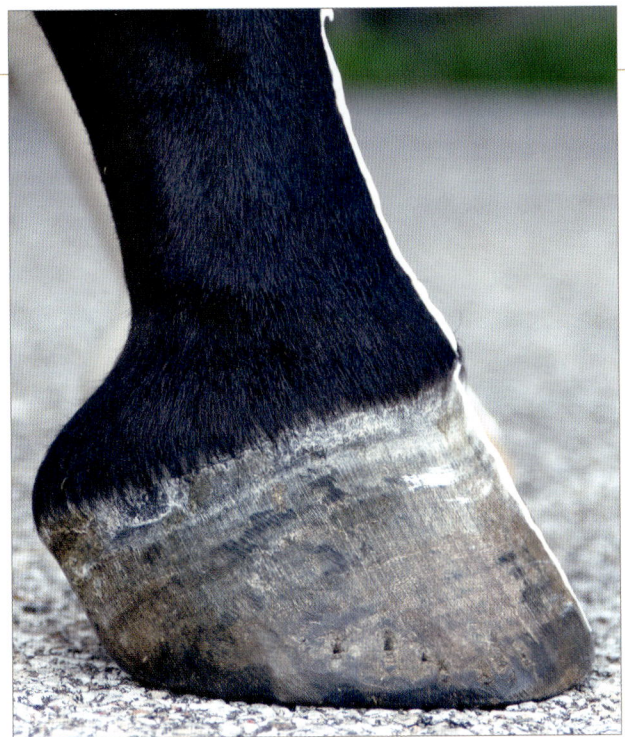

7.15 This grade 2 foot, like many low-grade clubs, is healthy and functions well, with a strong heel and good overall form and mass. The smart bet would be to maintain this foot as it is, but pay close attention to the lower profile feet, as they are probably more likely to have problems than this one.

instead of the club foot. Once the grade increases and the severity of the contraction force causes vascular compromise to sole and horn growth centers, the club foot poses a threat to gait, performance, and soundness. This is compounded by the crushed heel and often negative palmar/plantar angles of the two associated feet. This is a good reason to be alert to the ill effects of the club-foot syndrome and make every effort to minimize the DDFT tension as the foot develops. The mid-2 and higher grades require higher mechanical management, and the sooner it is applied, the better the overall results."

• From the front, the foot may be taller on one side than the other, with the hairline slanting upward, toward the taller side. The wall may have a markedly different angle on one side, sometimes due to *flaring* (see *Flares*, p. 99).

• From the bottom, the medial and lateral sides of the hoof may be quite different in width and shape. This is sometimes due to flaring.

• From the back, one heel may be wider than the other, or one may be pushed up higher than the other (sheared heels—see p. 73).

Like other forms of asymmetry, mediolateral imbalance can be a symptom of a variety of possible problems such as unbalanced trimming/shoeing or conformational faults, but it always relates to uneven loading of the hoof. It is the uneven loading that can damage the foot, as well as other parts of the limb. Problems associated with mediolateral imbalance include flaring, bone remodeling, joint pain, inflammation, arthritis, sidebone, ringbone, and tendon/ligament strain.

Dorsopalmar (or Dorsoplantar) Imbalance

In addition to seeing how the left and right halves of the foot are balanced, you also want to evaluate the hoof's front-to-back balance. We call this *dorsopalmar balance* when we're talking about the front feet, and *dorsoplantar balance* when we're talking about the hind. You may also see the term *anterior/posterior balance*, which is the same for both front and hind feet. Farriers and veterinarians may refer to this in shorthand as "DP balance" or "AP balance."

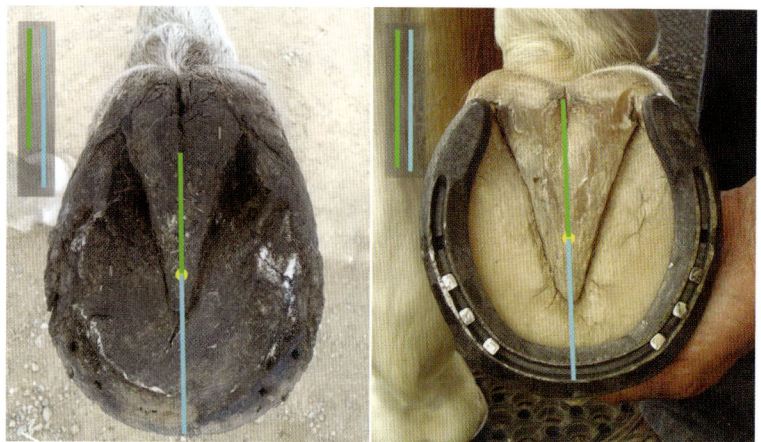

7.16 The foot on the left has poor dorsopalmer balance (DP), with much more mass ahead of the widest part of the foot (blue line) than behind it (green line). The foot on the right has nearly perfect DP balance. Note that the point of breakover on the right foot is where the bevel on the shoe sits.

What you ideally want to see is a foot with approximately ⅔ of its mass in the back of the foot, behind the true apex of the frog (usually located about ½ inch behind the front point of the frog), and ⅓ ahead of the apex. This also equates to a foot that has about 50% of its mass both ahead and behind the axis of rotation of the coffin bone, a point which corresponds to the widest part of the foot (fig. 7.16). A foot with these general proportions accomplishes two very important things. First, the foot will have a strong base of support, with the hoof set up well under the bony column of the leg, maximizing the hoof's ability to bear weight and dissipate impact forces. Second, good DP balance

Hands-On Activity:
Examine Your Horse for DP Balance

To check out your horse's feet for front-to-back balance, find the widest point of the foot, then draw a line across it with a marker. Next, measure from that line to the very back point of the heels that touch the ground and jot that measurement down. Lastly, measure from the line forward to the *point of breakover* (POB), which is the most forward point where the hoof would contact the ground if standing on a flat surface (see *Understanding Breakover,* p. 95). If there is any bevel in the shoe or toe, the POB is the spot where the bevel starts (fig. 7.17).

Now compare your measurements. If you find that your horse has more mass in the front part of the foot, talk to your hoof-care provider about it. If he or she is not concerned, it might be advisable to get a second opinion from another provider or your veterinarian. Repeat this exercise on all four feet. You can also use your measurements to compare the left front to the right front, and the left hind to the right hind. Note any disparities and discuss them with your hoof-care provider as well.

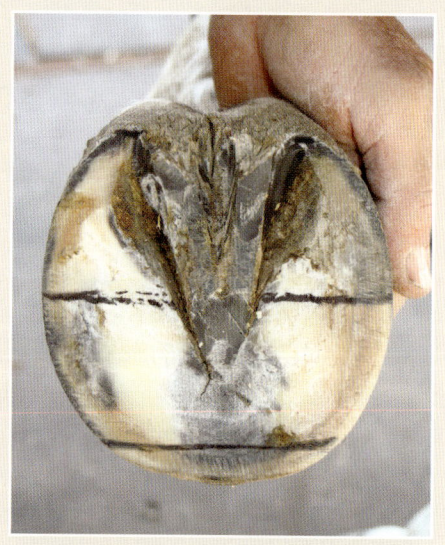

7.17 Master Farrier Gene Ovnicek shows you how to examine dorsopalmar/dorso-plantar balance (DP). This foot is prepared for the application of a shoe that has a bevel to facilitate breakover, so Ovnicek has drawn the front line where the point of breakover (POB) on the shoe will be.

allows for a *point of breakover* that puts minimal strain to the joints and soft tissues.

When the front part of the foot is longer than the back part, this is called *dorsopalmar* or *dorsoplantar imbalance*. An alarming number of domestic horses have this kind of imbalance, which most frequently takes the form of long-toe/low-heel syndrome, discussed in the previous chapter. When a foot has this conformation, breakover will be delayed, which can cause a variety of problems for the horse.

Understanding Breakover

The term *breakover* can be defined as the phase of stride that begins when the heel leaves the ground and starts to rotate around the toe, which is still touching the ground. The main direction of breakover is forward, but the foot also breaks over sideways to some degree when the horse is turning, and there can be a more significant amount of lateral breakover in horses with crooked limbs. The term "point of breakover" (POB) refers to the most forward point of weight bearing when the horse is standing with his foot flat on the ground. The POB may or may not coincide with the bottom edge of the dorsal surface of the toe wall. On a well-balanced, properly trimmed/shod foot, it will be a little way behind that plane (fig. 7.18). Most importantly, a correctly placed POB will be about ¼ inches in front of the leading edge of the coffin bone. The placement of the POB can be adjusted by how the hoof is trimmed and how shoes are applied, if the horse is shod.

Whether breakover occurs comfortably and easily—or with strain and difficulty—depends on the shape, balance, and length of the hoof. The

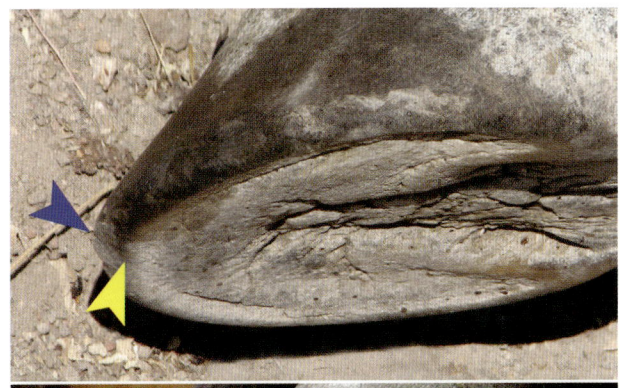

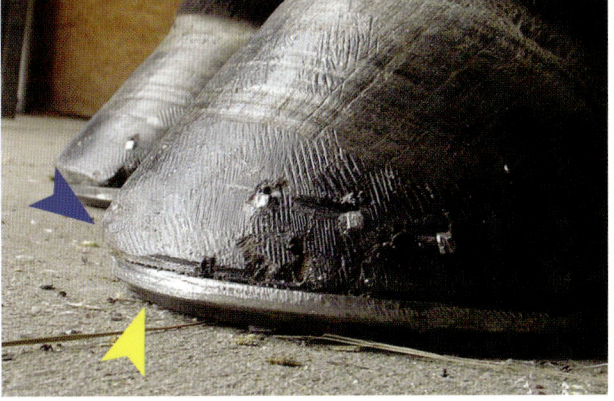

7.18 The yellow arrows indicate the POB on each of these feet, while the blue ones show where the dorsal surface of the toe wall ends. Naturally worn feet like the one above, and shoes designed to facilitate breakover like those below, both have a beveled edge that places the POB behind the edge of the wall.

placement of the POB is especially important, as it is this point that the foot will have to pivot over before the foot can be lifted up and forward in the stride. The most common problem with breakover is that dorsopalmar/plantar imbalance results in a toe that is too long, creating a POB that is too far forward. The result is excessive leverage and delayed breakover, which causes unnatural strain on all the structures attempting to get the foot to roll over the toe. This strain can result in various kinds of distortion and cracking in the hoof, soreness in the back part of the foot, or injury to the tendons and ligaments

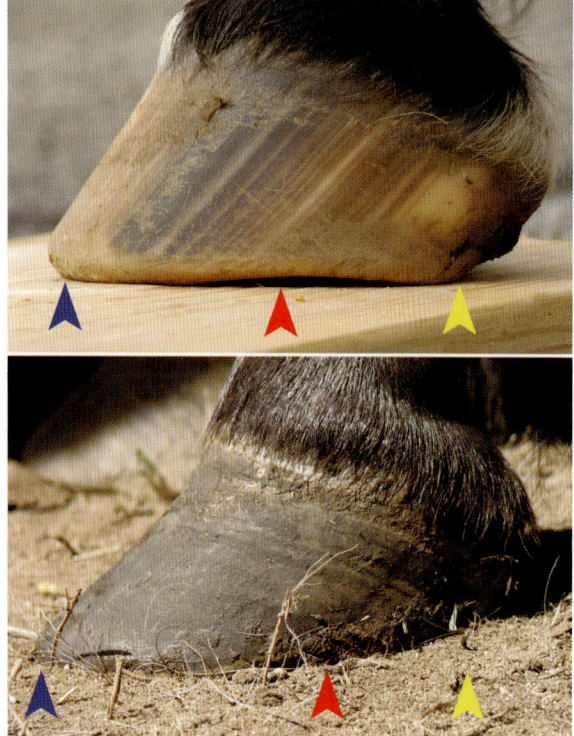

7.19 A well-balanced foot like the top one will have about half its length from the widest part of the foot (red arrow) to the POB (blue arrow), and half from the widest part of the foot to the back of the heels (yellow arrow). A foot like the bottom one, with much more length in front than in back, will experience significant strain every time the foot has to pivot over that long toe.

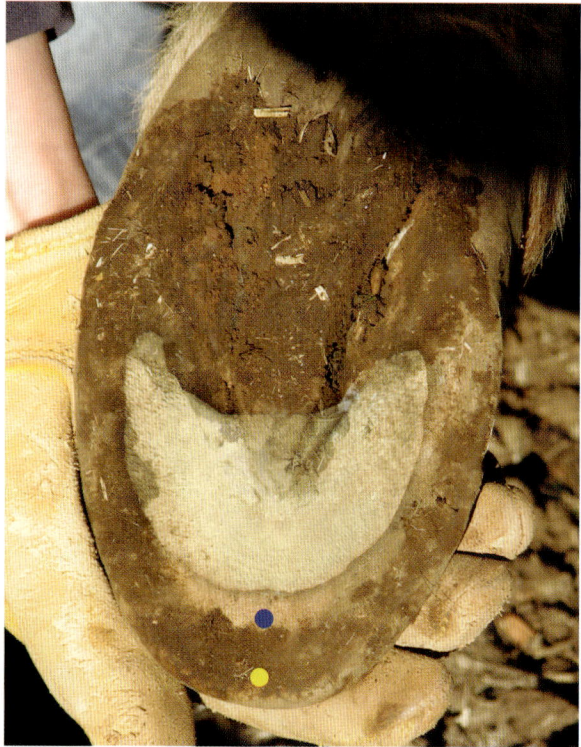

7.20 The toe of this foot is stretched far ahead of where it should be. If you were to place the POB just a bit behind the wall (yellow dot), it would still be well forward of its correct position relative to the coffin bone (blue dot). However, on a bare foot like this, moving the POB back to a more optimal position would be a process over time, as you simply can't cut away that much foot at one go.

in the limb. The longer the toe, the worse the strain (fig. 7.19).

However, breakover is not just about the hoof. The process involves a complex interplay between the tendons, ligaments, and muscles, as well as the internal and external structures of the hoof. Breakover starts higher up the leg with tension in the deep digital flexor muscle and the distal check ligament, both of which activate the deep digital flexor tendon (DDFT). That action combines with tension in the navicular ligaments, putting gentle pressure on the navicular bursa, which in turn acts on the navicular bone, then the impar ligament, and so on until the wings of the coffin bone begin to lift. This tips the coffin bone forward and begins the rotation of the foot. All of these actions begin before you see the heel even start to lift off the ground.

Unfortunately, there are a lot of misunderstandings about breakover, especially when it comes to correct placement of the point of breakover. A big part of the problem is that many people—including some hoof-care providers—think that the point of breakover is relative to the dorsal wall, when they should be looking at it as relative to the coffin bone. The reason this is so critical is that when you have dorsopalmar/plantar imbalance, the dorsal wall, in addition to the sole and frog apex, can migrate forward, leaving the coffin bone much farther back in relation to the dorsal wall. This makes the dorsal wall unreliable in terms of determining the correct point of breakover (fig. 7.20).

Another misconception has to do with heel height and the timing of breakover. Many people believe that if you are trying to make breakover happen sooner, you should increase heel height relative to the toe. The thought is that if the entire foot is already somewhat tipped forward, breakover will occur earlier in the stride. While this may seem logical, it is not actually what happens. Remember that tension on the DDFT that helps the foot to initiate lift off? When that is working correctly, the foot starts lifting up when the leg is close to the vertical position under the body. That only happens if the heel is the height it should be, close to the level of the functional sole.

Research has shown that when heels are taller, or when a wedge pad puts the foot in a similar position as a tall heel, the foot must actually stay on the ground longer, needing the leg to be tilted farther forward to increase tension on the DDFT enough to get the foot to lift off the ground. This causes a measurable delay in breakover, creating questions about such practices as raising the front heels of a horse in order to prevent forging (where the toe of the hind foot reaches forward and strikes the heel or sole of the front foot). While doing so might indeed stop the forging, the cause of the change is not accelerated breakover, as is commonly believed.

A similar but even worse delay occurs when the toe is too long. It is similar in the sense that the leg has to be farther forward to initiate breakover, but worse because the extra leverage created by the toe places unnatural strain on the tendons and ligaments in the back of the foot, especially the suspensory ligament (fig. 7.21).

7.21 In this illustration from Gene Ovnicek, the foot on the left has the POB ¼ inch ahead of the front edge ("tip") of the coffin bone (P3), and the process of breakover happens smoothly, without excessive flexion of the coffin joint. Notice the approximately 90-degree angle (A) formed by the coffin joint (P3, P2, and NB) as the foot begins to lift off the ground (B). Also note how far behind the perpendicular plane (C) the bottom of the cannon bone (D) is at this point.

Compare all of this to the foot on the right, which has delayed breakover due to a long toe. The coffin joint has to flex farther before the heel can begin to lift off, creating a tighter angle (A). This places strain on the joint and everything around it, including the deep digital flexor tendon and the suspensory ligament to the navicular bone, which are both pulled tighter by the navicular bone in this position. You can also see that the cannon bone (D) has to be leaning forward at a much greater angle before the foot starts to lift off (B).

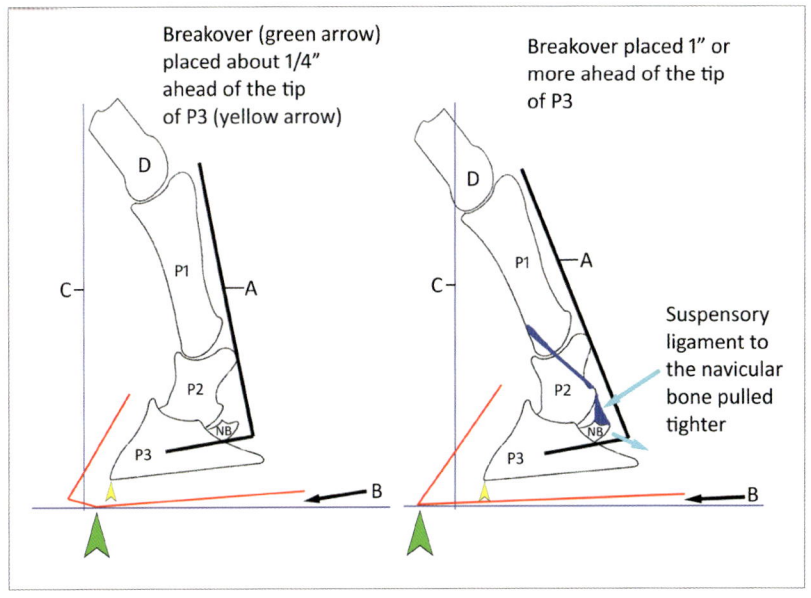

Breakover (green arrow) placed about 1/4" ahead of the tip of P3 (yellow arrow)

Breakover placed 1" or more ahead of the tip of P3

Suspensory ligament to the navicular bone pulled tighter

Hands-On Activity:
Finding Your Horse's Correct Point of Breakover (POB)

Master Farrier Gene Ovnicek explains how to locate the widest part of the foot, which allows you to determine where the front edge (tip) of the coffin bone is. This, in turn, allows you to determine the correct point of breakover. The widest part of the foot also shows you the center of rotation of the coffin joint, which should be approximately halfway between the toe and the back of the frog (remember that the frog is

7.22 A–C This foot has not been exfoliated and the tip of the frog has not been trimmed to reveal its true apex, both of which are recommended by Ovnicek to get the most accurate mapping. However, if the foot does not have much buildup of exfoliating sole, and you estimate that the true apex of the frog is about ¼ inch behind the visible tip, your mapping will still be reasonably accurate.

Step 1: Image A is marked with a red dot where you would estimate the true apex of the frog to be. Measure back 1 inch from that point and mark it with a line.

Step 2: The red dots on image B have been placed at the ends of the bars. Draw a line from dot to dot.

Step 3: Draw an arc on either side of the foot, as the red lines show in image C. Mark the apex or peak of each arc (blue dots), then draw a line across those marks.

If the three lines you have drawn are pretty much in the same place, you have successfully located the widest part of the foot. If one is a bit off but the other two are close together, go with the latter. Be aware that on a foot with poor dorsopalmar balance, the frog can be stretched quite far forward from its healthy position, making this the least reliable of the three markers.

meant to be part of the load-bearing surface of the foot). When the foot is balanced around the center of rotation, breakover is optimized and the foot is well balanced, with maximum support and minimum strain. Ovnicek says:

"The first and primary tool I use to evaluate the balance of the foot and find the correct placement for the POB is to locate the widest part of the foot, as established through studies done by the Equine Lameness Prevention Organization (www.lamenessprevention.org). The widest part of the foot study has shown that through the ELPO mapping process described here, you can fairly accurately locate the center of rotation of the coffin joint and you will consistently be able to find the tip of the distal phalanx (coffin bone) and balance the foot around the bony column. A combination of three approaches is used to accurately identify the widest part of the foot (figs. 7.22 A–C).

"The first step is to locate the *true* frog apex. This is not always easy because it generally requires some assertive

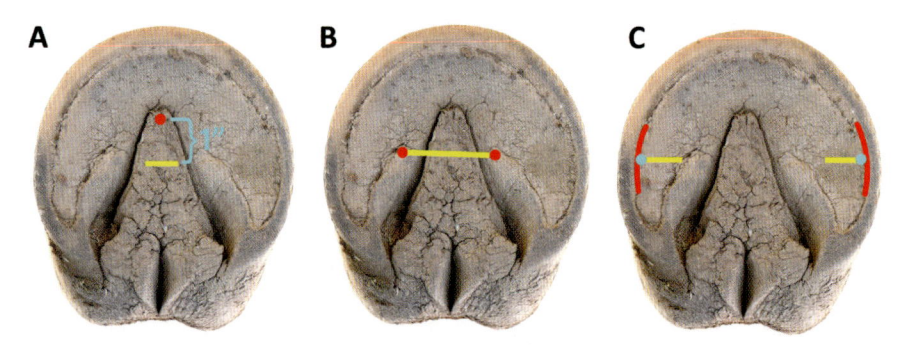

A　　　　　B　　　　　C

trimming to find the true origin of the frog from the sole. The widest part of the foot is generally about 1 inch behind the *true* frog apex. However, if the frog apex appears to be stretched and pulled forward, you must employ the other methods to get a more accurate assessment.

"The second method is to find the place where the bars terminate into the frog commissures (collateral grooves). If you run a pick along the commissures, you will feel or see a bulge or swell where the bars appear to terminate (fig. 7.22 B). A line across the foot at that point should be very close to the widest part.

"Third, and generally the most accurate, is to actually exfoliate the sole from the toe quarters to the heels on each side (meaning remove the chalky material until the waxy-appearing surface is revealed). Then, using a marker, draw a line at the wall/sole junction from the toe quarters to the heel. Mark a line at the apex or peak of the arc you've just drawn (fig. 7.22 C). Connect the mark from one side to the other. This line is reliably the widest part of the sole.

"If through the use of all three methods you find the lines you have drawn all fall on top of each other, you can rest assured that you are quite accurate with your assessment of the widest part of the foot. From this line, you can measure forward approximately 1¾ inch (on a number 00–2 size foot), to find the tip of the distal phalanx (give or take ⅛ inch to ¼ inch or so). The point of breakover should be approximately ¼ inch in front of that line, closer to the toe."

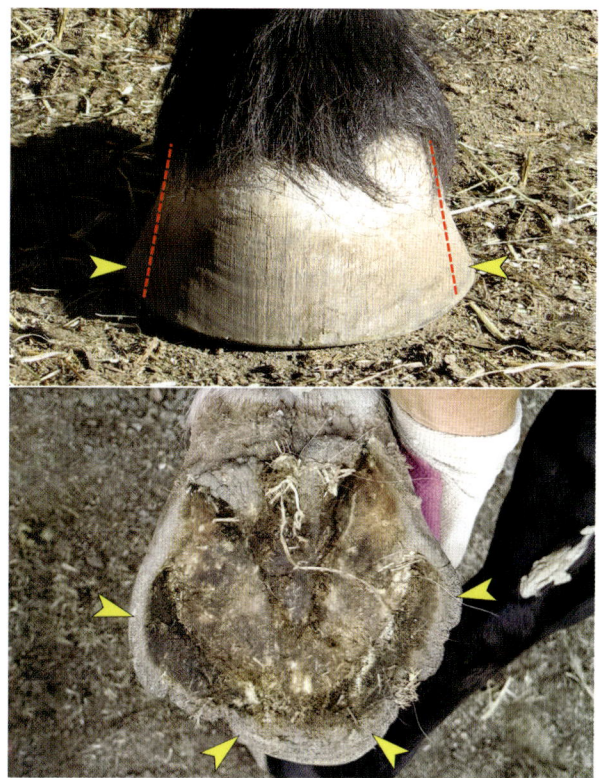

7.23 Flares can be seen by looking for deviation in the walls, either from the front, the side, or the bottom. The large foot in the upper photo has some minor flaring in the quarters (area outside dashed red lines), while the foot below has more severe flares all the way around the foot due to overgrown walls—sometimes referred to as "lack of farrier disease."

Flares

Flares are a type of hoof-capsule distortion where the wall horn is being stretched outward and pulled away from the coffin bone. As you recall, the wall of a healthy hoof should follow the same angle all the way from the coronet to the ground. Flares are present when part of the wall deviates or "dishes" outward from that angle. They can be observed by looking at the walls from the front (in the case of medial or lateral flares) or side (in the case of toe

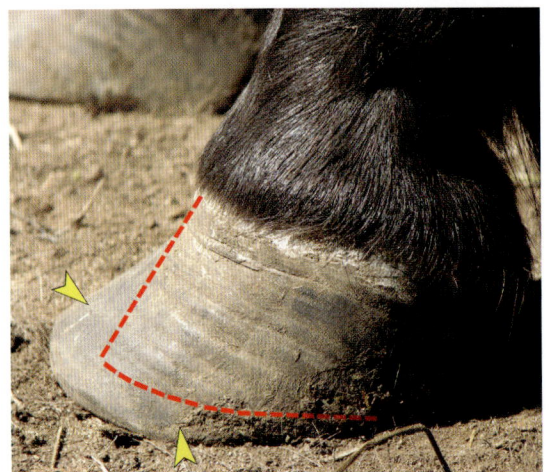

7.24 Flaring of the toe wall is a common consequence of laminitis. The toe flare can be so subtle that it is easily overlooked, or dramatically apparent, as it is in this miniature horse's foot. The dashed red line shows approximately what the shape of this foot would be without the flaring. Everything outside the line is flared hoof wall.

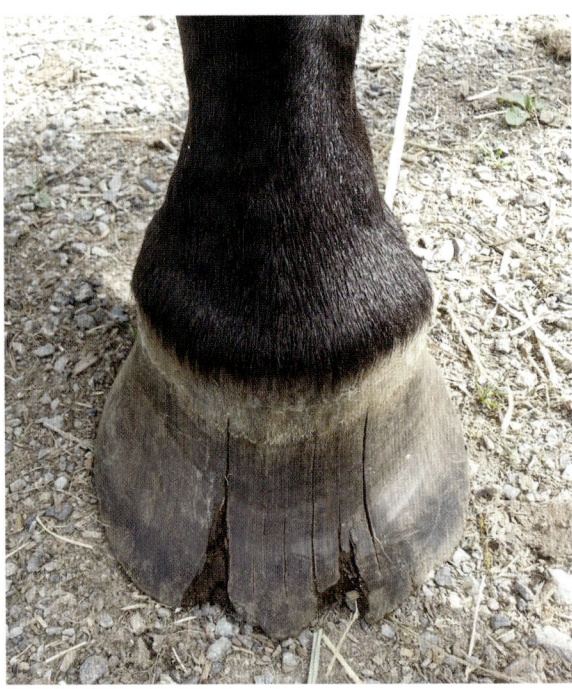

7.25 This foot ended up like this through a cascade of problems that likely started with some issue, internal or external, that led to flaring. This caused some separation that invited white line disease, which caused more separation and led to extensive cracking.

flares), and by viewing the foot from the bottom (fig. 7.23). Flares can show up in the toe or along the sides of the hoof, and they can develop for many reasons, sometimes in combination. These include:

• *Mechanical,* meaning that some form of imbalance or other issue is creating excessive physical pressure on part or all of the wall and forcing it outward. The pressure could be a result of conformation, poor trimming or shoeing, too much time between trims (overgrowth), pain, muscular imbalance, or injury.

• *Laminitis,* which leads to damaged laminae and separation of the hoof wall, which is then easily pulled away into flared shapes (fig. 7.24).

• *Nutritional,* meaning that something in the horse's diet—often too much sugar or starch—is weakening

the connection of the walls, leaving them vulnerable to flaring.

• *Metabolic,* meaning the horse has a metabolic condition such as insulin resistance or Cushing's disease that can prime the horse for physiological responses that may weaken the walls.

• *Infection,* usually secondary to walls that are already compromised due to weakened laminae. The stretched white line present in a flared section of wall allows debris to jam up into the area, which is an open invitation to bacteria and fungi (fig. 7.25).

Correcting flares can take time and often involves a multi-pronged approach. It is important to understand that once any part of the hoof wall has separated, it cannot reattach itself. Therefore, a flared hoof can only improve by growing down a new wall that is well connected to the coffin bone by healthy, tight laminae. In order for this to happen, the things that were causing the flare to occur in the first place have to be dealt with, and any leverage from contact with the ground that might keep the flare going needs to be addressed. When pressure from contact with the ground (or the shoe) is not relieved in the affected area, it will only continue to pull the wall outward and further weaken the connection of the laminae.

Fortunately, beveling the flared wall from below is often enough to relieve that pressure (fig. 7.26).

Beveling the wall actually changes the direction of the force experienced by the wall when it pushes against the ground, so instead of pressure levering the wall away, ground contact works to keep the wall tight (fig. 7.27). If you are concerned that beveling the wall will take away the support of the wall in that area, remember that any part of the wall that is flared is not well attached and is therefore not generally providing good support anyway.

That said, removing the flare should not make the horse uncomfortable. In most cases, a flare pulls painfully on the wall, and removing it provides relief. But there are instances where removing the flare can actually make a horse sore, and no matter what

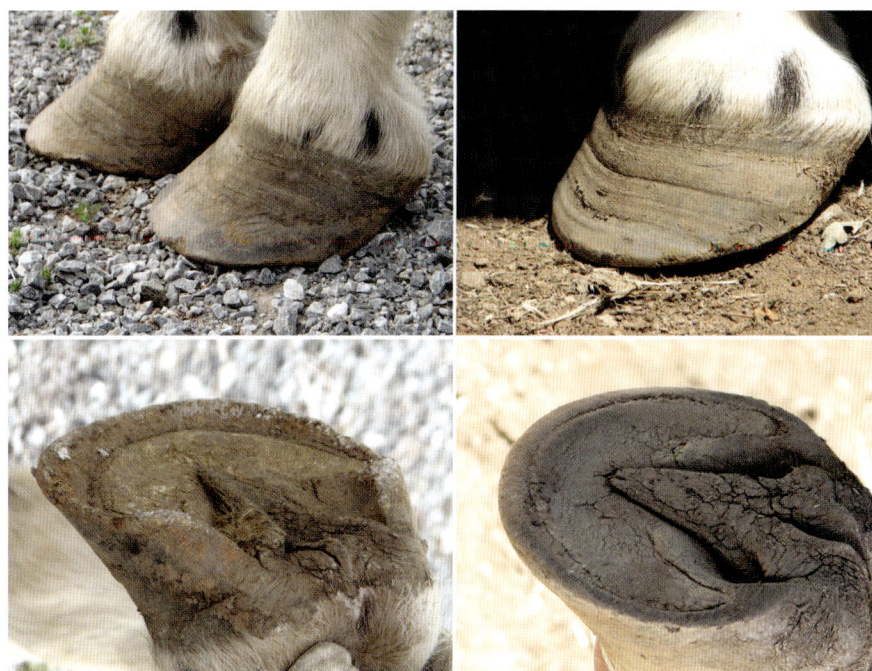

7.26 This pony was laminitic due to unmanaged insulin resistance, and her feet were neglected. Getting her flared toes on the right track involved a change to a low carbohydrate diet, an increase in movement, and regular, physiologically correct trimming. The images on the left show her left front foot before any changes were made, and the ones on the right show the same foot, three months later.

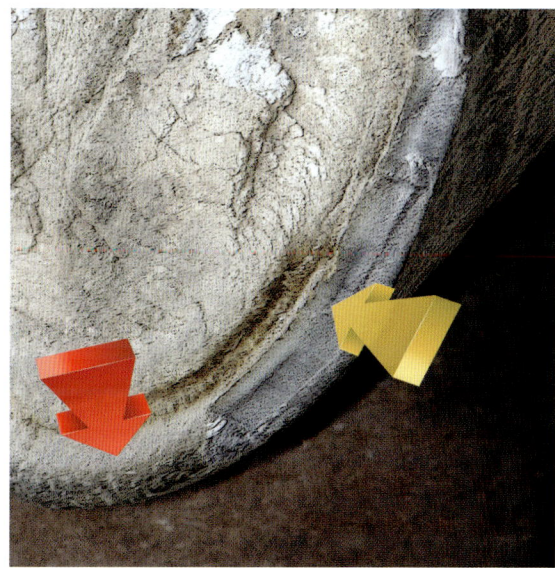

7.27 When all or part of the wall is long or flared, the pressure from ground contact creates leverage, pushing the wall outward (red arrow). When a beveled wall contacts the ground, any pressure it encounters—such as that during breakover—actually pushes the wall inward (yellow arrow). This wall is not very overgrown, but you can still see how much difference the beveled edge makes.

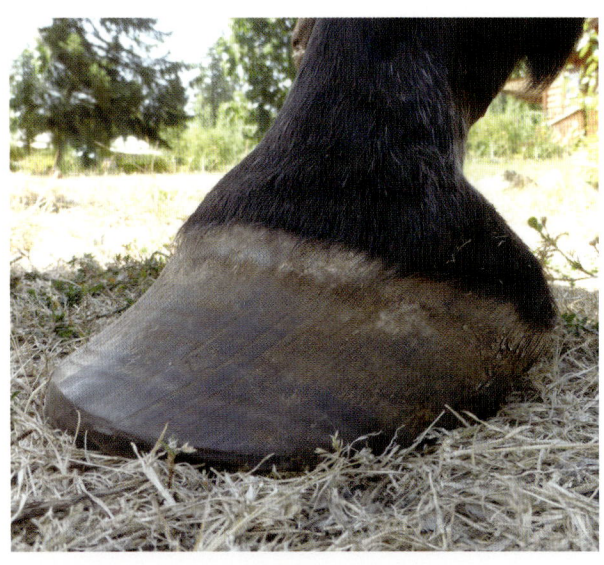

7.28 This horse has a flared dorsal wall resulting from demineralization and remodeling of the coffin bone. As the damage to the bone cannot be repaired, the flare cannot be "fixed"—only managed.

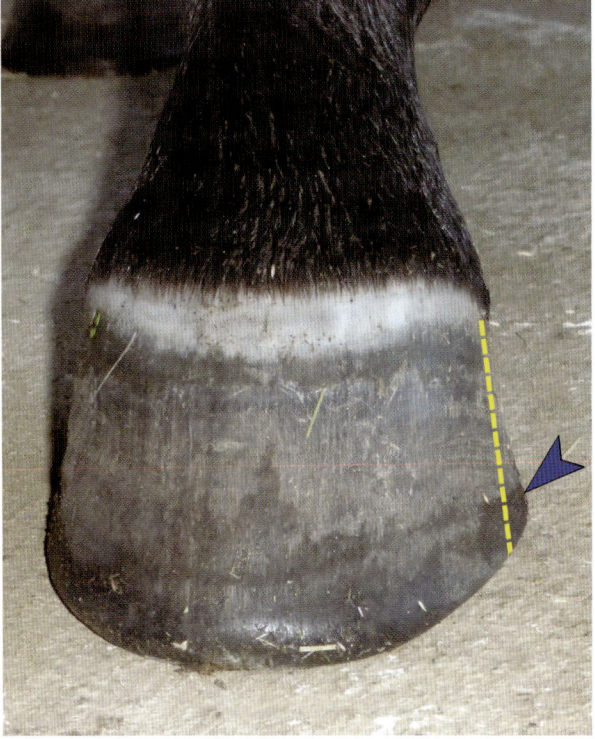

7.29 The minor flare in the lateral quarter of this hind foot is quite common and usually not cause for concern.

you try, it seems that the flare is the only thing keeping the horse comfortable. This may be especially true in horses with thin soles or damaged coffin bones. Thus, if you try correcting the flare and the horse gets sore, you may need to leave it be.

In addition to, or sometimes instead of beveling, your hoof-care provider might rasp the surface of a flared wall to make it more in line with the healthy sections of wall, the thought being that this will reduce levering forces and encourage the wall to grow down straighter, with better attachment. Other professionals disagree with this approach, believing that thinning the wall further weakens it, and is more likely to lengthen the time it takes to grow out the flare. Ultimately, both may be right or wrong, depending on what a particular hoof requires.

Whatever trimming methods are used to provide mechanical relief to a flare, if that is all you are doing, you may very well be missing important pieces of the puzzle. For instance, it is quite common for metabolic or nutritional factors to be at play in the weakening of the laminar connection, and if they are a factor in your horse's flaring, those issues will need to be addressed or the flaring problem is likely to continue. Hoof imbalances must also be corrected, if at all possible, or you will continue to "chase" the flare it is causing in the hoof. There are also going to be cases where the conformational defects or injuries that are causing imbalance are pronounced enough that it is impossible to get rid of the flares entirely (fig. 7.28).

Lastly, you should be aware that there are plenty of instances where flaring is not really anything to worry about, especially with minor flares in the quarters, as we see in the hind feet of many horses (fig. 7.29). While such flares do indicate imbalance,

Hands-On Activity:
Checking for Flares

Obvious flares are easy to spot, but horses often have more subtle flares that go unnoticed. Usually, minor flares are more of an aesthetic concern than anything else, but it is good to keep an eye on such things to be sure a problem isn't developing.

To check your horse for flares, you will need a short straight edge (if it is too long it may knock into your horse's cannon bone). Stand your horse on flat, level ground, and hold the straight edge against the hoof wall, starting at the center of the toe. You should see no gap under the straight edge. If you do see a gap, there is some flare in the wall—the bigger the gap, the greater the flare. Repeat on the sides, checking for medial and lateral flares. You can also put your horse's foot up on something like a hoof stand and check it there if that is more convenient (fig. 7.30).

One more tip: In most feet, the top ½ inch or so of the hoof wall, just below the hairline, is well connected, even when the rest of the wall is not. Looking at that top bit can give you a good idea of what angle the hoof wall "wants" to be, and will help you to see a flare (fig. 7.31).

NOTE: Only do this exercise if your horse is quiet and cooperative, and properly restrained. Try not to put your head in front of the foot or leg, as you could get a knock on the noggin if your horse moves.

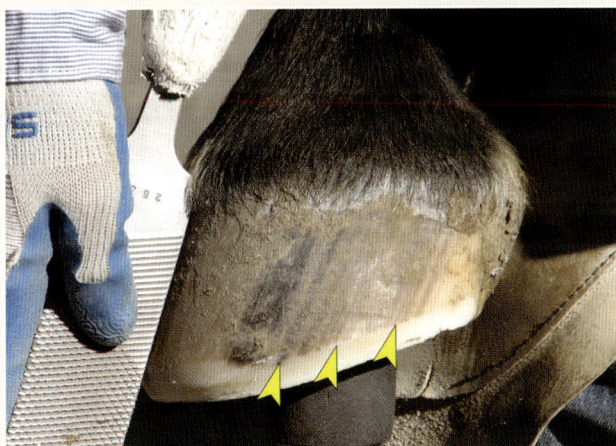

7.30 The straight edge on this rasp shows that the dorsal wall on this hoof has no flare whatsoever. Another sign that the wall is well-balanced and tightly attached is the straightness of the horn tubules, which you can see easily in the straightness of the stripes on the wall (yellow arrows).

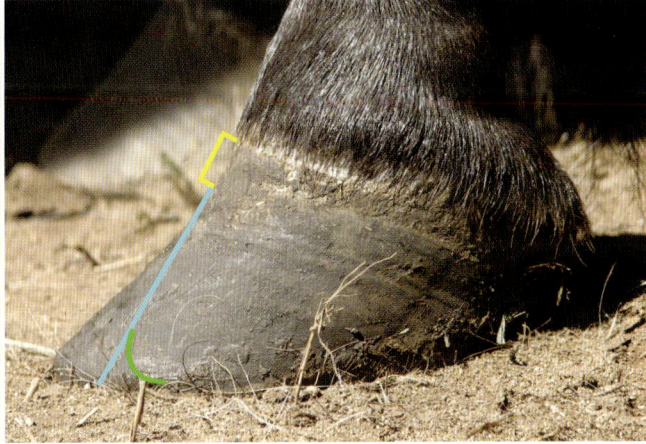

7.31 This hoof wall is seriously overgrown and flared, but the top ½ inch (yellow bracket) shows you what a healthy angle would look like for this foot. Follow that angle down (blue line), and you can start to see what the hoof would look like with the flare corrected. The green curve estimates what the edge of the toe would look like with a bit of a bevel and a rolled edge to help keep the flare from recurring.

the fact is that plenty of horses have minor imbalances that never actually cause a problem. If the foot is otherwise healthy and the horse is consistently sound, a minor flare is something to keep an eye on, but nothing to fret over. If, however, a horse never had any flare before but starts developing some, that indicates a change—most often in trim, diet, or an imbalance due to pain or injury somewhere in the body—and that is worth investigating.

Correcting Imbalance: A Few More Thoughts

If you note any kind of significant imbalance or asymmetry in your horse's feet, the challenge is to determine what is causing it, and figure out whether or not it can be fixed. If the problem is due to poor trimming/shoeing, which is, unfortunately, quite common, that is both a good and a bad thing. What's good is that the imbalance can very likely be corrected, but the bad part is either that the person that is doing your hoof care isn't performing the job very well—or that you, as the owner, aren't having the job done frequently enough to maintain hoof balance. Other causes of imbalance such as asymmetrical muscle development, injury, or skeletal malalignment can be more complicated to manage, but improvement is often possible through modalities such as physiotherapy, chiropractic adjustment, targeted training exercises, and veterinary care that address the underlying issues.

7.32 This very functional adult Mustang lives in the wild and has never had any care for her toed-in feet, which are the result of her conformation. Trying to significantly change the feet on a horse like this would very likely make this sound horse lame.

Unfortunately, some imbalances can't be corrected without causing other problems, especially in adult horses. For example, horses with crooked legs end up with hoof distortion due to uneven loading and wear. But, as we mentioned earlier, if you take an adult horse with such an issue and try to create a perfectly straight foot on a crooked leg through trimming or shoeing, you will actually strain the soft tissues and joints of the limb, which can't adapt to any significant degree once the limb's growth plates have closed.

We must recognize that there are many horses out there that do just fine with their "wonky" feet, and we don't necessarily need to mess with them (fig. 7.32). If you have an adult horse with a limb deformity, it may be that careful management to

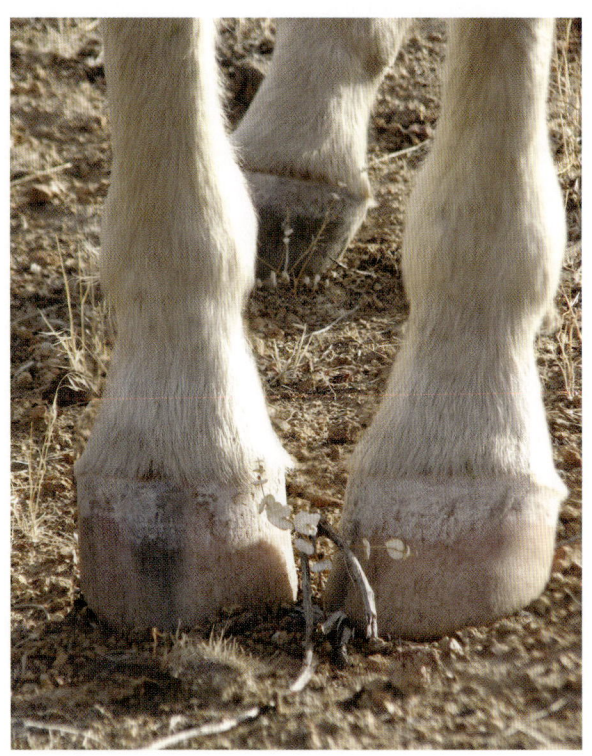

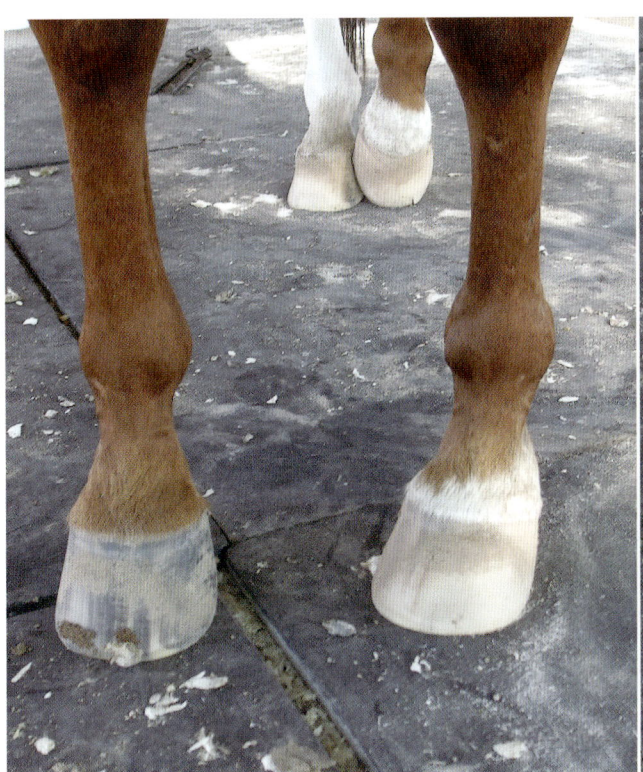
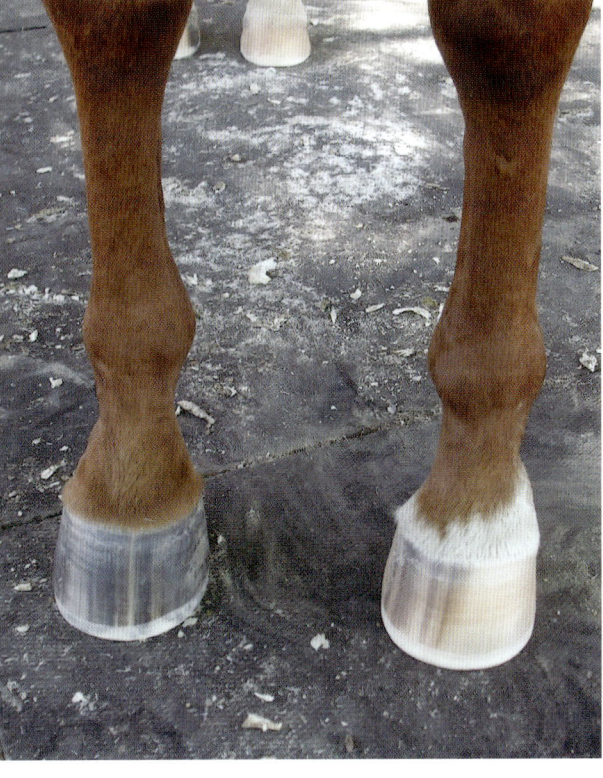

7.33 This is an example of a good trim to minimize distortion due to a crooked limb, without doing so much that the joints will get strained.

minimize distortion and prevent the hoof from deforming more, rather than trying to make it perfect, is the best option (fig. 7.33).

This is definitely not the case with very young foals whose limbs are still developing. Foals can have limb deformities that are present at birth (congenital) or that show up later (acquired). The most common types of deformities are classed as either *angular* (limbs bent sideways, either inward or outward), or *flexural* (limbs bent forward or backward due to excessive tightness or laxity of the tendons and/or ligaments).

Many kinds of limb deformities can be improved or entirely corrected when addressed early on, giving the foal the chance to develop normal feet

and legs. Traditionally, flexural and angular limb deformities have been treated with various kinds of splints and casts, but being completely inflexible, these have their dangers and they often cause pressure sores. Fortunately, a newer type of brace is now available, including an articulating model that allows the knee to flex (fig. 7.34). This provides the necessary support while avoiding many of the pitfalls of fixed splints and casts.

If you notice any kind of angular or flexural deformity in your newborn foal, get the vet out right away. He or she may tell you that the foal will simply grow out of the problem (often the case), but if intervention is necessary, your vet is the best one to determine what treatment options you should consider.

7.34 Even serious limb deformities, like the severe *carpus valgus* (outward deviation of the knee) seen here, can often be completely corrected if treated early. This foal was successfully treated with an articulated brace from Red Boot of Argentina.

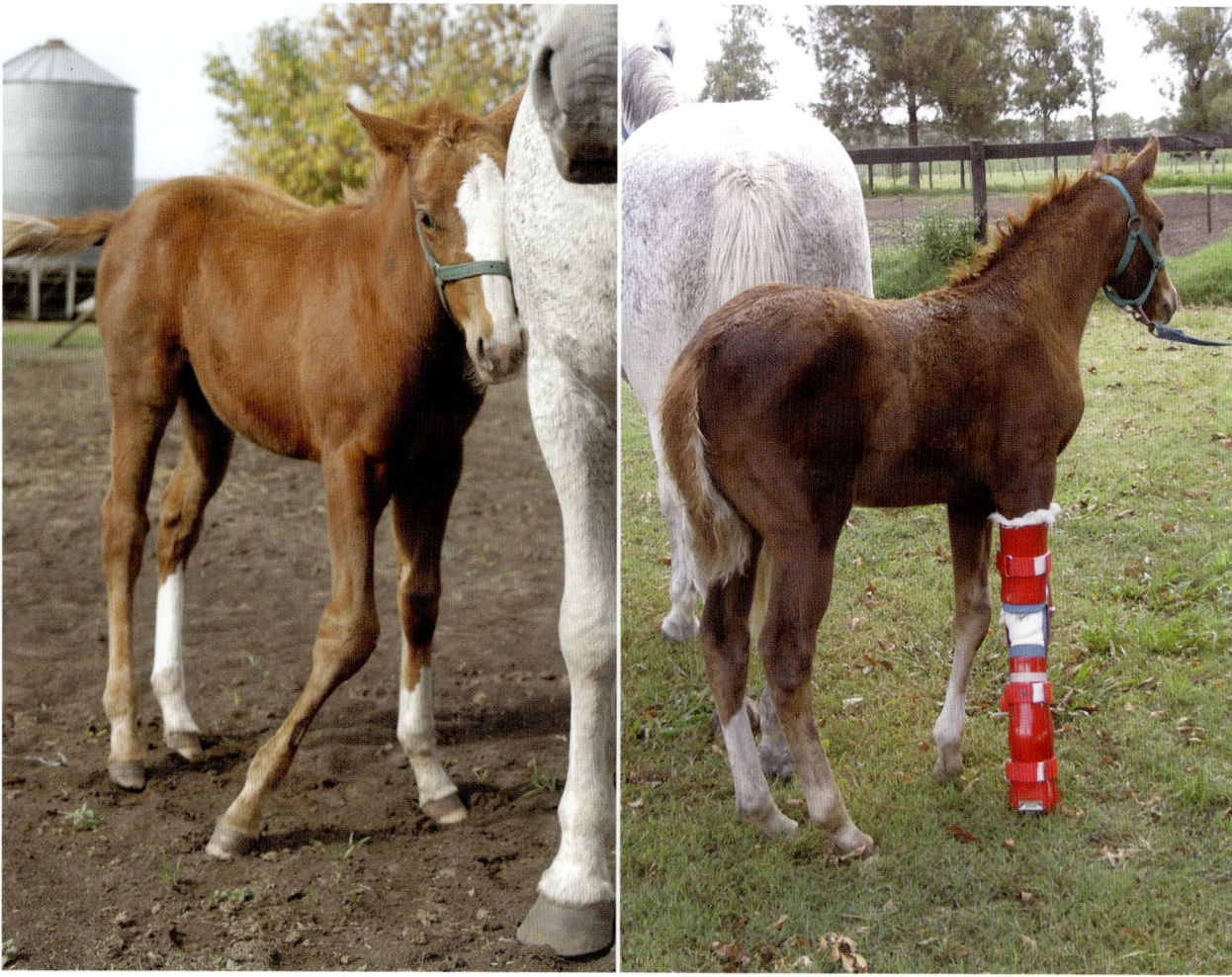

Even if you don't see any issue, it is a very good idea to have your vet and farrier check your foal early and regularly to determine if the wee one's feet and legs are growing properly. Though many people believe that the feet of a youngster can be left to their own devices, this can be a devastating mistake. The first two years of life are absolutely not the time to skimp on hoof care, because not only are the feet growing and changing rapidly, but all the bones above the hoof are growing and changing in relation to the platform (the hoof) they are based on. It is a simple but hard truth that horse owners frequently fail to recognize limb and hoof issues that can set a foal up for a lifetime of trouble, and by the time that trouble becomes obvious, it is often too late to correct the problem.

Toe Length—The Long and Short of It

Tall Toes

We talked earlier about the damage that can be caused by toes that are too long and have run forward. But, toes can also be too long and grow up instead of forward. Long, upright toes will be accompanied by long, upright heels, giving the overall hoof a "tall" look. Most of the time, tall feet are simply the result of overgrown walls. For this reason, tall feet are more often seen in shod horses because excess wall on barefoot horses tends to wear or break off. Barefoot horses with very strong, thick walls can also end up with tall feet, but whether the horse is barefoot or shod, a tall foot is definitely not an optimally functioning one.

The main problem with a tall, overgrown foot is that it loads the periphery of the foot and lifts the sole, bars, and frog off the ground, taking away their respective abilities to share in support, load bearing, and the dissipation of concussive forces (fig. 8.1). Through disuse, the structures in the back of the foot become weaker, the heels tend to contract, and you may start seeing problems like thrush invading unhealthy, atrophied frog tissue, especially since the excess wall length tends to lock in dirt and muck.

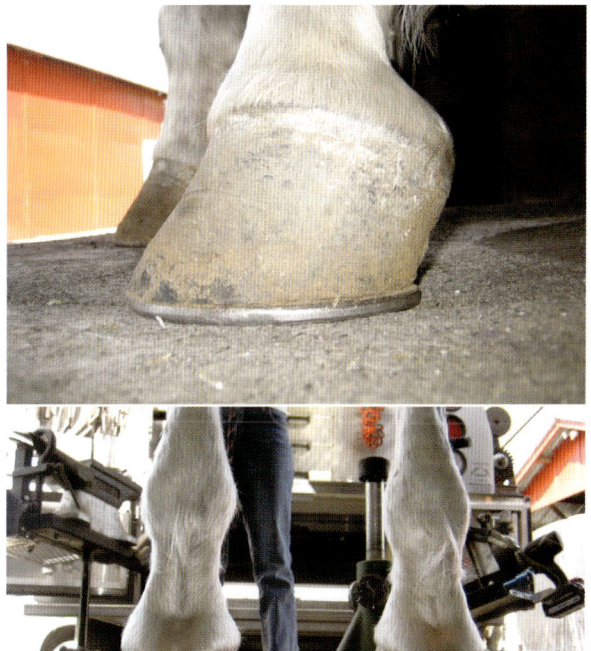

8.1 Chronically tall hooves like these can end up with numerous problems. This horse had a thrush infection that lasted for 11 years, despite the owner's diligent efforts to keep the feet clean and treat the infection. Fortunately, the problem was finally eliminated by a good farrier who understood that getting rid of the thrush would require not only treatment, but also getting the horse off his "stilts."

In addition, all the work of weight bearing and energy dissipation has to be borne by the walls, putting them under a great deal of pressure. This can lead to cracks, chips, and entire chunks of wall breaking off, and may also damage the laminar connection and the coronary corium, inhibiting good growth and leading to "shelly" (flaky), thin walls. Tall toes can also cause the horse's gait to become out of sync, creating problems such as tripping or forging.

Lastly, the coffin bone is left unsupported, which causes it to push down onto the solar corium with each step. This can damage the corium, cause thinning of the sole, and even lead to distal descent of the coffin bone, in some cases, which means the coffin bone has "sunk" within the hoof capsule (see p. 60), as it often does in cases of chronic laminitis. When this happens, you may see a tall foot with a

flat sole that is too close to the ground. In this case, the excess wall height is actually above the level of the sole, not below it (fig. 8.2).

Tall toes most often get that way because horses are not getting trimmed/shod often enough, or because they are being intentionally left that way. There seems to be a common misperception that a tall foot is a good foot, since it means the heels are not low, which is often equated with being weak. Nowhere is this mistaken view more clear than in the excessively tall feet used as models in many hoof-product advertisements. Once you understand enough about the equine foot to know what you are looking at, these ads are downright scary, as some very distorted feet are being held up as the ideal. Keep an eye out next time you flip through your favorite horse magazine—you might be shocked by what you see.

When a horse's feet are too tall, it is easy to blame the farrier, and sometimes the fault does lie there. However, in many instances, the problem rests with an owner who is simply not getting the farrier out frequently enough. Such owners often mention cost as the main reason why they don't have the horse's feet tended to more often. However, if they were more aware of the harm they could be causing by letting their horses' feet get so overgrown, they might realize that their short-term savings are likely to cost them plenty in the long run when their horse goes lame.

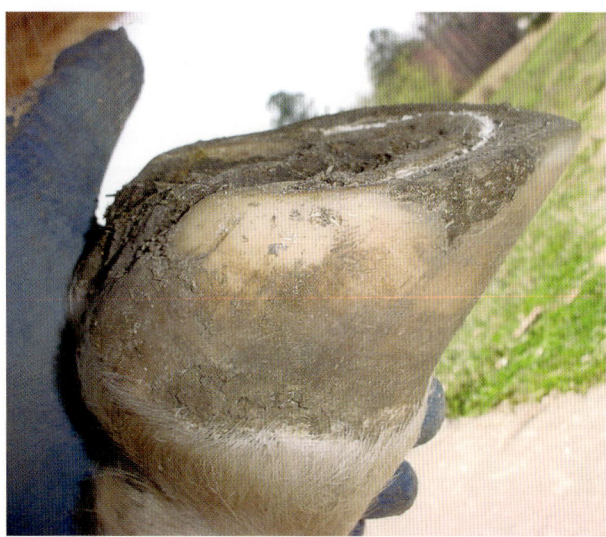

8.2 This tall, flat foot is the result of distal descent of the coffin bone. The front edge of this bone is very close to the ground, as shown by the white line that was lightly scraped onto the sole to highlight the bone's location.

Short Toes

You now understand some of the problems associated with long toes, so let's take a moment to talk about toes that are too short. Other than instances where a hoof-care provider takes off too much toe, or tips a barefoot horse onto his toes by leaving too much heel, this problem is actually quite rare and is usually associated with some kind of flexural deformity (a club foot, for example).

Even so, one of the main reasons people cite if you ask them why they choose to shoe their horses is the concern that the horse, if left unshod, would wear his toes down to nubs and get sore. While it may be true that their horse's toes would get shorter if allowed to wear naturally, that would probably be a good thing, in many cases. Why? Because many domestic horses are running around with toes that are too long, as we've mentioned earlier. The fact is, we have become so used to seeing excessively long toes that many of us believe this is normal. Therefore, when we see toes that are a healthy length, we get alarmed, thinking they are too short.

The ideal length for an individual horse's toes will vary depending on the size of the horse and his conformational angles, but as a general rule, domestic light horse breeds with healthy feet seldom have a toe length greater than 3½ inches measured from the center of the coronet to the ground (fig. 8.3). This is not as short as we see in some Mustangs' feet, but it is shorter than many domestic horses. Large Warmbloods may be a healthy length at closer to 4 inches, and heavy drafts a bit over that.

As for barefoot horses, if their feet are healthy and properly trimmed, they usually don't wear their toes or any other parts of the wall too short, as very few domestic horses work hard enough or get enough movement on abrasive terrain to wear their feet down excessively. Some also assert that a healthy, well-functioning hoof actually responds to the stimulation of work and abrasion by getting

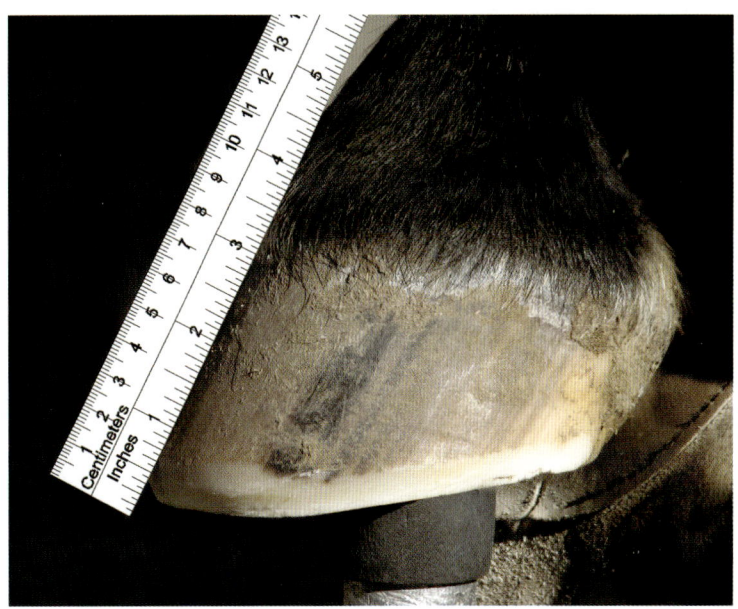

8.3 The toes on the healthiest feet in the light horse breeds generally measure no more than about 3½ inches. This 16-hand gelding's toe measures 3¼ inches.

stronger and growing faster, which makes it more than capable of keeping up with the demands of domestic use. Most barefoot horses actually require regular trimming, as their feet grow faster than they wear them down. It is true, though, that the toes of a well-maintained barefoot horse might look short to those used to seeing the too-long ones often assumed to be "normal."

If a barefoot horse is actually sore because he is wearing his feet down faster than they can grow, it may be that adjustments to trimming, diet, environment, or lifestyle could improve that, or some form of protection might indeed be in order. This does not necessarily mean that the horse needs shoes, as there are now many styles of hoof boots that can provide extra protection when needed (see *Going Barefoot,* p. 265).

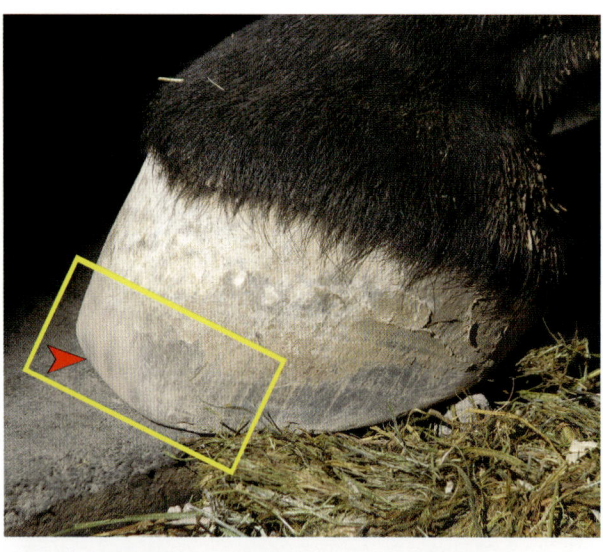

8.4 This hind foot belongs to a very old horse that has some arthritis in his hind end. As a result, he sometimes drags his toes, causing them to become dubbed. The area inside the yellow rectangle shows where the lower dorsal wall has been abraded away, leaving a square edge on the bottom of the toe (red arrow).

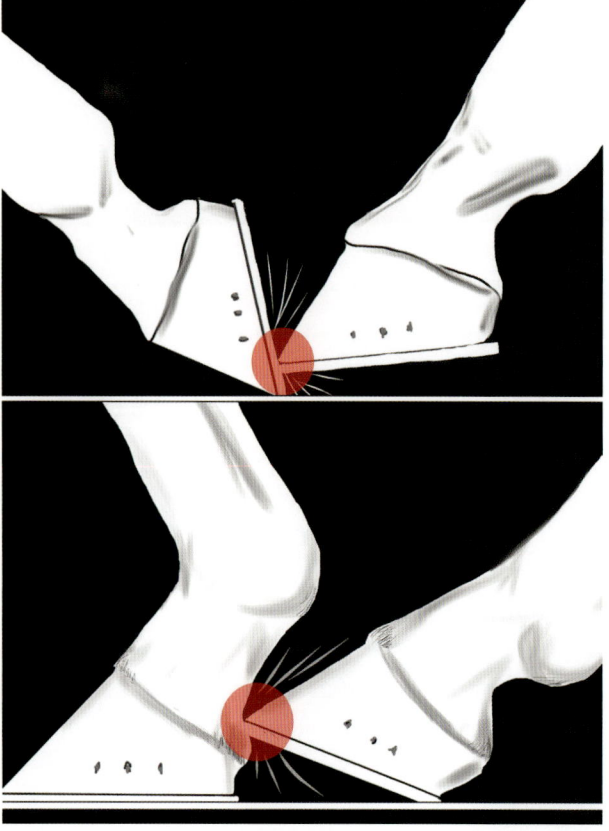

8.5 Both forging (upper) and over-reaching (lower) can injure the horse, so hoof-care providers will sometimes dub a horse's hind toes in an effort to prevent these forms of interference.

Dubbed Toes

There is another hoof shape that sometimes gets labeled as a short toe when it may not actually be one—the dubbed toe. When a toe is dubbed, the lower part of the dorsal wall has been abraded, giving the hoof a convex appearance (fig. 8.4). In addition, the bottom edge of the toe will often appear to be squared off, rather than rounded. With a dubbed toe, the toe may indeed be short, but a long toe can also be dubbed, and some dubbed toes look shorter than they actually are if measured from the coronet to the ground.

Toes can get dubbed in two ways: by a hoof-care provider, or because the horse wears them into that shape. A farrier or trimmer might dub a horse's toes for several reasons. When the hind feet get dubbed, it is often an effort to correct over-reaching, where the toe of the hind foot reaches up and makes contact with the front heel or limb. Similarly, it may be done in an attempt to prevent forging, which as we've mentioned is where the toe of the hind foot reaches forward and strikes the sole of the front foot (fig. 8.5). Either way, dubbing the hind toes is usually not the best solution.

On either hind or front feet, dubbing may be an attempt to help the walls grow out a flare, to make the toe fit a slightly setback shoe, or to "cheat" a dished toe into appearing straighter. Some people will dub the toes in an attempt to shorten them, though toes are more effectively shortened from the bottom, not by rasping the dorsal surface. In many instances, a farrier will run the rasp over the toe and lower dorsal wall for a few light strokes to simply finish the foot after the shoe is put on, creating a slightly dubbed profile.

What you, as the owner, should be aware of is that dubbing the toes, for whatever reason, is actually thinning the dorsal wall, and a thinner wall is a weaker wall. A light finishing stroke or two is not likely to make a significant difference, but take any real thickness off the wall and it is more likely to distort, crack, or chip, and is also more likely to tear around nail holes or lose a shoe. While dubbing may be called for in certain circumstances, it is probably done far more often than is beneficial, and sometimes causes more problems than it solves.

There are also instances where the horse dubs his own toes. This is more commonly seen in the hind feet, but it can happen in front as well. When a horse is dubbing a toe, something is causing him to either drag that toe when he moves, stand with that toe pointed into the ground, or both. The reason could be soreness due to an injury, or arthritis—particularly in the hocks or stifles. In some instances, horses drag their toes as a result of a neurological problem. Then again, some horses have nothing wrong with them at all, but drag their toes when they simply lack the motivation to move actively.

"Bullnosed" Toes

You will sometimes hear people referred to a dubbed toe as a "bullnosed" toe. However, a true bullnosed hoof is not the result of an abraded dorsal wall. Instead, it occurs when the dorsal wall takes on a convex shape, typically due to the coffin bone having a *negative palmar/plantar angle* inside the hoof (fig. 8.6). As we discussed earlier, a negative palmar/plantar angle means that the coffin bone is tilting up in the front and down in the back,

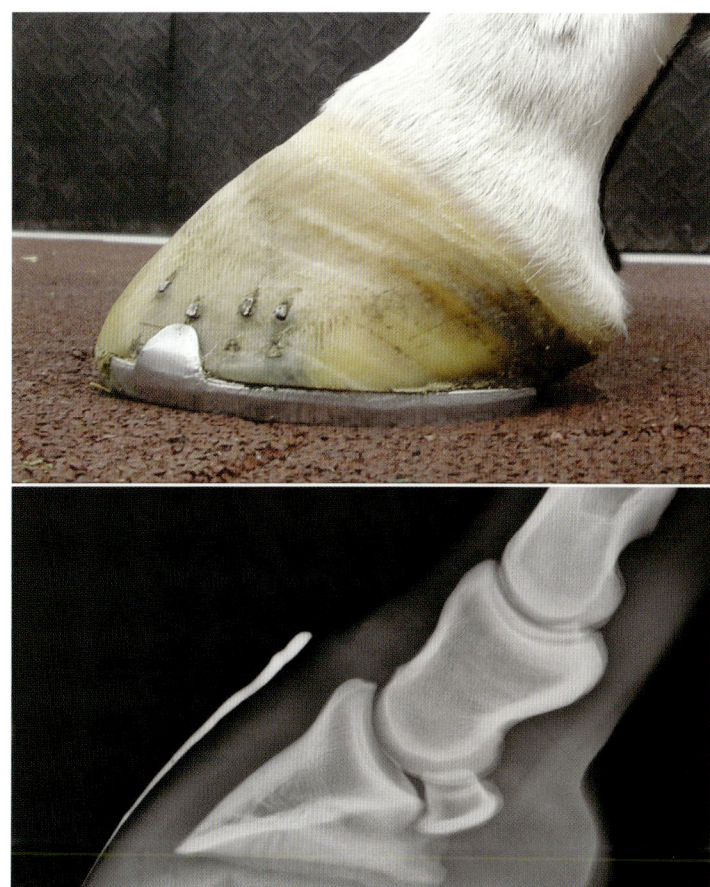

8.6 A negative palmar/plantar angle causes the tip of the coffin bone to lift up, which changes the shape of the hoof wall. Looking at this "bullnosed" hoof (above), it would be a safe bet that the angle of the coffin bone is negative, and the X-ray confirms it (below).

the opposite of what it should be (see the sidebar on p. 25 where *palmar angles* are discussed). This can cause remodeling of the dorsal wall due to the front of the coffin bone pressing up against the inside of the wall. What you end up with is a wall that bulges outward in the middle. This is different than the artificially thinned bottom portion of

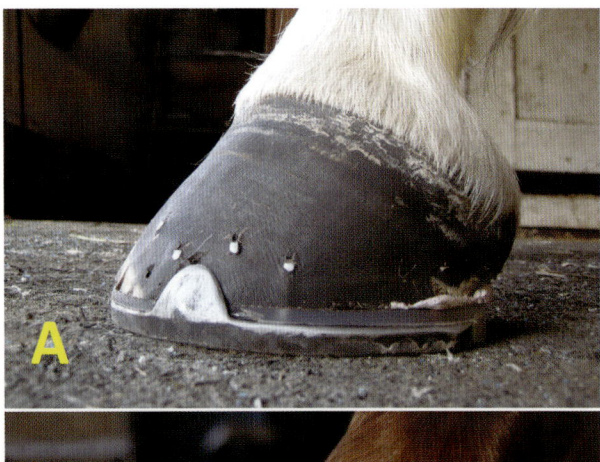

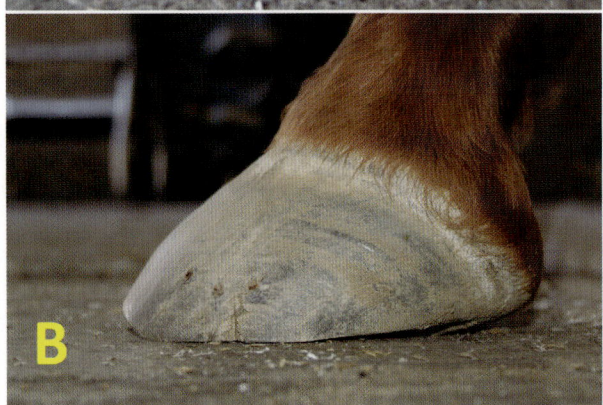

8.7 It can sometimes be hard to distinguish between a dubbed toe (above) and a bullnosed toe (below), but the heels can give you a good indication. The hind foot above has heels of reasonable height, which do not suggest a negative plantar angle. The hind foot below has crushed heels, which are strongly associated with negative palmar/plantar angles. Also note that the convex curve starts right at the hairline, whereas on foot above, the wall is straight for quite a way below the hairline.

the wall of a dubbed toe, but the profiles of both types of hooves look somewhat similar (fig. 8.7).

Bullnosed walls on the front feet are generally associated with heels that are too low, underrun, or collapsed, as it is the problems in the back of the foot that cause the negative palmar/plantar angle to occur. However, bullnosing seems to be more common on hind feet, where it can be a result of leaving the toes too long. It can also be a symptom of poor conformation, or may be associated with lower back/hock/stifle problems.

If you are trying to determine whether a horse has a dubbed toe or a bullnosed wall, check to see if the lower part of the wall is abraded or not, and take a good look at the structure of the heels. A foot with a healthy heel of reasonable height is not likely to be bullnosed.

Bottom Line: Toe length should typically be no longer than 3½ inches, unless the horse is larger than average.

Frog, Sole, and Bar Health

Frog Health

As we mentioned in the anatomy section, the frog is a critical player in overall hoof and limb health, with its tough but elastic tissues absorbing concussion and cushioning the structures inside the hoof. In order to accomplish this, the frog must be robust and healthy, and make contact with the ground at the back of the foot. You may also recall that the appearance of the frog can vary quite a bit depending on the environment the horse lives in. In moister environments, a healthy frog has a more "plump" appearance and a smoother surface. In extremely dry climates, the frog will not be as plump and is likely to have a rough, dry-looking exterior surface. This is an adaptation that allows the foot to function optimally in an environment that probably has hard, rocky ground.

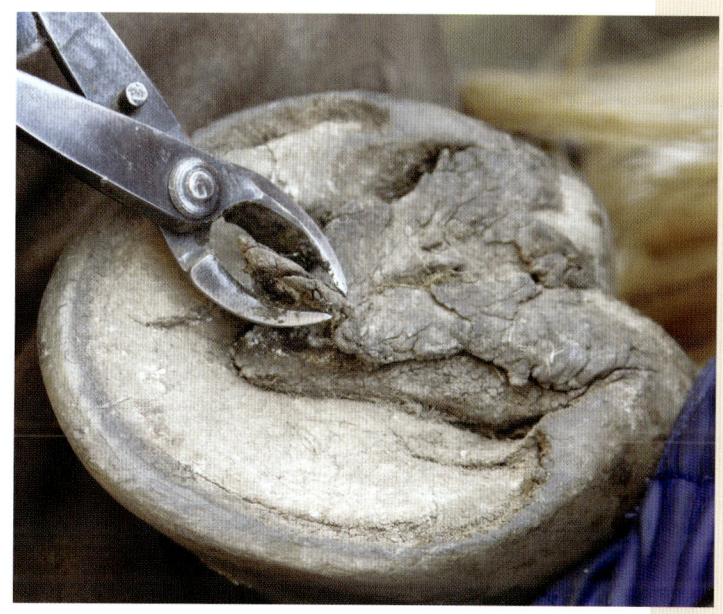

9.1 When the frog is naturally exfoliating, like this foot, it can form flaps and shreds that can trap muck underneath them, providing a perfect environment for bacteria and fungi. Loose bits are therefore best removed.

Exfoliating vs. Trimming

Regardless of climate, it is natural and normal for the frog to exfoliate excess material, and at certain times of the year, some horses will shed quite a bit of frog in a short period. When this happens, the frog may rid itself of excess material in the form of shreds, or it may peel off in layers. This is nothing to worry about, as the foot is just naturally making room for new frog to grow in. Still, it is a good idea to remove loose shreds and peeling pieces of dead frog so that they don't trap moisture and muck (fig. 9.1).

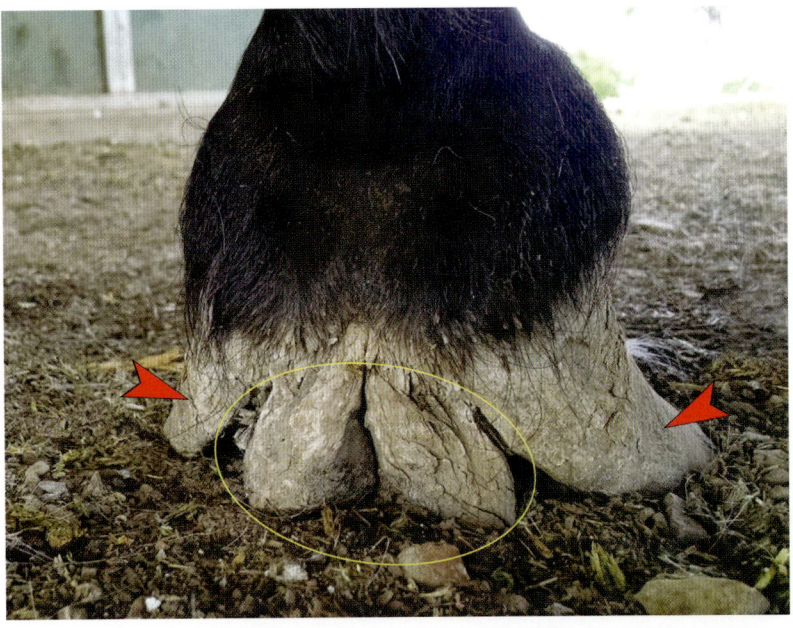

9.2 This massive frog (circled), photographed from the back of the foot, grew to these proportions as the foot's attempt to support itself while saddled with terribly overgrown, flared, weak walls (red arrows). When the walls were trimmed down, the frog had to be trimmed as well or it would have stuck out far past the walls.

Otherwise, removing frog material is generally a no-no, with a few exceptions. It is okay to remove the flaps that can form near the heel buttresses if they tend to trap crud. The same goes for very small amounts on the edges to keep the collateral grooves open, making them easier to clean in environments where that is necessary. Necrotic frog tissue, such as may be seen in some cases of thrush, should definitely be removed, and it is sometimes necessary to take material off a frog that is too tall in relation to the hoof wall or shoe (fig. 9.2).

However, some hoof-care providers will attempt to make the frog "neat and pretty" by cutting off significant swathes of perfectly healthy frog material, not realizing that they are seriously weakening the foot in the process, and possibly starting the horse down the long, dark road of foot pain. At the very least, removing live frog can make your horse sore and leave the foot vulnerable to bruising, as the outside of the frog is similar to the calluses a person forms by walking around barefoot. Think about what it would do to that person if you cut off those calluses (ouch!), and you'll get an idea of what it is like for a horse to have his frogs thinned. Far too many horses are thought to "need" shoes or hoof boots due to tenderfootedness, when all they really need is for their frogs (and sometimes soles) not to be continually carved away. Leave the healthy frog material alone, and such horses often become "miraculously" sound (fig .9.3).

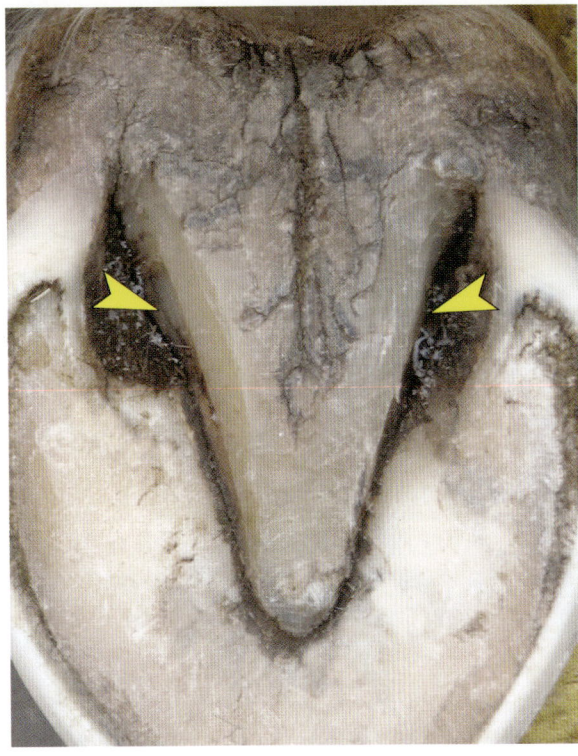

9.3 Trimming the frog should be done as minimally as possible. The hoof-care provider caring for this foot has removed only the merest amount to help the collateral grooves (yellow arrows) stay open so that they are easy to clean.

Thrush

Thrush is an infection of the frog that can also invade the collateral grooves, and it is particularly likely to take up residence in the central sulcus (see p. 20). The main culprit behind thrush is the *Fusobacterium necrophorum* bacteria, though other bacteria may assist in the disease process. Thrush is so common that many people think it is "no big deal," but left untreated, it can penetrate deep into the dermal layer of the foot where it can cause serious pain, lameness, and sometimes permanent damage to the frog corium and other internal structures. One clinician at a major university veterinary hospital believes that thrush is a factor in a majority of the lameness cases he sees.

In obvious cases of thrush, you will notice a foul, rotting smell, may see a blackish, greasy discharge in the affected areas, and there will be patches of black or missing frog tissue (fig. 9.4). The frog and central sulcus often become tender and will sometimes bleed if scraped or prodded, and the central sulcus is likely to be deeper than normal. Horses with thrush might be reluctant to have their feet cleaned or handled, may stand and lean their weight slightly forward to relieve the pressure on their tender frogs, and may be sensitive to walking on uneven surfaces such as gravel.

However, thrush often presents in a way that is not so obvious, especially in the early stages, as

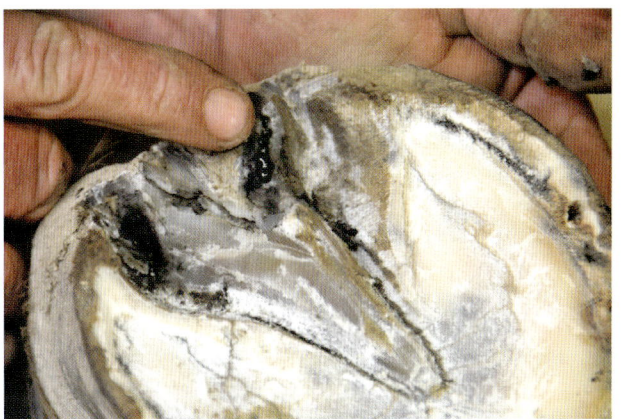

9.4 The farrier has cleaned up the ragged superficial layer of this frog with his hoof knife, revealing deep pockets of thrush. The greasy, blackish discharge is a classic sign of the infection, but one that is not always present.

there may be no discharge, obvious damage, or horrific odor. Quite often, the only clue that a thrush infection is present is a central sulcus that looks a bit deeper than it should be, and maybe has a dark or "punky" appearance (fig. 9.5). Often, you can discover how unhealthily deep that crevice actually is by putting the tip of a hoof pick in there and

9.5 The two top images are examples of healthy central sulci, the left from a moist environment, and the right from a dry one. The two below both have thrush infections. The left one has the moist, somewhat gooey appearance we generally associate with thrush. The right one, from a dry climate, doesn't look like much of a problem, but a hoof pick inserted into the sulcus showed that the infection was much deeper than it appeared, which is often the case.

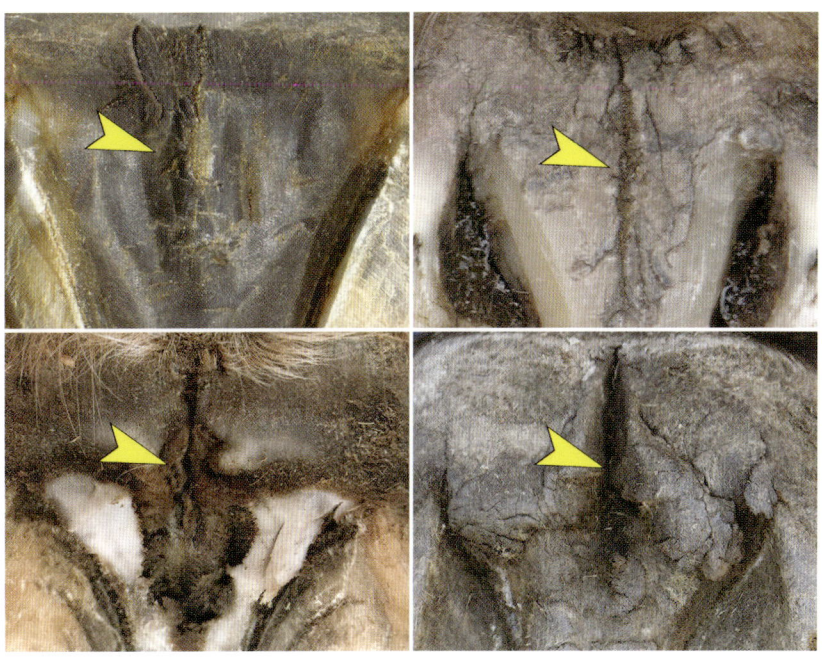

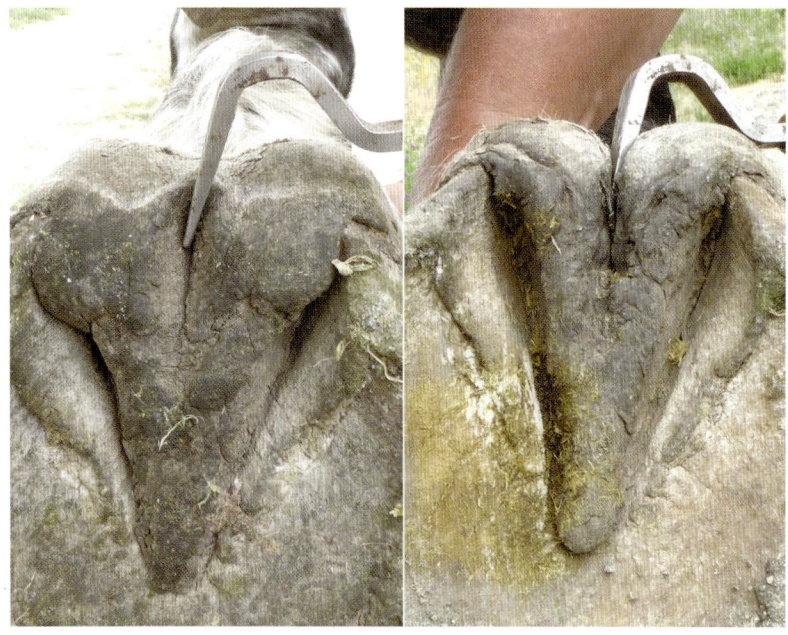

9.6 The shallow, healthy central sulcus on the left provides no port of entry for the tip of a hoof pick, but the pick sinks deeply into the thrush-infected sulcus of the frog on the right.

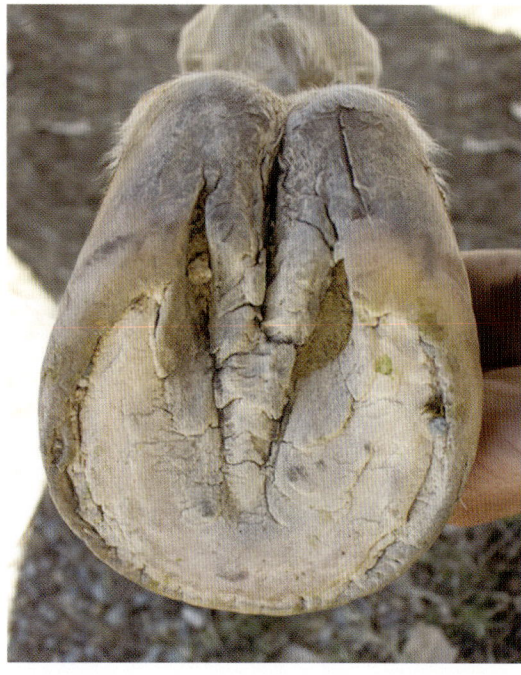

9.7 This dry, hard frog does not have the typical moist, rotting appearance we envision when we think of thrush, but the very deep central sulcus shows that it is there, nonetheless. Contracted (unhealthily narrow) feet like this one are highly vulnerable to thrush infections.

watching it disappear, something you can't do in the shallow sulcus of a healthy frog (fig. 9.6). If you try this, keep in mind that you are poking an area that might be quite sore, so tread carefully. If you wiggle the hoof pick in such a frog crevice and your horse flinches, there is definitely a problem brewing.

It is especially easy to miss thrush in dry climates or at low-moisture times of year, as we tend to look at a dry, hard frog and not imagine that it could have a thrush infection (fig. 9.7). The conventional wisdom is that thrush is a problem brought on by moisture in the environment, but it is important to know that it can affect horses in dry climates as well by getting up into small cracks that lead to the moist, anaerobic environment just below the leathery exterior of the frog, and by hiding deep within the central sulcus.

Whether they live in a wet or dry environment, some horses seem prone to thrush infections, and some never get them. While there are many factors that influence this, the bottom line is that a healthy, correctly functioning hoof that gets plenty of movement in a clean environment is likely to remain thrush free, even if that environment is very wet for long periods of time. Let's take a closer look at that statement, as it contains all the various factors that make a horse more or less vulnerable to thrush:

• A *healthy hoof* means one that is not suffering from contraction, imbalance, heel pain, metabolic distress, mineral deficiencies, excessive carbohydrates in the diet, or any other issues that can compromise the frog, leaving it more prone to infection.

• A *correctly functioning* hoof, in this context, means that the foot is able to flex as nature intended, which allows the sole to pop out packed in material that is likely to harbor harmful bacteria. Anything that limits hoof flexibility or encourages the foot to trap and hold muck makes it more difficult for the foot to self-clean (fig. 9.8).

• A *hoof that gets plenty of movement* is much more likely to pop out built-up muck, and it is also going to have better circulation and be more robust over-all, making it more resistant to disease.

• A *clean environment* is one in which the horse is not forced to continually walk or stand in manure and urine. Continual exposure to these substances is damaging to the hoof, and especially to the tissues of the frog, where it creates fissures that give bacteria easy entry. And, to make matters worse, areas soiled with manure and/or urine are a veritable stew of thrush-causing organisms.

If you think about all of these factors, it becomes clear that keeping thrush at bay requires multiple considerations. First, you want to do everything possible to ensure that your horse's feet are healthy and functioning well. Contracted feet, in particular, are highly vulnerable to thrush. The frogs on such feet are unhealthy to start with, plus the contraction makes the collateral grooves narrow, which traps muck, making self-cleaning less effective. In addition, the central sulcus on a contracted foot may form a tight, deep cleft that is difficult to clean, providing a perfect environment for thrush bacteria. This is one of the many reasons why it is so important to prevent contraction, and to work diligently to try to get rid of it when it is present.

Next, you want to make sure your horse gets plenty of movement. If at all feasible, give your

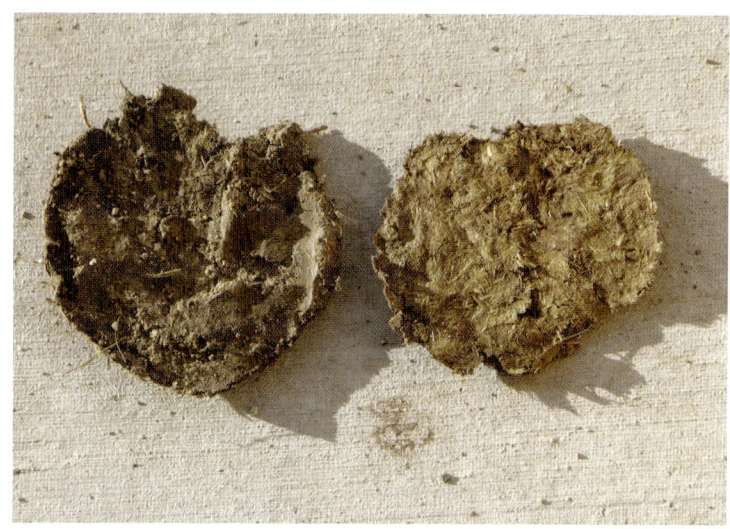

9.8 These "pads" of dirt are the result of "self-cleaning" in the feet of a couple of barefoot horses. They have some mucky areas in their paddock, but enough room to run around, which causes their feet to flex and push out the dirt.

horse access to turnout 24/7, in as large an area as you can arrange. And, whatever your horse's living arrangements are, keep the area as free of manure and urine as possible. Lastly, if your horse does tend to pick up muck in his feet, clean them out thoroughly at least once a day. Remember that the thrush bacteria are anaerobic, so removing muck and getting air up into the collateral grooves and central sulcus will discourage the growth of these organisms.

Unfortunately, the realities of modern horse-keeping mean that hoof health, housing, and management practices aren't always ideal, and even when they appear to be, some horses still get thrush. When your horse has thrush, treatment should be implemented as soon as possible. If the infection hasn't penetrated deep into the tissues, treatment is fairly straightforward. Any shreds or

Diet and Thrush—A Kind of "Hoof and Mouth" Disease?

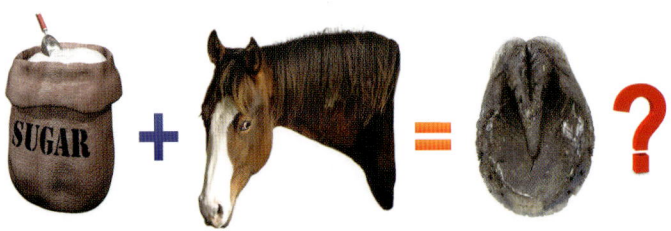

9.9 Too much sugar in a horse's diet can be a contributing factor in thrush infections.

We are learning more all the time about how a horse's diet can affect his feet, but many people still don't know that diet can be a major contributing factor in many cases of thrush. This is particularly true when the infection seems to linger endlessly or continually recur, despite the owner's best efforts to eliminate the problem. Diets high in sugar and starch are a major factor, but unbalanced mineral uptake can also be a problem. Either of these dietary issues can make treating thrush a truly uphill battle in some susceptible horses.

If thrush is a continual problem for your horse, it may be worth looking at your feeding program, and perhaps try cutting down on the carbohydrates to see if that helps. Give it at least a few months, as it takes the body some time to heal from the effects of a carb-heavy or imbalanced diet. People are often pleasantly surprised and greatly relieved to find that something as simple as cutting out grain and getting their horse on a low-carb hay got rid of the chronic thrush they battled for so long.

flaps of dead material should be trimmed away, and then an appropriate topical product can be applied. If the central sulcus has become deep, it may be beneficial to use a syringe to help the medication reach the affected tissues. The medication must come in contact with the affected tissue or it is not going to work. Most treatments need to be repeated daily until the infection clears.

There are many commercial products available for the treatment of thrush, as well as plenty of homemade preparations, some of which can be

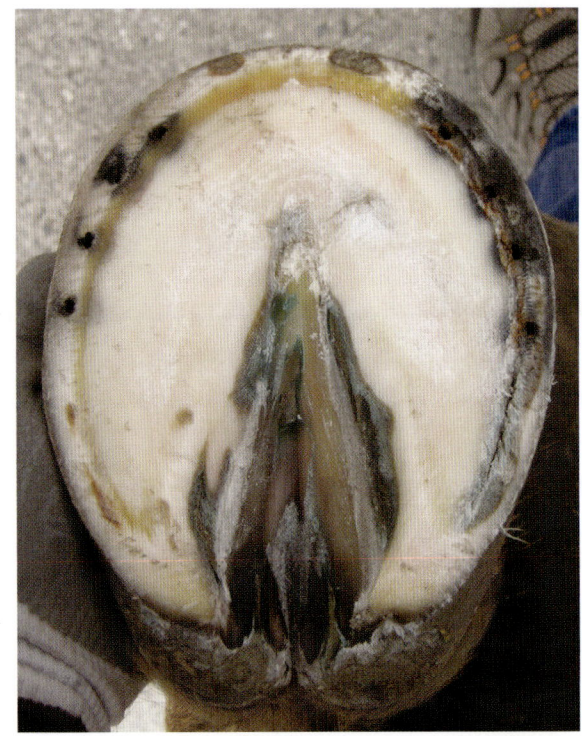

9.10 This horse had a very longstanding thrush infection that had eaten deep into the tissues. This is what the foot looked like once all the necrotic material was cut away by a skilled farrier. You can see how easy it would be to damage the corium (blood vessel rich layer of tissue) under the frog if this was done incorrectly.

quite effective. Unfortunately, what works on one horse in one environment might not have the same effect on another horse in a different environment. It seems that all thrush remedies work some of the time, but there probably isn't one that is going to work all of the time. If it is working, improvement could be evident within a few days or it could take weeks, depending on the severity of the case, how effective the medication is, and how it is being applied. If a thrush infection is not responding to a particular treatment in 4–6 weeks, it may be advisable to change to a different remedy.

When you are dealing with an infection that has gotten deep into the tissues, consult with your hoof-care professional or vet to get their advice on how best to treat the problem. Areas of dead tissue may need to be carved away to allow air and medication to get in, a process that requires a knowledgeable hand (fig. 9.10). Keeping areas of deep infection open and clean can be a challenge but one you must stay on top of if your horse is to recover.

It is important to understand that in most cases, there are underlying factors that predispose a horse to getting thrush, and if those factors are not addressed, the infection is likely to linger or recur. Many people find themselves fighting thrush repeatedly, not realizing that whatever is setting their horse up for thrush is still going on. For this reason, it can be helpful to think of thrush as a symptom of another problem, rather than as the main problem itself.

9.11 This foot has very nice concavity that helps it to function well in both arena work and on rugged trails.

Sole Health: Through Thick and Thin

The sole of the horse's foot is a critically important structure, but one that is often misunderstood or even abused—albeit unknowingly. As the largest part of the hoof's interface with the ground, the sole deals with tremendous forces, both from within and from the ground. To function well, the sole has to be thick and strong to protect the coffin bone from damage, well-callused so that it can resist abrasion, yet flexible enough to allow the foot to expand and contract for good circulation and shock absorption.

Concavity

Part of how it achieves all these things at the same time is through the natural concavity of the sole (fig. 9.11). Nature designed the bottom of the equine

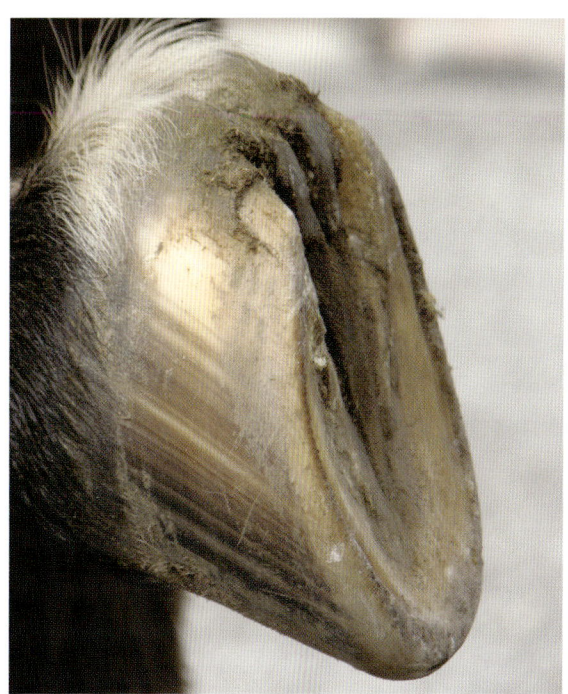

foot to be higher in the center than it is around the rim and the back, creating a cupped surface. Having that concavity protects the foot by lifting the coffin bone higher away from potentially damaging contact with rocks and such, and it also enhances the foot's ability to flex, all while providing excellent traction. However, horses vary in how much concavity their feet have, for a number of reasons.

To start with, as we mentioned in the anatomy section, the concavity of the live sole on a healthy foot generally reflects the shape of the vault on the bottom of the coffin bone, with the arc of that vault being related to the horse's size (see p. 24). Surprisingly, healthy coffin bones generally have about the same distance from the plane of the solar margin to the highest point of the arc on the solar surface, regardless of the size of the horse—but the *width* of that arc changes in relation to size. The result is that a larger coffin bone (and foot) will typically look less concave, even though the height of the arc is actually the same (fig. 9.12).

Concavity can also be affected by hoof-health issues, particularly anything that causes thinning of the sole, distal descent, or both, as the two quite often occur together. When the coffin bone moves down in relation to the hoof capsule, the bone puts

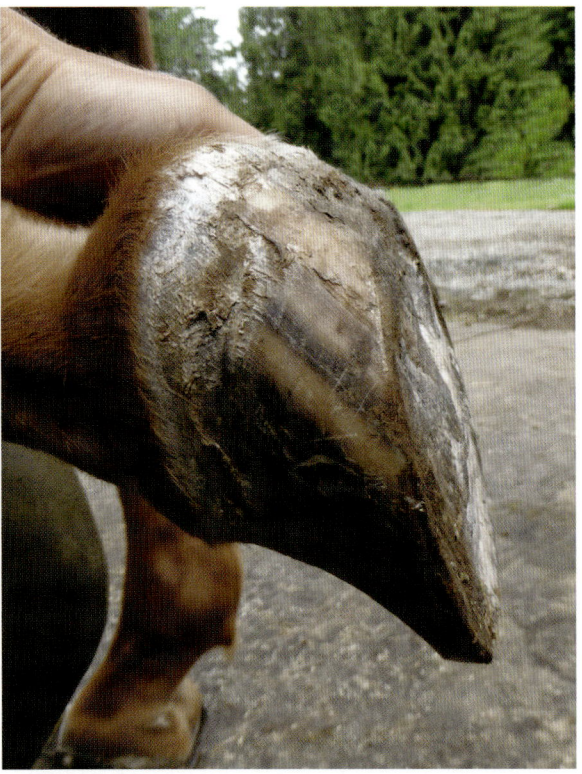

9.13 The bulging sole on this laminitic foot indicates that the coffin bone is pushing down on the sole from within.

pressure on the sole from within, causing the sole to lose concavity, as well as squeezing the solar corium, which in turn can cause the sole to become thinner. Conversely, a thin sole can't provide adequate support from below, which can lead to distal descent—one of the many chicken-and-egg scenarios in the hoof world. Whichever way it starts, a loss of concavity from distal descent can sometimes get so bad that the sole may actually bulge outward, which is called a *prolapsed sole*. This is a dire situation, as it means the coffin bone is very close to the surface and may break through (fig. 9.13).

9.12 These two hoof representations have the same measurement from the ground (blue line) to the highest part of the foot's arc. However, the large foot on the right looks flatter because the width of its arc is greater.

Thin Soles

Fortunately, most horses will never experience the agony of their bones coming through the bottom of their feet, but it is a sad fact that many domestic horses are walking around on soles that are too thin to provide all of the comfort, support, and protection they need. Such horses are tender walking on rough or hard ground, they may be prone to bruising or abscessing, and their feet will have little to no concavity. Horse owners are often told that "this is just the way the horse is" and that the only way to help the horse is by shielding the bottom of the foot with shoes (often with pads added), or with hoof boots if the horse is barefoot.

However, while putting something between the foot and the ground might make the horse less ouchy, it may not be addressing what is causing the ouchiness to occur. To make matters worse, some hoof wear meant to offer protection may actually work against the development of a healthy sole in the long run if it causes peripheral loading.

This may all sound pretty grim, but it is important

Dr. Ric Redden on
Why Sole Depth Matters

"Sole depth is defined as the vertical distance between the palmar/plantar margin of P3 and the outer surface of the sole (fig. 9.14). It is routinely measured at the distal tip, or apex, of P3. A normal, healthy foot has a sole depth of at least 15 millimeters. Based on venographic (radiography of the vein) studies in a wide variety of horses, I consider a sole depth of less than 15 millimeters to be clinically significant. In a normal foot, the papillae (see p. 38) of the solar corium appear to need a space of at least 10 millimeters between the palmar/plantar surface of P3 and the cornified (hardened through the process of keratinization) layer of the sole for adequate vascular filling; and at least 5 millimeters of cornified sole is required to protect the solar corium. Venograms in horses with a sole depth of less than 15 millimeters show solar papillae that are bent, compressed, or even absent. This distortion or compression surely inhibits sole growth, creating a vicious cycle of thin, tender soles."

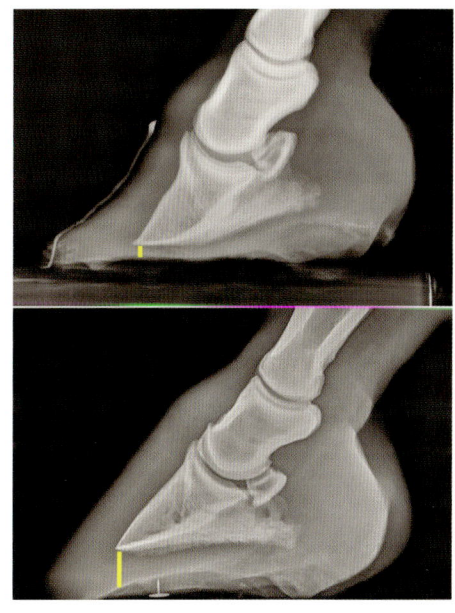

9.14 On an X-ray, you can measure from the bottom of the tip of the coffin bone (the palmar/plantar margin of P3) to the bottom of the sole to get the sole depth. The laminitic foot in the upper X-ray has only 4–5 millimeters of sole, whereas the healthy foot in the lower one has about 16 millimeters.

to know that in many instances, a thin-soled horse can grow a healthier, thicker sole if changes are made to correct the underlying issues. The first step in making those changes is to understand why the horse's soles got thin in the first place. The most common reasons why this happens include:

• *Compromised blood flow:* Since the sole gets its nutrients from the blood that flows through the solar corium, anything that negatively affects the solar corium can affect the growth of the sole. A compressed or damaged corium means less blood flow, resulting in slower production and possibly poorer quality sole material, which may abrade away faster than new material is produced. Laminitis, peripheral loading, and hoof imbalance are the most frequently encountered problems that negatively affect the solar corium in the foot.

• *Invasive trimming:* While it should be obvious that cutting away live sole material makes the sole thinner and weaker, far too many hoof-care providers do it anyway. Farriers sometimes carve away sole material to make the sole blend with a wall they have taken down, instead of using the callused sole plane as a guide for trimming the wall. In other instances, the provider removes sole in a misguided attempt to create more concavity in the foot, a practice that is counterproductive and downright dangerous (see *Concavity*, p. 119). Trimming the sole near the toes or heels is also done at times with the aim of shortening a hoof capsule that is too long or doesn't have the angles the provider thinks they should have. When the sole is already thin, as is often the case, this can be a disaster.

• *Dorsopalmar/plantar imbalance:* Horses with long-toe/low-heel syndrome often suffer from thin soles. This may be due to changes inside the foot affecting the health of the solar corium, or it may be that when the toe migrates forward, it pulls the sole with it, so you end up with the same amount of sole stretched out over a larger area. However it happens, long toes usually mean thin soles.

• *Flaring:* A flared-out hoof wall is a sign that the wall is no longer well connected to the coffin bone. When this happens, the coffin bone sags in the hoof capsule a bit, causing the sole to flatten out.

• *Lack of movement:* The hoof needs movement in order to develop and function properly. A horse that is not moving is at an increased risk for developing all sorts of hoof problems, including thin soles. Moving incorrectly—meaning landing toe first—will increase these risks as well.

• *Coffin bone damage:* Horses with damage to the coffin bone often have a hard time growing thick sole, quite possibly related to compromised blood flow. If the coffin bone has been exposed to enough trauma that it has sustained damage, it is very likely that the solar corium has also been affected. When both the coffin bone and the corium have been damaged, the prognosis for the development of a healthy, robust sole may be guarded.

• *Genetics:* Just as some people don't have the thickest or strongest fingernails, some horses aren't genetically designed to have the thickest soles. Often, these horses have fine coats, refined cannon bones, and a thinner hoof wall in addition to soles that aren't terribly stout. Still, while their genes may be working against them to some degree, there is

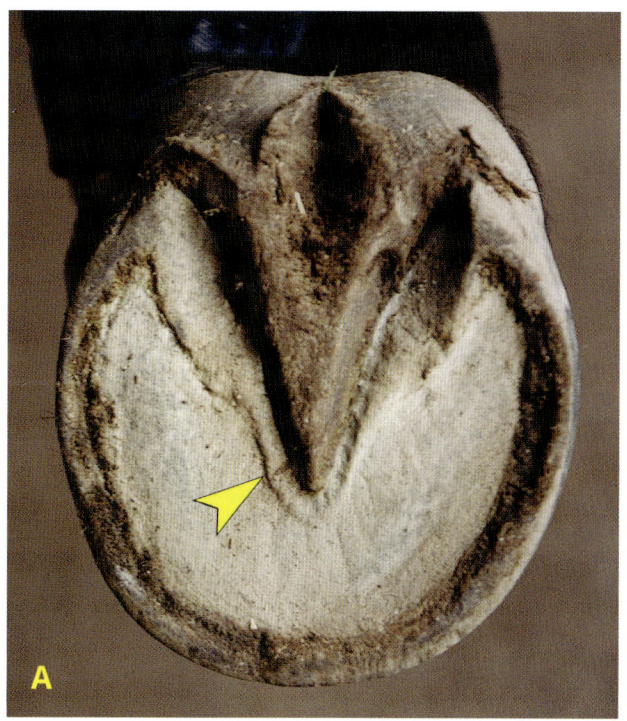

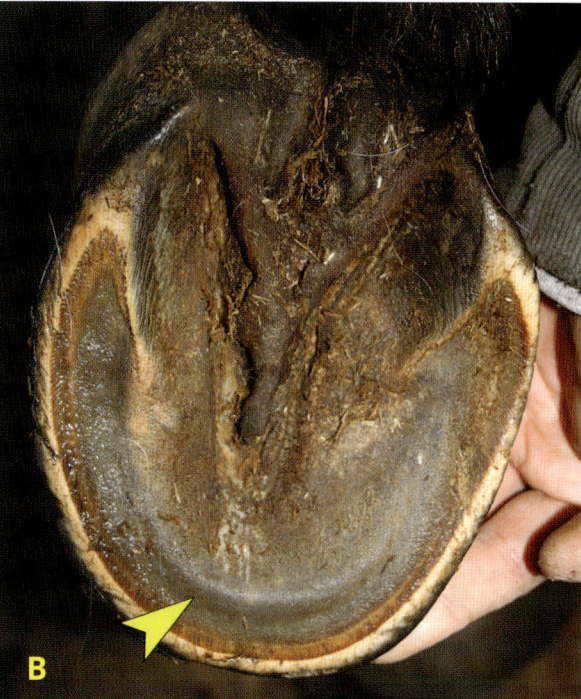

9.15 A & B While many hoof-care professionals would be tempted to pare away the ridge of sole this foot has grown all the way around the frog, the fact that it is there may mean that the foot needs it for support and protection of the coffin bone (A). A ridge of sole around the toe is often seen in a recovering thin sole (B). There can be other reasons for a ridge, but if the sole has been thin due to excessively long toes, it may make a ridge like this one as the toe migrates back and the foot snaps back together. Once the sole has achieved good thickness, the ridge typically disappears.

a lot that can be done to help such horses achieve their maximum potential sole thickness.

Building Better Soles

If a horse's soles have become thin for whatever reason, the length of time it takes for that sole to recover will vary. Under optimal conditions, the sole can regain a significant amount of thickness in as little as a few months. If the underlying causative factors are still at work, or existing damage is severe, recovery can be slow or simply impossible.

A sole that is attempting to regenerate can go through some interesting interim phases where it puts out lumps, bumps, or ridges that seem like they shouldn't be there (figs. 9.15 A & B). In many cases, it appears that such protuberances are the

hoof's attempt to provide extra protection and support where it needs it, and as such, they should not be trimmed away. If they are removed but reappear quickly, it is a safe bet that the foot requires extra support in that area. Usually, such lumpy bits will gradually smooth out and disappear on their own as the sole achieves full thickness.

As for what you can do to actively promote sole growth, a multi-pronged approach is most likely to produce good results. First, you need to look at the horse's environment, and how much movement the horse is getting in that environment. Moving around on firm (not hard) terrain improves overall hoof health and stimulates both wall and sole growth, and thus it can make a huge difference in sole health. Riding, longeing, and hand-walking can

Pete Ramey on
"Excess" Bars and Sole

"I trained Alex Sperandeo to trim some years ago and he took off on his own, constantly maintaining hundreds of horses. Although I was initially his instructor, Alex has ended up teaching me plenty as well, especially when it comes to reconsidering the need to shave down 'excess' bars and sole. This case is from his files.

"A Warmblood had built a tremendous ridge of sole around the frog (fig. 9.16). The material was attempting to travel to the previously thinned sole under P3. Alex trimmed this hoof with a Mustang roll (beveling and rounding of the edges) on the walls, but the bottom of the foot was left alone.

"Neither the bars nor the sole were ever trimmed, but when the hoof achieved adequate sole thickness at the toe, the 'excess' formation of sole from the bars stopped on its own. This horse stayed in dressage competition throughout this process, never missing a beat.

"For those of you who might think you need to carve down a sole ridge like this horse had, you need to forget everything you 'know' and look at the left photo in figure 9.16 with a fresh perspective. Can you see that 'excess material' as a repair attempt? This foot had no lamellar integrity and very little sole. Can you see that the horse was trying to support himself and push much-needed protection forward to pad P3? This foot was trying to 'start over,' and once the man-made impediments to its progress were removed, it was able to do just that, with minimal interference.

"While there are times when you do need to trim away excess growth, a basic guideline I'm starting to embrace is this: If more than ¼ inch of any part of the foot 'needs' to be removed at a four-week maintenance trim, that spot was likely over-trimmed at the last visit—not by any *expert's* standard, but by the *horse's* standard, in his given terrain, and given the current health of the internal structures. The horse will work overtime to replace needed material when it is removed. This is a strong statement, I know, but I'm learning to trust it more every day.

"How do you apply this? *Not* by just leaving all of the excess, but by always leaving anything that excessively pops back ⅛ inch longer than you took it down at the last trim. You'll be amazed as you watch the excess growth immediately slow down, and you'll see the hooves start to move toward self-maintenance."

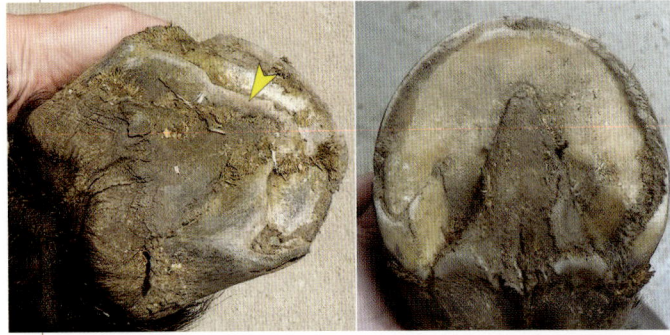

9.16 Sole ridge, before and after. The photo on the left was taken just after pulling the horse's shoes, before trimming. The right picture is the same foot four months later, post trim.

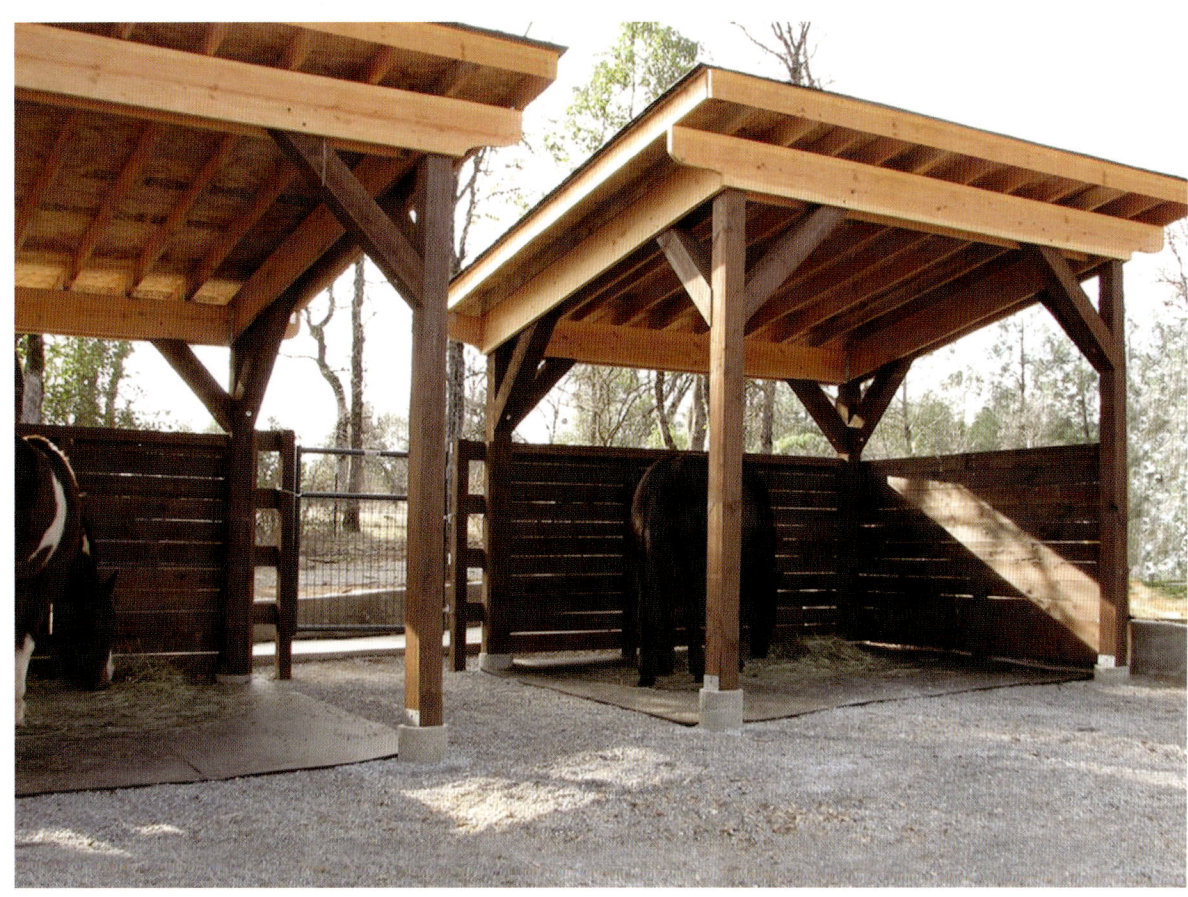

9.17 Adding pea gravel around shelters and other high-use areas can stimulate the foot and promote better hoof development.

all help, but it is best if the horse can live in a place that affords 24/7 turnout in a large area with at least some firm footing. If your horse's environment is too soft to provide the pressure and release that encourages good hoof growth, adding some areas of pea gravel to vary the footing can be very beneficial. Placing the gravel in high-use areas is often particularly helpful (fig. 9.17). One caution: when the horse's soles are so thin that movement is uncomfortable, forcing the horse to move can be counterproductive until he has recuperated further.

Diet can also work for or against your horse's soles. Proper nutrition (see *Feeding the Foot,* p. 238) provides the solar corium with the nutrients the horse needs to produce good quality sole. When a horse has dietary deficiencies, the sole will not grow as well as it should. Likewise, if a horse is consuming an inappropriate amount of certain feeds or nutrients—a much more common situation—it becomes harder to grow a healthy sole and wall.

An equally important component of growing a healthy sole is good hoof care. Reaching optimal sole thickness just won't happen when a horse has peripherally loaded or unbalanced feet that cannot function properly, so any such issues must be addressed before you can expect improvement in the sole. Hoof-care providers also often make the mistake of paring the sole when they shouldn't, not realizing that they are harming the horse through their actions. Very often, the best possible thing your hoof-care provider can do for the sole is simply *leave it alone*. Many of our domestic horses desperately need every hair's breadth of sole they can manage to grow, and taking off even a little will often perpetuate the very problems you are trying to solve.

Perhaps nowhere is inappropriate trimming more of a problem than it is in relation to concavity. While most hoof-care providers understand that concavity is important for a foot to function well, some don't understand that you simply cannot create concavity on a thin, flat sole by carving away

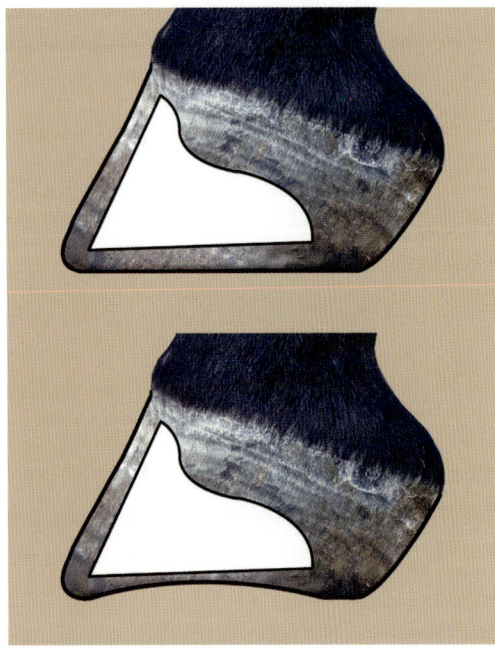

9.18 If you attempt to create concavity in a flat foot (above) by carving into the sole, you will only succeed in thinning the sole and bringing the coffin bone closer to the solar surface (below).

live sole horn. Any attempt to do so only makes the sole thinner and encourages it to flatten even more, possibly damaging the nerves and the blood supply in the solar corium and very likely making the horse sore (fig. 9.18). Tragically, many cases where the coffin bone does end up penetrating the sole are due, at least in part, to the sole having been excessively thinned by the knife of some well-meaning hoof-care provider.

The correct and only way to increase the concavity of the sole is to encourage the foot to build an adequately thick sole and create a strong wall attachment, both of which work together to "lift" the coffin bone within the hoof capsule, creating more concavity. Once a person understands that a truly flat sole (not a build-up of exfoliating sole) or a flat area on a sole equates with a lack of adequate sole thickness, it becomes clear that trying to improve concavity by carving into those already thin areas is a serious mistake.

Retained Sole: Should It Stay or Should It Go?

Sometimes, a sole that isn't actually flat can look that way if it gets filled in with retained exfoliating material, often called *dead* or *false sole*. As you learned in the anatomy section, the live sole of a healthy hoof will have a fairly uniform thickness of about ½ inch in most domestic horses, possibly as much as ¾ inch in a really fabulous foot. Once it achieves the maximum thickness of which it is capable, the outermost cells die and shed off, making room for the new cells that are continually being produced. If, however, the dead cells pack together instead of falling off or abrading away, they can form a substantial layer that will make the sole

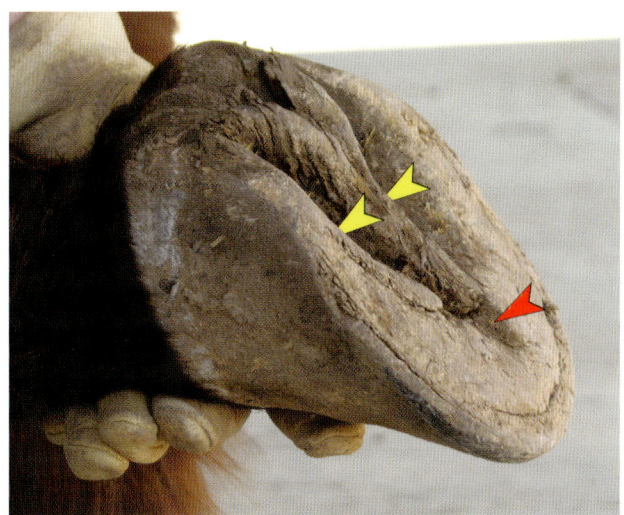

9.19 The unusually deep collateral grooves (yellow arrows) extending into a deep depression in front (red arrow) of the frog show us that this apparently flat foot is actually just filled in with exfoliating sole material.

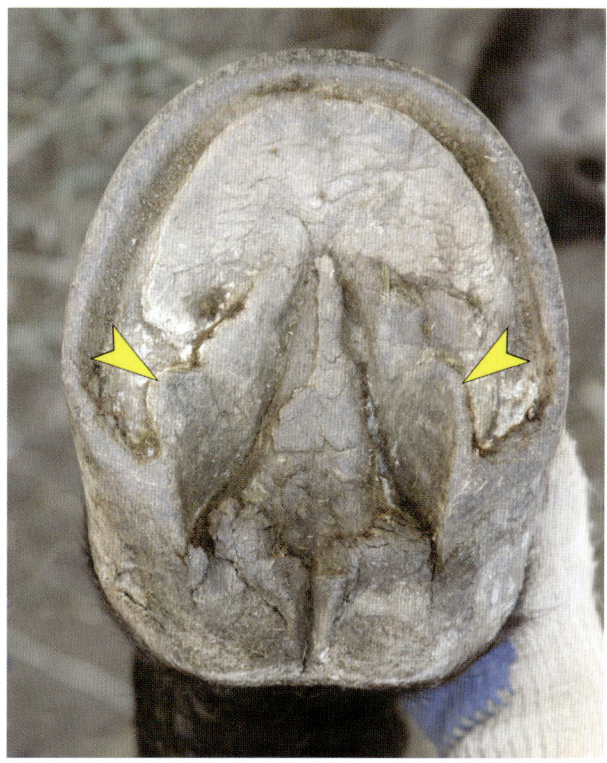

9.20 This foot is starting to lose its accumulation of retained-sole material. The chalky look and missing pieces are quite typical, and the peeling frog is also perfectly normal. The bars (yellow arrows) are long now that the sole is starting to chunk away from them, so if they didn't soon wear away on their own they would need to be trimmed.

appear thicker and likely flatter than it really is (fig. 9.19). In such cases, the texture of the sole will often appear chalky or cracked, there may be pieces that have flaked away, and the collateral grooves may be abnormally deep and appear to extend around the tip of the frog. All of these are clues that what you are looking at is retained sole (fig. 9.20).

Horses that live in dry areas are much more likely to retain exfoliating sole because the material is quite porous and will tend to absorb water, become very soft, and slough off in a wet environment. Horses that don't get much movement are also more likely to build up dead sole than those that are moving miles every day, as movement increases abrasion, and flexion of the hoof can encourage the dead sole to pop off. That said, even wild Mustangs that get plenty of movement on very abrasive terrain sometimes retain dead sole in the

dry seasons. This may be an adaptive mechanism that acts as a natural "hoof pad," providing extra protection for their feet when the ground is at its hardest.

When exfoliating material does build up on a domestic horse, deciding whether to leave it on the foot or remove it can be a real conundrum. In most cases, letting the retained sole remain in place is perfectly fine and possibly even desirable, as it may give your horse the same kind of extra protection that appears to benefit the arid land Mustangs. Indeed, many domestic horses seem to "want" their retained sole during dry times of year, and they travel much more comfortably over rough terrain if you leave it alone. Though every case is individual,

Hands-On Activity:
Measuring Sole Thickness

Sole thickness is one of those things that is hard to determine just by looking, especially if you don't know what to look for. Radiographs are the only way to get a 100% accurate measurement of sole thickness, but we do have several ways to get a good idea of where a horse is on the sole-thickness spectrum.

The first indicator is function. If your horse can move freely and easily over hard terrain and surfaces like gravel, chances are good that his soles are at least adequately thick. If your horse flinches, stumbles, or slows down on such terrain and veers for softer

ground whenever possible, he is telling you that his soles are too thin for comfort or that there is inflammation present in his feet. Try walking your horse over a patch of gravel and note if there are any changes in his gait.

The second is feel: if you take your thumb and press into the sole using 5–7 pounds of pressure (you can test how much pressure this is by pressing down on your bathroom scale with your thumb), a thin sole will have some give or flex to it, while a thick sole is not going to flex under such light pressure.

Of course, retained sole can skew matters quite a bit. As you just learned, retained exfoliating material can mask the concavity of the sole, making the bottom of the foot appear flatter than it actually is. If there is too much retained material, it has the potential to create problems and may have to be removed. But you also learned that removing sole material from a truly flat foot can seriously harm the horse. Before taking action, you need to be able to tell the difference between a filled-in foot that can be safely pared down, and a thin-soled one that shouldn't be touched.

Fortunately, barefoot specialist Pete Ramey has discovered that you can use the depth of the collateral grooves to reliably gauge the thickness of the sole, allowing you to make sound decisions about whether or not it is safe to trim it. Says Ramey, "Nature gave us a trustworthy guide in the collateral grooves. If we learn to read them, we will never have to wonder what needs to be done—or not done—to the bottom of the foot."

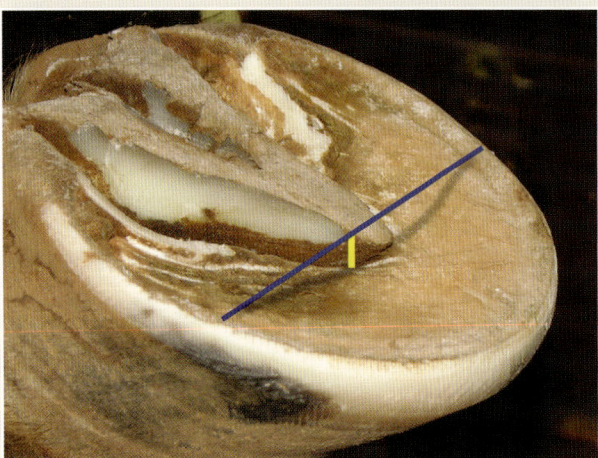

9.21 The blue line in this picture shows where you should place your straight edge to find the depth of sole at the true apex of the frog, which is usually about ¼ inch behind the tip of an untrimmed frog. The yellow line shows what the ruler would measure.

Ramey explains that the collateral grooves are very consistent in their depth to the underlying inner structures, about ⅜ inch from the bottom of the groove to the sensitive corium, regardless of whether the rest of the sole is too thick or too thin.

"This means," says Ramey, "that if a horse has too much sole, the collateral grooves will be too deep. If there is not enough sole thickness, the collateral grooves will be too shallow. Only a sub-solar abscess can push the grooves farther from the coffin bone, and I have never seen or heard of a situation that brings them too close."

To get your horse's measurements, start by laying a straight edge across the wall over the apex of the frog (usually about ¼ inch behind the tip of an untrimmed frog), then use a thin ruler to see how deep it is from the straight edge to the bottom of the grooves (fig. 9.21).

Explains Ramey: "If the measurement to the bottom of the groove is ½–¾ inch, there is probably a correct amount of sole covering the internal structures. If it is ¼ inch, you can very safely assume that there is not enough sole between the coffin bone, its sensitive corium, and the outdoors. It must be allowed to build. If this measurement is 1½ inches deep, you can very safely assume material could be removed."

Keep in mind that these measurements include a wall height of approximately ⅛ inch above the sole, so if your horse's walls are longer or shorter, or he is wearing shoes, you will have to factor in the difference.

a good rule of thumb with such horses is that it is okay to pop out any areas of shedding sole that come off easily (with light prying with a hoof pick), but parts that are still tightly attached can be left in place.

However, there are some instances where retained sole can fill in too much of the foot, effectively negating its natural concavity. This can cause bruising (which may lead to abscessing), and inhibit flexion of the hoof, thereby affecting circulation. Occasionally, a horse will get a buildup of retained sole so thick and dense that it mimics the appearance of live sole. This material can make it quite difficult for a hoof-care provider to gauge the correct height for the walls, heels, and bars, resulting in a foot that ends up growing too tall and becoming less functional. When this is the case, carefully removing some or all of the dead sole, then trimming the walls appropriately, may immediately improve the feet.

One other possible problem with leaving retained sole in place is that it will eventually start to crack and flake, which can trap gunk and allow fungal or bacterial infections to set up shop. If an infection is suspected, the dead sole should be removed to expose the infection to the air and allow the application of medication, if necessary. While it is wise to keep an eye open for such issues if your horse has retained sole, remember that most horses do just fine and many do even better than they would otherwise when you leave the retained sole alone and allow the foot to find its own equilibrium.

Bar Health

The bars on the bottom of the hoof are another amazing part of the complex support system that nature gave the equine hoof. They are also the source of much disagreement among hoof-care providers. While everyone concurs that the ideal bar is straight and upright, as this is the position that allows them to assist most in weight bearing, this is where universal agreement comes to a grinding halt (fig. 9.22).

Trimming the Bars: Listen to the Horse

One of the main areas of controversy is when to trim the bars, and how much to trim them if and when you do. Opinions are all over the map, ranging from aggressive trimmers who dig the bars down below the level of the live sole, to those who believe in trimming the bars flush with the callused sole, to those who say that the bars will usually grow the way the horse needs them to be with minimal, if any, interference from the trimmer.

So, who is right?

While carving the bars out below the level of the sole is very likely to make the horse sore and can cause serious harm, every other idea on the spectrum is likely to be right in some cases, and wrong in others. A bar that is harmfully tall, lumpy, or laid over on one horse might be exactly what keeps another horse comfortable. Factors like the degree of concavity a foot has, the type of footing it travels on, how much moisture is in the environment, and how healthy the other structures of the foot are, all play a role in determining the optimal bar height for a particular horse at any given time. Generally speaking, though, most horses appear to be comfortable when the bars are fairly close to the level of the sole, perhaps a couple of millimeters longer than flush.

Some instances where bar material may need to be removed include bars overgrown enough to cause excess pressure inside the foot, or bars that have laid over and are putting pressure on the sole—the latter being more likely to cause a problem on a flatter foot than a concave one (figs. 9.23 A & B). Such bars can cause bruising and subsolar abscesses under the bar area, and if this state continues long-term, the corium can be permanently damaged (fig. 9.24).

Long bars can also grow inward at their terminal ends and pinch the frog, affecting its growth and function, as well as the comfort of the horse.

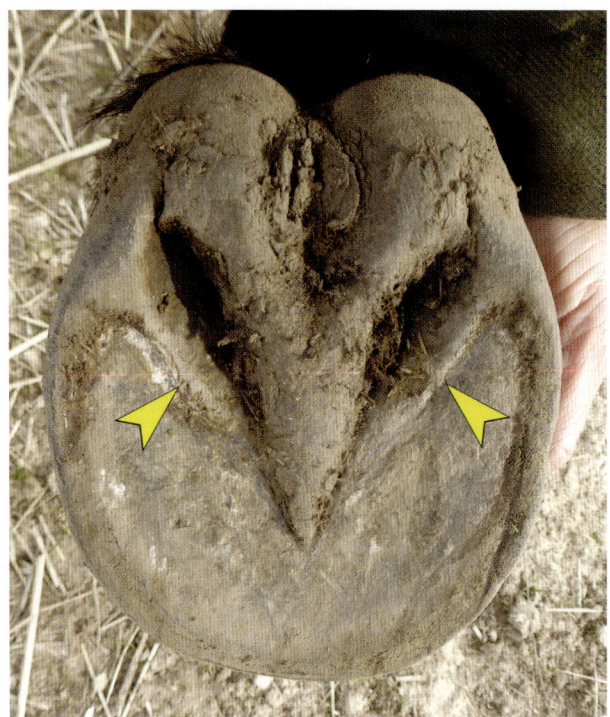

9.22 This horse has nicely straight, naturally short bars that require little, if any trimming.

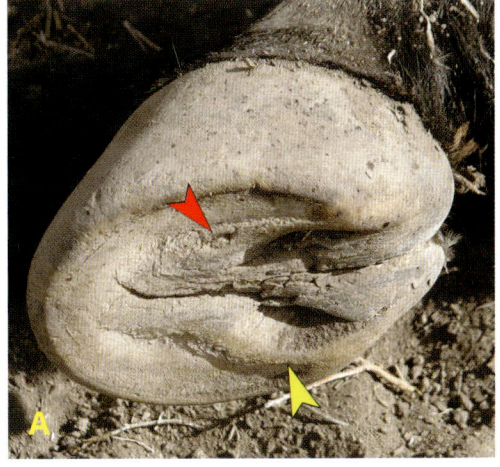

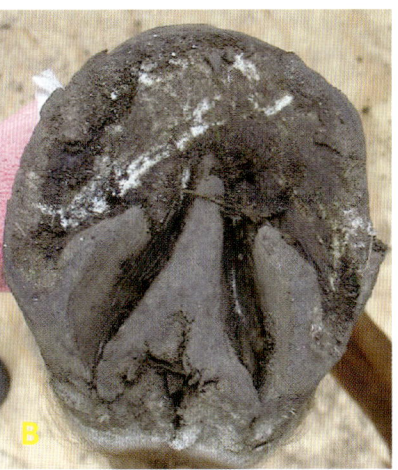

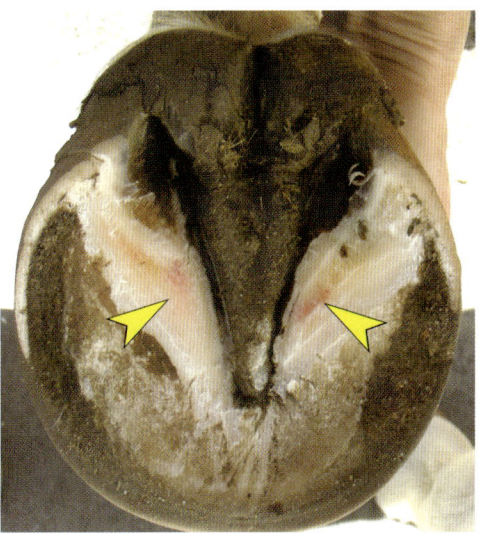

9.23 A & B The wild Mustang's foot in A has one bar that has grown large and thick (yellow arrow), and one that has "laid over" (folded sideways) and spread downward (red arrow), a difference likely due to some degree of mediolateral imbalance. Due to the significant concavity of this foot, these bars are probably not bothering the horse, and may even be an adaptation that gives the foot some extra protection during the driest part of the year when the frog is desiccated and the ground exceptionally hard. The overgrown bars on the rescue horse's flattish foot in B were causing so much pain that she could hardly move and could not hold up a foot for trimming. The owner's boyfriend supported the horse's weight on his back (someone give that man a medal!) while the hoof-care provider worked quickly to get the bars down. Once the trim was done, the mare was immediately comfortable.

9.24 Before this foot was trimmed, the bars were overgrown and laid over. The trim revealed bruising (yellow arrows) in the sole underneath the area where the excess bar material had been. While taking the bars down this far might be too aggressive in many instances, it can be a beneficial step in the healing process when the bars have been badly distorted, causing damage and sometimes infection in the tissues below.

Another potential problem with bars that have laid over is that they can trap unhealthy muck that can be impossible to get at and clean out. The result can be a cesspool of "bungus" (bacteria plus fungus) that may lead to abscesses if the undesirable organisms invade the white line of the bars (fig. 9.25).

But, it is critical to understand that the hoof can and often does attempt to support itself where it is weak by growing extra bar and/or sole material that can look like it shouldn't be there. If overall management is helping the foot recover from that weakness, such anomalies usually go away on their own. Taking away this extra support before the foot is ready can cause pain and slow its recovery. This may be why we

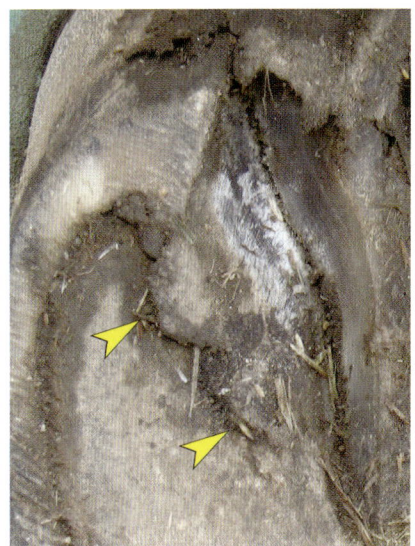

9.25 The bars on this foot are slightly overgrown and beginning to lay over. This would not be bothering the horse at this point, but it is starting to trap bits of material and moisture underneath.

9.26 A–D The bilateral flaring on the quarters of the foot in A has pulled the bars outward, causing them to curve. See the yellow lines, which follow the curve of the bars. The healthy, functional foot in B has a bit of medio-lateral imbalance that causes the lateral half to be larger than the medial half, pulling the lateral bar into a stronger curve. The sloping pasterns on the horse in C make his feet want to "run forward," meaning his toes tend to get long and his heels want to migrate ahead of where they should be. Regular hoof care keeps his feet in relatively good shape, but the curve in his bars is a reminder of what those heels would do if left untended for very long. The foot in D is quite contracted in the heels, which has pushed the back of the bars closer together, causing them to curve. If those heels widen out, the bars should get straighter.

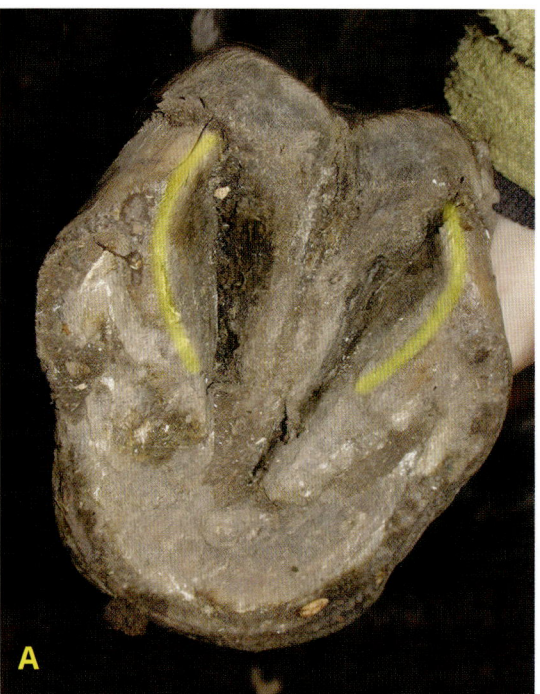

A

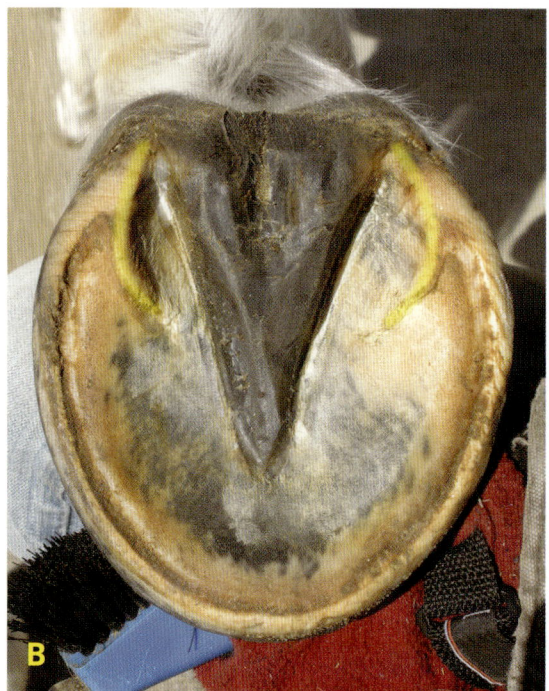

B

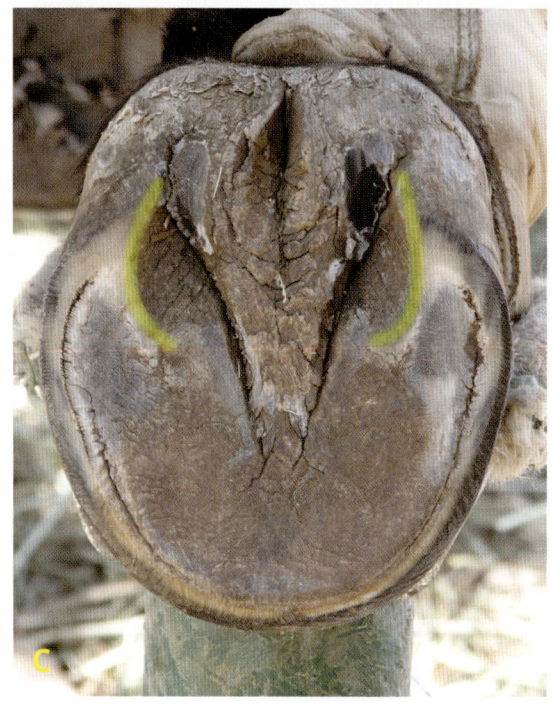

C

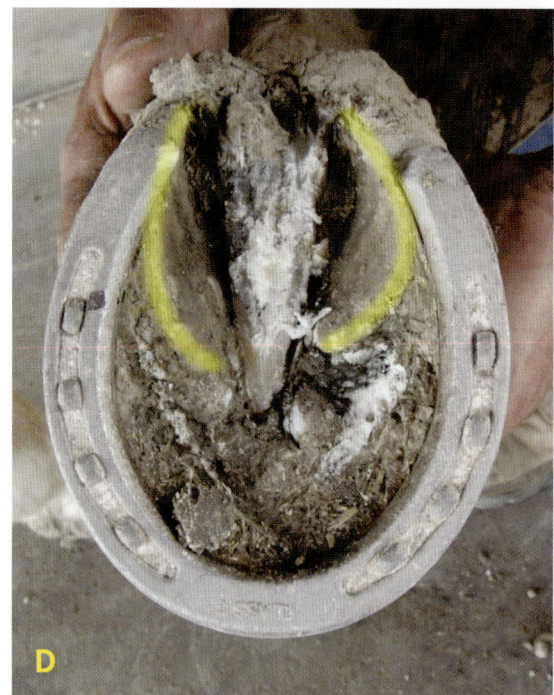

D

often see big, ugly-looking bars in feet with thin, collapsed heel regions. Such non-textbook bars may look like they should be pared down, but they are providing some support to very weak structures. As soon as the heels get a little healthier, the ugly bars may be able to go or may disappear on their own.

It can definitely be hard to know what should or shouldn't be done when you see bars that are not ideal. Therefore, when modifying the bars, don't forget to listen to the horse. Trimming is supposed to take the horse closer to optimal, and should therefore make him more comfortable, not make him sore. If the bars are being taken down and the result is that your horse is in pain, it might be best to rethink your trimming strategy. Also, if bar material seems to be growing back very quickly after a trim, this is an indication that the foot needs it there. It is not due to "compacted" bars popping out of the foot—the bars simply don't grow that way.

Curved Bars

Curved bars are extremely common. A slight degree of curvature is within the range of normal and is likely nothing to be concerned about, especially if the foot looks otherwise healthy and functions well. However, a number of very common issues can also lead to curvature of the bars, so when there is curving, it can be a clue that something else is going on (figs. 9.26 A–D). The main reasons why bars distort into a curved shape are:

- Flares in the quarters, which can pull the bars outward, causing them to curve. This can happen on one side of the foot or both.

- Overly long or laid-over bars, which result in pressure that pushes the bars outward, creating a similar distortion.

- Contracted heels, which push the backs of the bars inward.

- Heels that have migrated forward, which can push the entire bar into a shorter and thus more curved frame.

- Mediolateral imbalance, which can cause the foot to grow wider on one side than the other, usually causing a curve in the bar of the wider half. It is more common to see the lateral side wider with more curve in the bar.

If the bars are simply overgrown and laying over, regular trimming is likely to help them straighten out. However, if the curvature is due to another problem with the foot, you will have to address and correct that problem before the bars will be able to become straighter. Once again, listening to the horse is helpful in regards to how hard you need to chase this problem. If the horse does his job happily with no soundness issues, the curved bars are probably not worth getting gray hairs over.

10

Cracks, Bruises, Abscesses, and Puncture Wounds

The hooves of a horse have a pretty demanding life that can be more than a little rough at times. When we look at what nature requires of them, then factor in all that we ask them to do, as well as all the problems we cause for them, it is no wonder they sometimes end up worse for wear. Cracks, bruises, abscesses, and puncture wounds are all common problems that can hit any horse as he makes his way through life, so we need to know what we can do to try to prevent these problems, and how to handle them when they do occur.

do. One universal truth about cracks is that they cannot reattach or knit back together. Getting rid of a crack is, therefore, a matter of growing it out and preventing the wall from cracking again.

The first step in dealing with a crack is figuring out what kind of crack you are looking at. Once you know that, you must determine what is causing the crack so that you can address the problem. Attempting to manage a crack without removing the underlying cause of the crack is likely to be an exercise in frustration. The most common types of cracks you are likely to encounter are on the pages that follow.

A Crack in the Armor

When it comes to hoof cracks, some are superficial and have no effect on the hoof whatsoever, while others can be full thickness, penetrating all the way through the wall and into the sensitive tissues below, and possibly up into the coronary band as well. Full-thickness cracks can cause tremendous pain and may bleed or become infected. In terms of treatment, some cracks will resolve on their own, others need intervention, and some will be permanent, no matter what you

Grass Cracks and Sand Cracks

Grass cracks are superficial fissures that typically *start at the ground and head upward* (fig. 10.1). *Sand cracks* are the same thing, but they *start at the coronet and move downward*. Both types of cracks form when the molecular bonds between the outermost layers of tubules get weakened by repeated cycles of exposure to moisture followed by drying, which eventually causes them to split apart. Hoof walls that are already weakened by poor nutrition or other factors will be more likely to present with grass and sand cracks.

Grass cracks get their name because the problem is often seen in horses turned out on grass that is wet and dewy in the morning, but dries up later in the day. However, any environment where the feet go through alternating periods of wetness and dryness can lead to grass cracks or sand cracks, even if there is not a blade of grass or speck of sand in sight. For example, horses turned out in muddy paddocks then locked into stalls with dry shavings at night can develop these kinds of cracks, as can horses that are bathed frequently. The good news is that grass and sand cracks are not generally a problem and should grow out on their own. However, if something that first appeared to be a superficial crack develops into a deeper one, there is likely more than just the wet/dry changes going on, and you will want your hoof-care provider to take a look.

One mistake people often make when dealing with grass and sand cracks is to believe that the hoof is actually too dry and therefore needs moisturizing. It is important to realize that while the cracks may indeed make the surface of the hoof look dried out, it was too much moisture that started the problem in the first place, so applying anything that adds moisture is only likely to make the problem worse. Hoof dressings can also seal in bacteria and fungi, creating an anaerobic breeding ground that promotes infection and further damage to the hoof.

Preventing grass and sand cracks is best accomplished by avoiding exposure to the conditions that cause them. This means providing "high and dry" areas where horses don't have to stand in mud and puddles, and waiting until grass is dry if you are having a problem with your horse on pasture. Sealants designed to keep excess moisture from penetrating

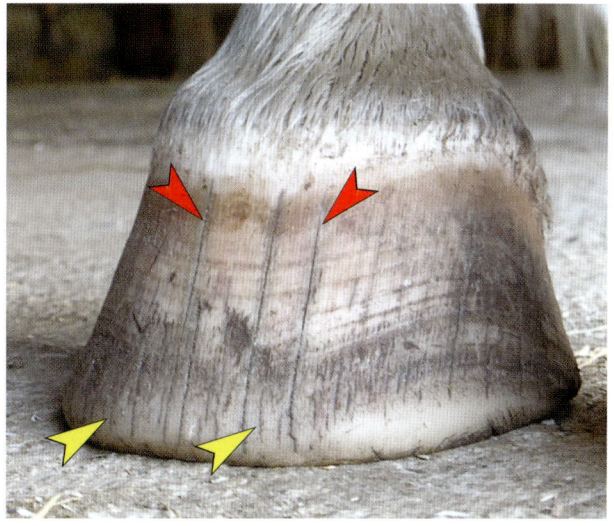

10.1 There are two different kinds of superficial cracks on this hoof. The short cracks in the lower part of the wall (yellow arrows) are grass cracks, but they may have started due to poor nutrition. The cracks that run the entire height of the wall (red arrows) are the result of overgrown, flared walls that are now being managed, but it will take some time for the cracks to grow out.

the hoof wall can sometimes help, but they can also make things worse by sealing in bacteria and fungi, especially if applied when the foot is already wet.

Toe Cracks

While *toe cracks* can appear for many reasons, they are most often due to a combination of mechanical stresses in the toe region paired with compromised laminae that cause a lack of good connection between the wall and the coffin bone (fig. 10.2). The reason these two factors so often work in tandem is that poorly connected walls are more vulnerable to mechanical stresses, but mechanical stresses can also weaken the laminar connection. So, whichever one happens first, it opens the door for the other one to follow. Mechanical stresses on the toe may

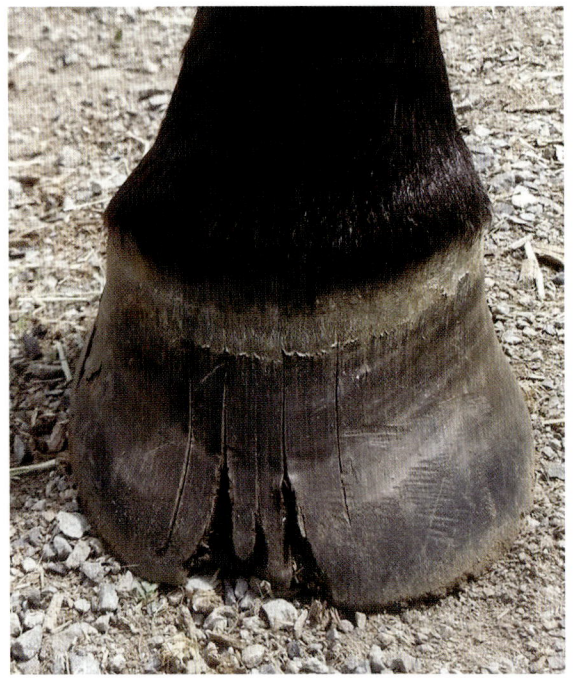

10.2 The connection between the wall and the coffin bone of this foot was weakened by both white line disease and the mechanical stresses that result from flaring. When the wall simply couldn't take any more, it cracked and split. Fortunately, a good hoof-care professional was able to get rid of both issues, and the foot grew out to be perfectly fine.

include compressive, shearing, and tensile forces—basically anything that pulls, pushes, twists, levers, or loads the wall horn (fig. 10.3).

These stresses are not normally a problem for a healthy foot, but they can easily start or worsen a toe crack when the toe wall is already set up to fail for any of the following reasons:

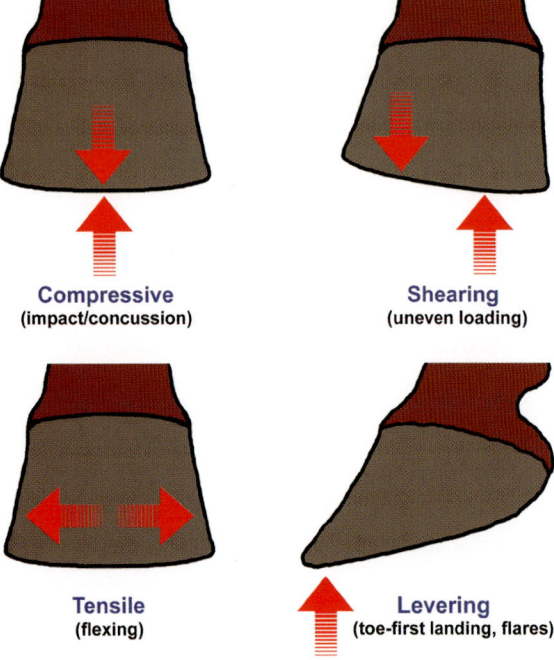

10.3 The mechanical forces the hoof regularly encounters do not typically cause problems for a healthy, well-balanced foot, but they can wreak havoc when the foot is already compromised.

Compressive
(impact/concussion)

Shearing
(uneven loading)

Tensile
(flexing)

Levering
(toe-first landing, flares)

• *Dorsopalmar/plantar imbalance:* This common hoof capsule distortion typically manifests as the front part of the foot having more mass than the back, which means you have a long toe and a point of breakover that is too far forward. With every step, the toe on such a foot experiences tremendous levering forces as the rest of the foot tries to roll over the toe to get off the ground. The levering forces weaken the laminar connection and put tensile stress on the bonds holding the tubules together—a double whammy of crack-causing potential.

• *Toe flares:* Dorsopalmar/plantar imbalance and problems like laminitis can lead to toe flares, which are a sign that the toe wall is not well connected and is being stretched and bent. If toe flares go unchecked, cracking is likely to follow (fig. 10.4).

• *Medial-lateral imbalance:* This side-to-side imbalance exerts shearing forces on the toe when the hoof lands unevenly, with one side of the hoof being pushed up upon impact while the other is still descending. It can

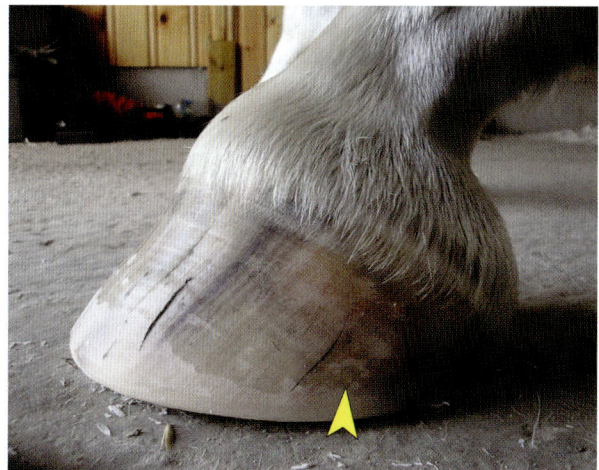

10.4 Before it was trimmed, this toe was even more flared than it is in this picture. The toe wall was dishing from the stress of the leverage caused by the flared wall pushing against the ground with every step, and cracks followed. Note the crack and bruising in the quarter as well (yellow arrow), a reminder that long toes stress the entire foot.

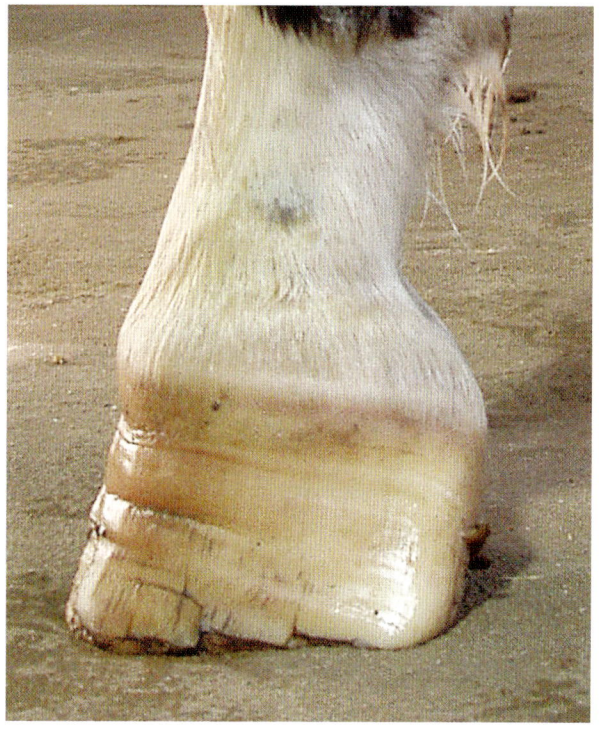

10.5 Excessive loading of the toe, like you see in this club foot, can cause cracks as well as chipping and other kinds of damage to the hoof wall.

also cause tensile stress if one side of the hoof flexes outward more than the other.

• *Compromised laminar connection:* The connection between the toe wall and the coffin bone can be damaged by laminitis, white line disease, metabolic problems, inappropriate diet, and mechanical stresses.

• *Toe-first landing:* Pain in the back of the foot can cause a horse to land toe first in an attempt to protect the painful area. Unfortunately, toe-first landing interferes with the biomechanics of the entire limb and subjects the toe to an unnatural amount of concussion, which can lead to toe cracks.

• *Toe loading:* A horse that stands with his toes loaded more than his heels due to pain or an issue like a club foot will also be more prone to toe cracks

(fig. 10.5). Horses that travel heavy on the forehand will also tend to stress their toes, making them more vulnerable to cracking.

• *Overgrown walls:* As you've learned, the hoof wall is simply not designed to support the weight of the horse on its own. This is why overgrown walls—meaning walls that have grown well past the level of the live sole (see fig. 7.23, p. 99, bottom photo)—tend to crack, split, and otherwise fall apart. This truth applies to the entire wall, not just the toe.

• *Presence of a crena:* A *crena* is a notch in the center solar margin of the coffin bone, which can

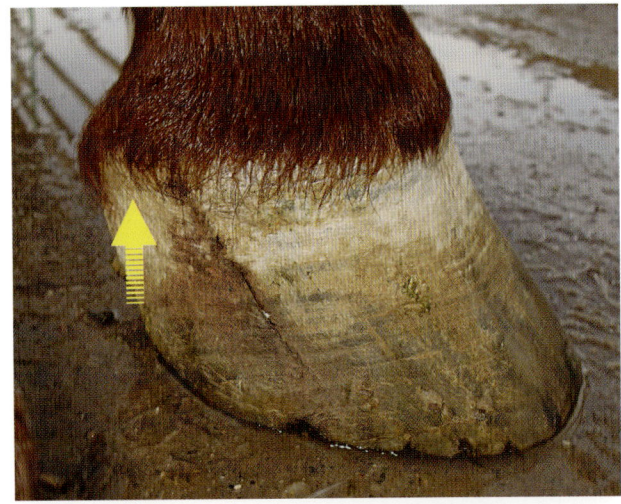

10.6 This horse's overgrown, tall hooves with their jammed (pushing upward) quarters caused this deep, bleeding crack to open up in the coronet and work its way down.

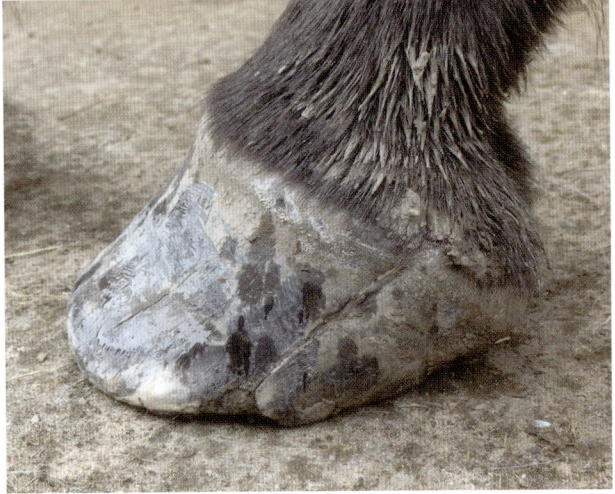

10.7 While this horse's feet are now in the process of being rehabilitated, they had previously been allowed to develop long toes, underrun heels, and flaring, all of which contributed to the formation of this quarter crack.

sometimes result in a corresponding disruption in the sole-wall juncture that you can see on the bottom of the foot at the center of the toe (see fig. 4.5, p. 24). This disrupted area gets filled with material that is not as strongly organized as normal material, similar to the lamellar wedge (wedge-shaped area of keratin proliferated by the laminae) that often grows between a wall and coffin bone that have separated due to laminitis (see p. 182). A crena can sometimes

make the hoof wall more prone to cracking due to this weakness, but this is usually manageable with good, timely hoof care.

Quarter Cracks

Quarter cracks, as their name implies, occur in the quarters of the hooves. They generally start at the coronet and spread downward, penetrating through the full thickness of the wall and into the tissues under the wall. As such, they can easily become inflamed and infected, and they are often quite painful. Because quarter cracks occur near the heels, they are affected by the continual flexing of the heel region, which leads to instability and makes them potentially difficult to manage.

Quarter cracks are most often caused by uneven loading of the foot, whether that is due to medial-lateral imbalance, dorsopalmar/plantar imbalance, overgrown ("jammed") quarters, injury, or a conformational defect (fig. 10.6). They can also result from shoes that are too short or too long, injury to the coronet, or damage to the coffin bone. Horses with long-toe/underrun heel syndrome are quite susceptible to quarter cracks, as their weak heels can't dissipate impact forces the way they are supposed to, transferring excessive concussion to the quarters (fig. 10.7).

One theory about quarter cracks proposes that they don't really start out as cracks at all, but rather as a defect in the hoof wall produced from damage to the coronet. In this model, the excessive forces caused by the problems mentioned above cause damage to the tissues under the stressed part of the wall, resulting in bleeding and a buildup of fluid. This fluid gets squeezed upward, creating pressure that damages the coronary corium, which then produces abnormal, weak tubules. The defective tubules cannot hold together as well as healthy ones, and so split apart easily. The fact that quarter cracks are often preceded by swelling and soreness in the coronet over the stressed area adds weight to this theory.

Cracks Due to Abscesses (aka "Blowouts")

When an abscess forms under the hoof wall, the pus and exudate (fluid containing protein and cellular debris) usually can't break through the hard, dense wall material to drain. But, that yucky gunk has to go somewhere, so it often ends up migrating upward until it "pops out" at the much softer material of the coronet, or backward where it will emerge in the pliable heel area. The good news is that the horse will generally feel much better when this happens. The bad news is that the hoof wall is likely to develop a hole or crack at the spot where the abscess emerged due to a temporary disruption of the coronary corium. The cracks that form in this way are often referred to as "blowouts" (fig. 10.8).

But, here is some more good news: the cracks caused by abscesses usually cause no problems for the horse. They will simply grow down as the hoof grows and disappear on their own. It is possible for damage to the coronary corium to be permanent, creating a defect in the wall that most often shows up as a vertical groove growing down the entire length of the wall, but this is not typical when the problem is a simple abscess.

Sometimes, the portion of wall below a blowout crack crumbles away or chunks off (fig. 10.9). This most often means that the wall was not well connected in that area due to the abscess migrating upward under the wall before it blew out. While this

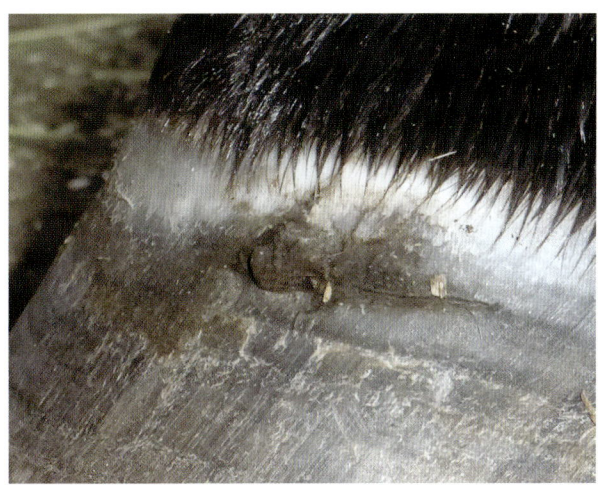

10.8 Cracks like this that form when an abscess pops out at the coronet usually just grow down and disappear with no permanent harm to the hoof wall.

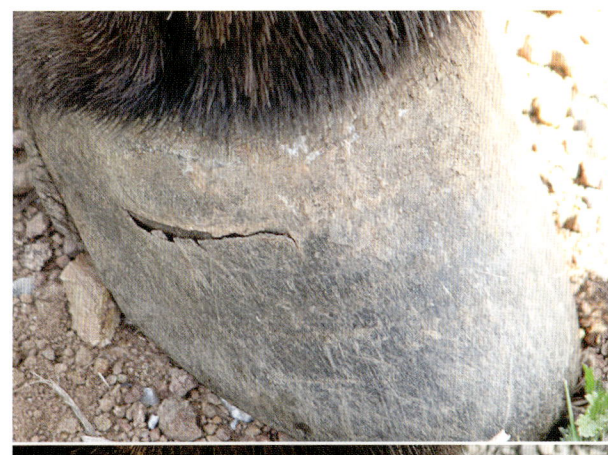

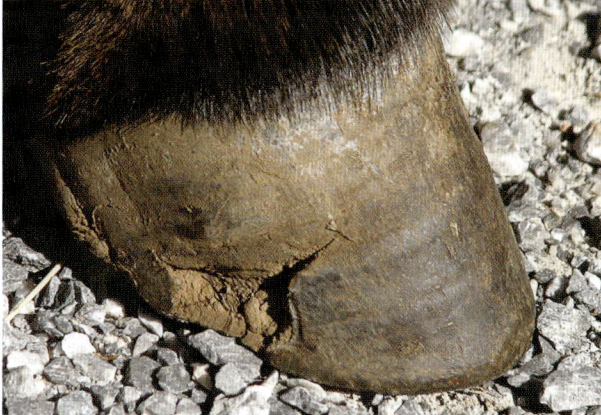

10.9 This Miniature Donkey's hoof had an abscess blowout that created a horizontal crack in the wall (above). The damaged wall below the blowout eventually chunked away (below). When this happens, it usually looks worse than it is. This section of missing wall grew down and disappeared within a few months or so, with no lasting damage.

10.10 This horse sustained a minor injury to the hoof wall. The worst trouble with it was that it was initially pestered by flies, so the owners covered it with a bell boot that kept the flies away. Once they did that, the wound healed over quickly, and the crack grew down and disappeared.

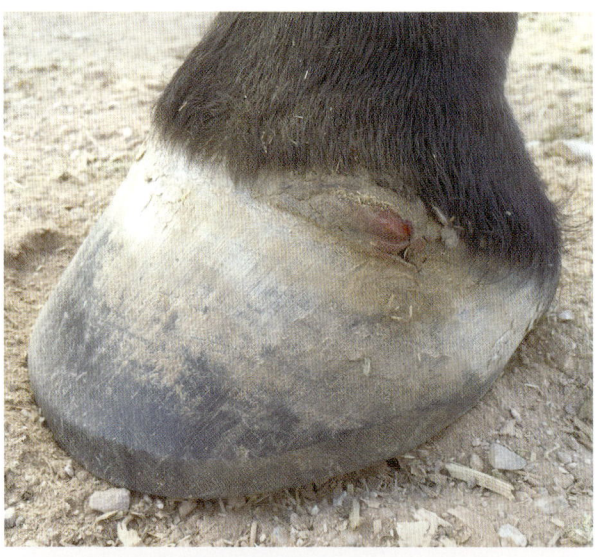

10.11 Serious injuries to the coronet can sometimes affect the growth of the hoof wall permanently, causing a perpetual crack, as seen here. Note the broad scar above the crack on this foot, indicating that the area once sustained a substantial amount of damage.

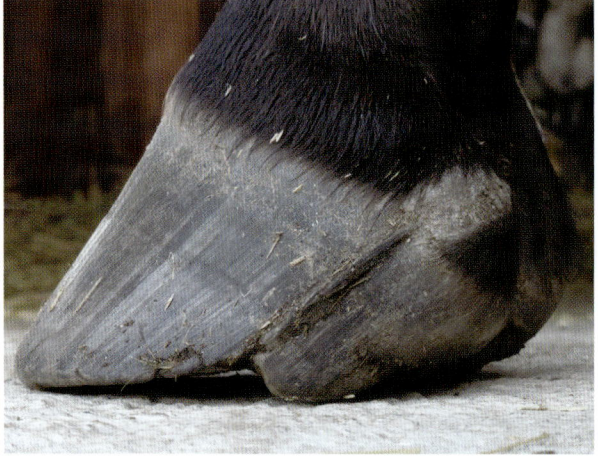

can look very alarming, the damaged portion of the wall will most often simply grow out and not cause any permanent problems. It is certainly worth keeping an eye on and discussing with your hoof-care professional if you have any concerns, but hooves tend to recover very well from this sort of problem, especially if there are no underlying problems leading to repeated episodes of abscessing (see more on abscesses on p. 148).

Cracks Due to Injury

The hoof wall, heels, and coronet can all end up with cracks due to injury. Sometimes a horse will hit a hoof against something hard enough to cause a wall to crack, or another horse may kick or step on him. A coronet injury can happen from an impact as well, but the coronet may also be damaged by getting a foot getting caught in a fence or hooked over a wire. The disruption to the coronet can then cause the hoof wall in that area to grow in a disorganized manner, leading to a crack.

If a crack results from a minor injury, it is likely to heal just fine and grow out without issue (fig. 10.10). However, a more serious injury can result in a crack that is difficult to get rid of (fig. 10.11). Any injury that causes substantial damage to the hoof wall or coronet should be looked at by a vet because preventing infection and stabilizing the foot quickly may help the foot mend better, thus preventing a crack from becoming a permanent feature of the foot.

Treating and Preventing Cracks

The most appropriate treatment for a crack is going to depend on its location, severity, and cause. Any contributing disease condition, injury, nutritional problem, or hoof imbalance will need to be addressed if possible, and the mechanical forces working to cause or perpetuate the crack will need to be relieved. In most mild to moderate cases, and even some pretty bad ones, the latter can be accomplished by getting the foot balanced, removing any overgrown wall, and putting a strong bevel on the cracked wall area so that it is free from ground-contact forces.

Doing this generally negates the need for additional stabilization, though some hoof-care providers prefer to add mechanical stabilization in the form of a shoe or hoof cast. When a crack is severe, it may require more intensive treatment best performed by a veterinarian or very qualified farrier. They may use a variety of techniques including stainless steel lacing, debridement of infected areas, and patching with special materials.

Chronic cracks—the ones that seem to never want to go away or that disappear for a while but then come back—may or may not be truly permanent. Sometimes, what is a chronic crack in one hoof-care provider's hands can be successfully grown out by another who uses different methods (fig. 10.12). If your horse has a crack that is an ongoing problem, it may be worth talking to another hoof-care provider or two to see if they think they might be able to do something to fix the crack. Tell them what has been tried thus far, and ask what they would do differently. If it sounds reasonable, you might want to consider giving them a shot at it.

Preventing cracks from happening in the first place is always better than trying to fix them after the fact. Make sure that your horse doesn't suffer from "lack of farrier disease," as overgrown,

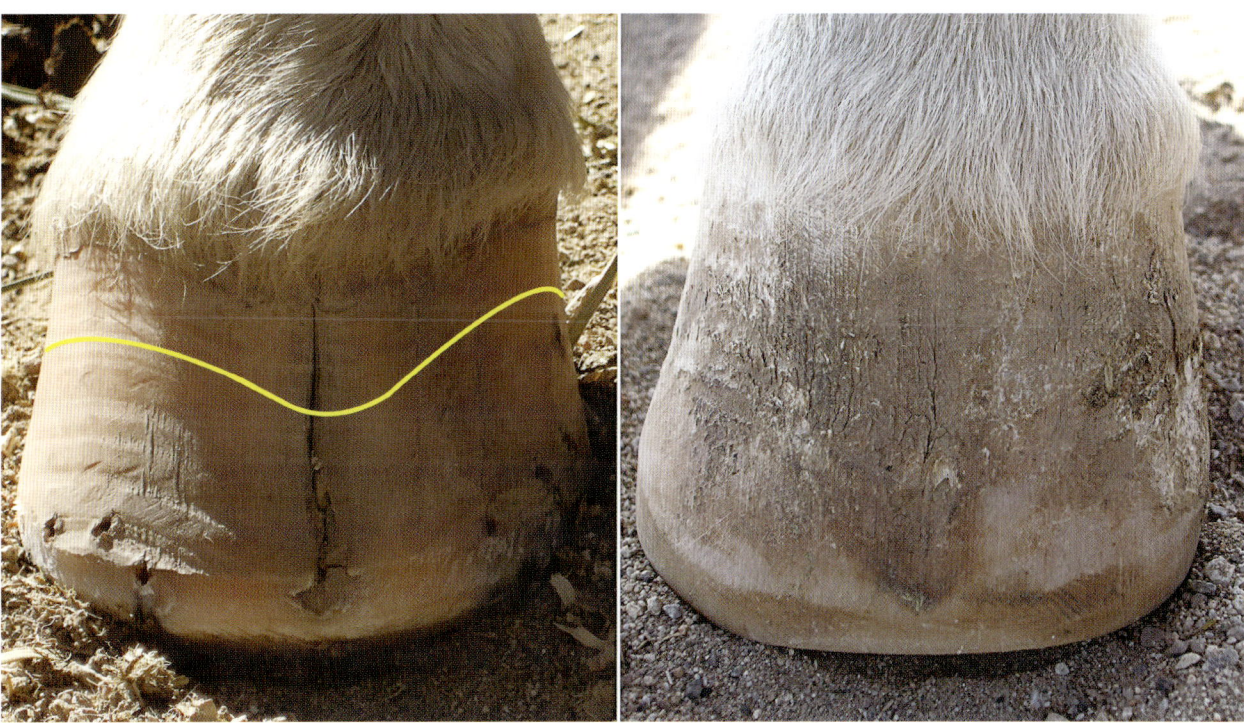

10.12 This foot had a "chronic" toe crack that was treated unsuccessfully for years by a veterinarian and farrier using orthopedic shoeing and pads. Despite their combined expertise, the distorted growth lines on this foot (yellow line) show that their methods were putting unnatural pressure on the hoof wall, contributing to the perpetuation of the crack. A different professional treated the crack by dispensing with shoes, reducing peripheral loading (especially in the quarters), beveling the hoof wall to relieve pressure on the crack, and increasing movement to improve overall hoof health. These photos show what the foot looked like after the new hoof-care professional's first trim, and what had been achieved only seven months later.

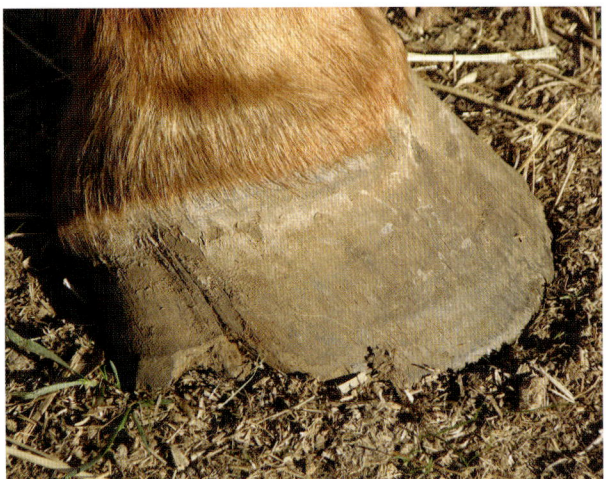

10.13 This foot was allowed to get underrun, which distorted the entire foot, weakened the heels, and put excessive pressure on the quarters. The resulting crack has been made much worse by the continued lack of care.

neglected feet are highly vulnerable to cracks (fig. 10.13). But, while regular hoof care is one of the most important crack-prevention strategies, just having the feet tended regularly doesn't necessarily mean they are being tended well. You need to stay on top of the quality of work being done by your provider, as so many cracks are caused by man-made hoof imbalances. Don't be afraid to pick up a foot and check the balance of the trim. If you see a problem, politely call it to the attention of your provider. If your horse is barefoot, make sure your trimmer puts a good bevel on the walls, which will go a very long way to prevent cracking.

Also take a look at your horse's diet to see if what is going into his mouth could be setting his feet up to crack. Think about potential hazards like excessive moisture and exposure to repeated cycles of wet and dry. Study how your horse moves and stands, as there could be imbalances or soreness

somewhere else in the body that are causing uneven loading that could lead to hoof cracks.

One thing you don't need to worry about is a dry environment causing the foot to crack. The hoof gets all the moisture it needs from the fluid circulating within the hoof, and the moisture in the inner and middle layers of the hoof wall—the layers that are supposed to be moist—simply has no way to exit the foot. That means that as long as there is still blood circulating through your horse's body, it will produce enough moisture for his feet, and that moisture cannot be "sucked out," even if your horse lives in the desert. The equine foot actually loves a dry environment and is extremely well adapted to thrive in one. It is ironic that so many people believe that their horse's feet get too brittle and crack in the summer because the weather has turned dry, when in fact, it is the damage the hoof sustained during the wet season that actually causes the foot to crack once it fully dries out.

Bruising

When you think about the tremendous force coming down on each foot with every step your horse takes, it is not surprising that he sometimes ends up with bruises on his feet. Almost every horse will end up with a "stone bruise" at some point, the result of him stepping on something hard that causes a bruise in any of the structures on the bottom of the foot (fig. 10.14). While such bruises are indeed the most common, bruises are not always caused by the foot coming down on something hard, and they are not always confined to the bottom of the foot.

A *bruise* is the result of some form of trauma that ruptures one or more small blood vessels, allowing blood to seep into the surrounding tissue. This causes localized inflammation, pressure, and pain, with the degree of pain depending on the severity and location of the bleeding. Bruises in most parts of the hoof show up as reddish or purplish discolorations, though they can be hard or impossible to see on dark feet. Whatever their color, by the time discolorations are visible, the event or problem that caused the bruising is usually long past, as the discolored spot you can see is tissue that has grown out from an internal area that was damaged weeks or months earlier.

The location of the bruise can often give you an idea of what may have caused it. Bruises on the bottom of the foot are most often caused by the horse stepping on a hard object, but they can also be the result of pressure from something like an overlaid bar or a buildup of exfoliating sole material, or concussion caused by working on a hard surface or a jumping horse landing heavily on his feet (figs. 10.15 A & B). We can also see bruising on

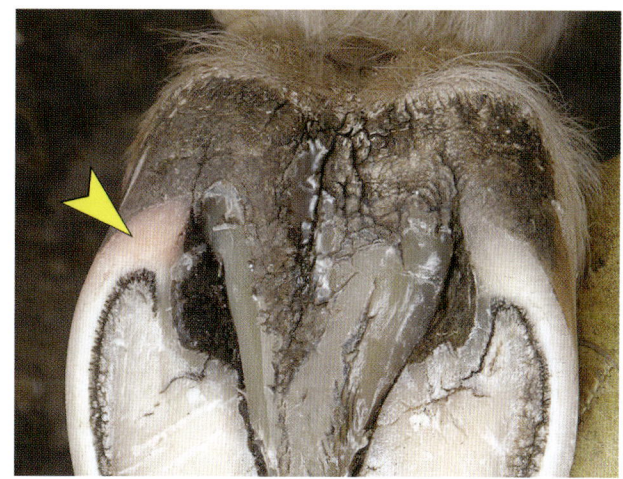

10.14 The stone bruise that showed up on the heel when this foot was trimmed resulted from the horse stepping on something hard weeks or months earlier. A minor bruise like this usually causes no lameness and so goes unnoticed at the time it happens.

the sole in horses with laminitis, high heels, or long-term peripheral loading, any of which can lead to the coffin bone pressing down on the solar corium. Excessive trimming anywhere on the bottom of the foot can also lead to bruising.

When bruises show up on the wall, they are most often due to the horse knocking his foot against an unyielding object such as a fence or stall wall.

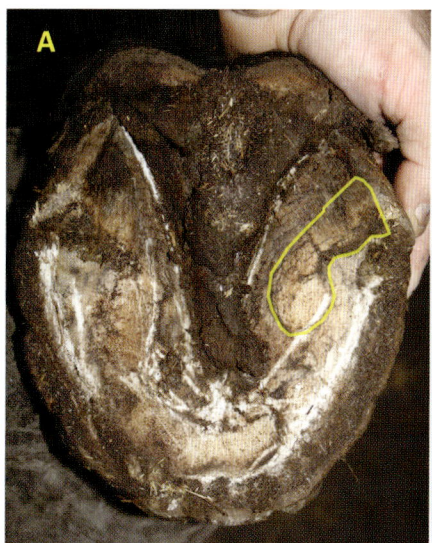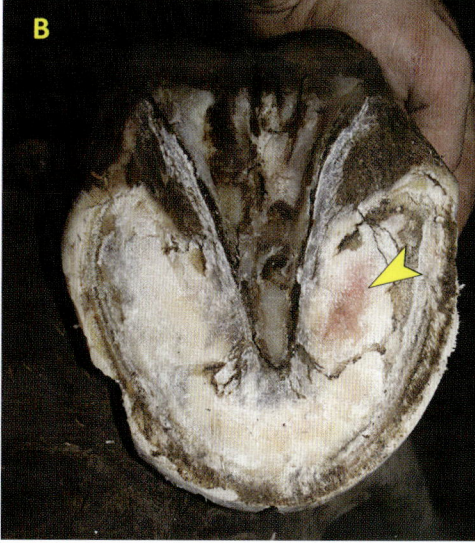

10.15 A & B In A, you can see the laid over (folded down) bar on this foot circled in yellow. This excess material put pressure on the sole underneath, leading to a bruise that become apparent only after the bar was trimmed back, shown in B.

Horses that habitually paw or stomp often end up with bruises in their walls. Horses that strike their own feet or shoes when they move may also exhibit bruising on the walls, as can horses whose feet load unevenly enough to put excessive pressure on part of the coronary band (fig. 10.16). And sometimes, horses will develop bruising in concentric circles parallel to the coronet. This indicates that there was some bleeding at the coronary corium, a situation that most often results from too much work on hard surfaces, or possibly from laminitis (fig. 10.17).

Bruising in the white line can also be a consequence of laminitis, though there are other possible causes as well. Anything that results in overloading of the toe, including heel pain, high heels, traveling heavy on the forehand, or a conformational problem, can injure the laminae and cause a bruise (fig. 10.18). Long toes that experience excessive leverage can also get tearing in the laminae that causes bruising.

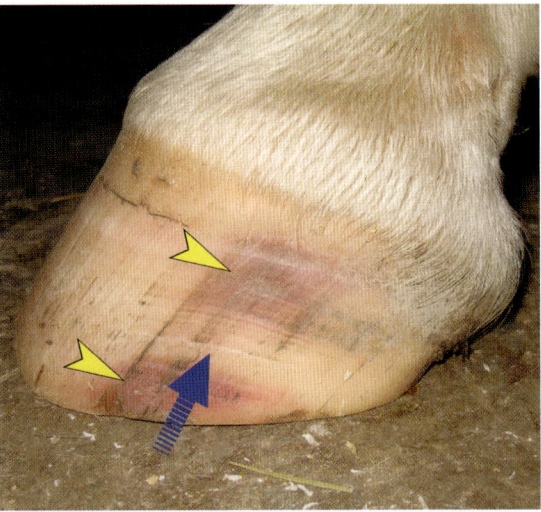

10.16 Uneven loading, indicated by the upward wave in the growth lines (blue arrow), may have contributed to the bruising in the wall of this hoof (yellow arrows).

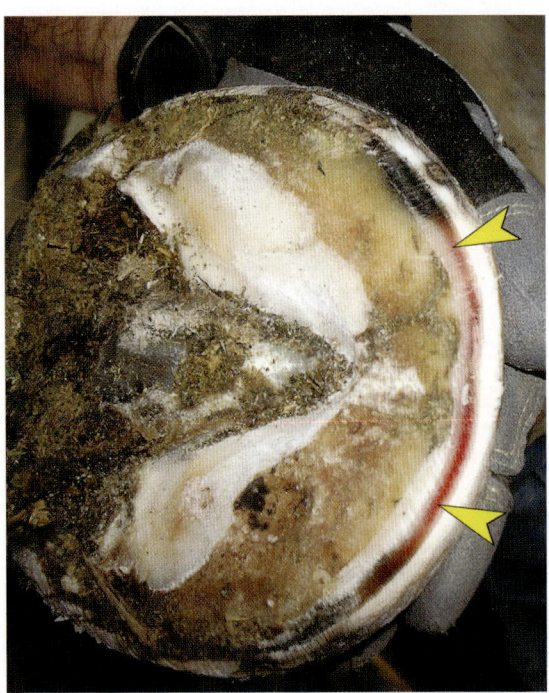

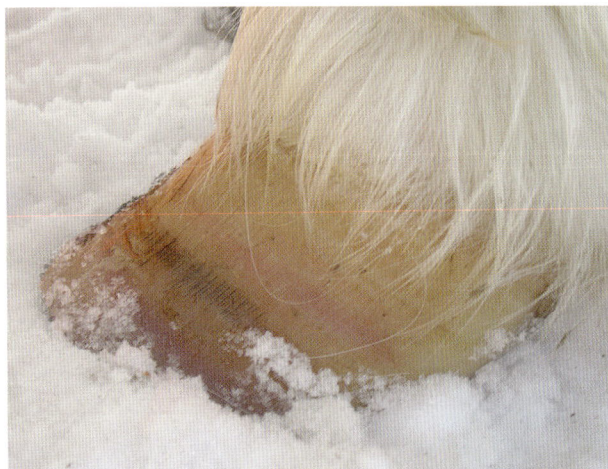

10.17 The concentric bruise rings on this foot are most likely due to repeated bouts of laminitis, which is also making the hoof wall flare forward.

10.18 Heel pain caused this horse to land and stand heavily on his toes, which led to significant bruising in the white line.

As already mentioned, many bruises are mild enough that you don't even know they have happened until the visual evidence shows up later, but some bruises are so painful that the horse will come up extremely lame. When this happens, it is always best to get the vet out to determine what is actually going on, as the pain that may be due to a bad bruise could also be the result of another problem such as a fractured coffin bone, strained ligament, or laminitis.

If you are dealing with a severe bruise, the horse may require rest, and pain relief can be provided through the use of non-steroidal anti-inflammatory medications such as phenylbutazone ("bute") and icing. Temporary protection in the form of pads or hoof boots may also provide some respite from pain, but be aware that these can make some horses more uncomfortable, not less, so you want to be attentive to how your horse responds to them. You will also want to check the bruised area for any fissures or cracks that could admit bacteria and potentially lead to an abscess (see p. 148). But regardless of whether you see any external openings, be watchful for the signs of abscessing, as they can occur after a bruise even when there is no external pathway for bacteria.

Fortunately, most bruises are not cause for concern and will heal on their own as the damaged tissue grows out. However, if a horse is getting bruised repeatedly, especially in the same area of the foot, something is making that foot vulnerable and the problem should be investigated. Chronic bruising can be due to a number of factors, including:

• *Imbalance*: An imbalanced hoof causes the horse to bear more weight than he should on part of the foot, and the greater load means that area is coming down harder than normal on whatever it encounters on the ground. If the overloaded part hits a stone or anything else raised and hard, it is more likely to bruise than it would have been otherwise. Just the weight of the horse can be enough to cause bruising when the imbalance is bad enough, as is often the case with heel bruises that result from long toes and underrun heels. Imbalance can also cause stretching and pulling of the laminae, leading to bruises in the white line. Long toes, for example, put excessive leverage on the laminae, so it is not uncommon to see white line bruises in feet with long toes. Shoes cover the white line, so if your horse is shod, you may not be able to see these bruises until the foot is being trimmed.

• *Thin soles*: Even a horse with thick, tough soles can get the odd stone bruise. However, when the sole is thin, the blood vessels are already under stress, plus they are just that much closer to all the things the foot has to travel over. It is not surprising, then, that horses with thin soles are prone to bruising. Unfortunately, thin-soled horses are not just more likely to get bruised soles—they are also more likely to get bruises of the coffin bone, which can be extremely painful, slow to heal, and may be a precursor to bone disease. Making sure that your horse has an adequate depth of sole, and avoiding any paring or thinning of the sole unless there is some specific, medical reason for it, is an important part of protecting against sole bruises.

• *Shoeing/trimming issues*: Poor or overdue shoeing or trimming can cause or contribute to bruising (fig. 10.19). For example, shoeing long or short puts excessive pressure on the heels, and this can lead to a type of bruising called a "corn." Shoes that have been on the hoof for too long can lead to contraction, which can cause bruising as the heels crush together and the bars pinch in on the frog. They can also cause the foot to migrate forward, causing imbalance that can result in bruising. Devices meant to increase traction (for example, toe grabs, borium, studs, caulks) may delay breakover and put stress on the laminae, which can lead to bruising, and some can put added pressure on the heels that can be a problem. And, bare feet are not immune to bruising by any means. Overgrown or unbalanced bare feet have many of the same issues as their shod counterparts. One common issue with bare feet is bars that have been allowed to distort and/or lay over, which can cause bruising in the adjacent sole.

• *Hoof conformation*: The shape of some horses' feet make them vulnerable to bruising. Flat feet are more prone than normal feet to bruising on the bottom of the foot, while upright feet often take a pounding on the toe and white line, making those areas more likely to get bruised. And, as we've mentioned, long-toe/low-heel conformation increases the risk of both heel and white line bruising.

• *Contraction:* Whether caused by poor shoeing or other issues, contraction compromises circulation and puts pressure on the structures in the back of the foot, both factors that make bruising a more likely occurrence.

• *Terrain:* Hard, rocky ground makes stone bruises on the sole more likely for any horse, but horses kept in soft footing and then asked to head out on rocky trails are especially at risk. Such horses should be given extra protection in the form of pads (if shod) or hoof boots (if barefoot) before being asked to work on rough footing they are not accustomed to. Working on hard surfaces like asphalt or compacted road base, even without rocks, can cause bruising too, but this will tend to show up in the walls rather than the sole. Keep in mind that it is harder to see wall bruises in horses with black feet, but this doesn't mean they don't get them.

• *Environmental conditions*: Exposure to moisture in the form of rain or mud softens the sole, which increases the chances of bruising in two ways. First, just being soft makes the sole less able to protect the foot from impact with anything hard, but a soft sole also wears away more easily, so it can become thinner. Ice and snow can be an issue as well, as they not only create hard, lumpy ground, but can also pack into the bottom of the foot, negating the foot's natural concavity and filling it in with hard material. Shod horses are more vulnerable to collecting ice balls in their feet, so if you have a shod horse in snow country, you might want to consider

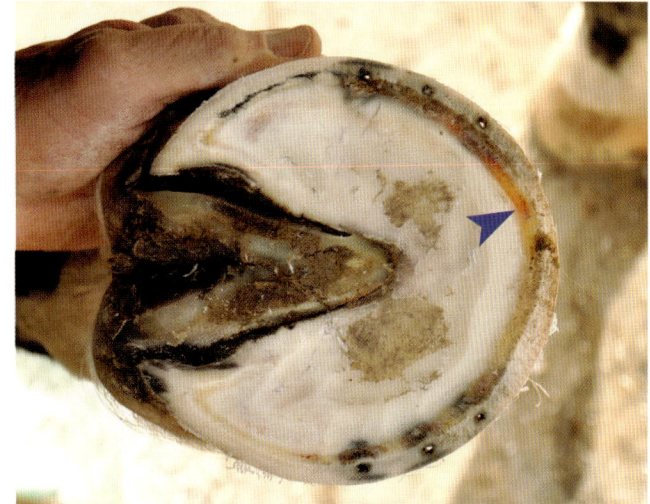

10.19 The minor bruising in the white line on this foot (blue arrow) was caused by dorsal wall distortion that is now being corrected with good farriery. The bruising will continue to grow out over time.

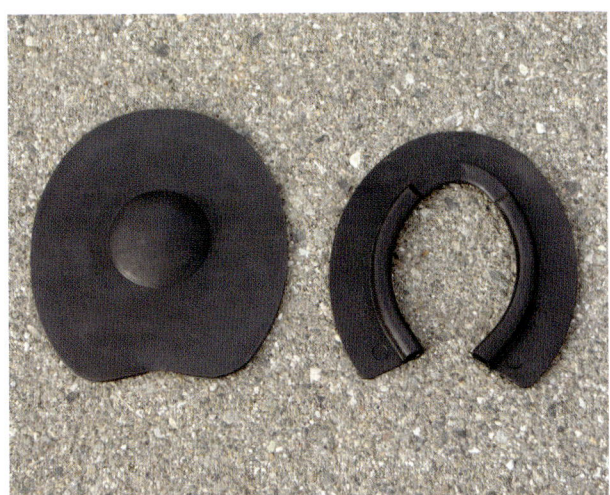

10.20 If you live in snow country and have a shod horse, snow pads, either the bubble type (left) or the rim type (right), can help your horse avoid bruising by preventing snow from building up under the foot.

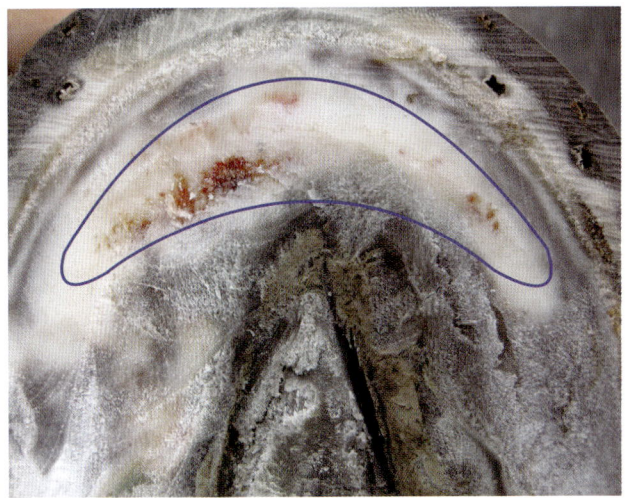

10.21 Displacement of the coffin bone can cause it to press down on the solar corium. When it does, you will sometimes see bruising in the sole echoing the shape of the front edge of the bone (circled area).

using snow pads or snow rims that help prevent the cold stuff from building up inside the shoe (fig. 10.20). A note on manmade environmental problems: Standing in muck and urine weakens the entire hoof but particularly the sole, leaving the foot more likely to bruise.

• *Laminitis*: When the laminae are not holding the coffin bone to the hoof wall, the front edge of the coffin bone may end up pressing down into the solar corium. This can cause bruising, which typically appears in a crescent shape, echoing the shape of the bone in front of the apex of the frog. Be aware that by the time this bruising is visible, the bleed that caused it happened months earlier. It may be tempting to your hoof-care provider to trim down the bruised area to see if the bruise is very shallow, indicating that the bleed was brief, but thinning the already compromised sole even a millimeter at such

a time can be extremely detrimental (fig. 10.21).

• *Weight and hoof size*: The weight of the horse in relation to his feet can play a part in how likely that horse is to get bruises. Heavy horses tend to have flatter feet, giving them less clearance when they step on a rock or whatnot. And, when a horse is heavy but has small feet for his size, the pounds per square inch (PSI) of pressure exerted every time those hooves touch the ground can be enormous. Selecting horses with large, strong feet and making sure your horses don't get overweight can help minimize the chances of bruising.

• *Interfering*: A horse that steps on or strikes his own feet can bruise himself by doing so.

• *Behavioral problems*: Horses that continually paw the ground or strike their hooves against a gate or wall can bruise their feet.

The best strategy in the fight against bruised feet is to be aware of the issues that can leave your horse more likely to sustain bruises, and do what you can to prevent those problems. As always, a healthy, balanced foot is far more able to cope with whatever it encounters, so good nutrition and good hoof care are your perpetual allies.

Abscesses

An *abscess* in the hoof is a pocket of infection or necrotic tissue that can cause a buildup of pressure underneath the hoof wall or sole, often resulting in extreme pain and dramatic, sudden lameness. The most common form of abscess forms when bacteria get into the foot, most typically through the white line, a misplaced shoe nail, a fissure in the sole, or a puncture wound (fig. 10.22). Another type, called a *sterile abscess,* does not generally involve infection, but forms instead when a loss of circulation, combined with compression, leads to tissue death in a localized area. This type of abscess is often seen with cases of laminitis where the coffin

bone is displaced and pushing down on the solar corium (fig. 10.23). More rarely, bacteria are carried to the foot through the bloodstream, creating an infected abscess even though there is no external entry point. This most often happens when the foot experiences a trauma that causes a bruise, as the damaged tissue creates an environment amenable to bacteria, which proliferate at the site of the bruise and form an abscess.

Left untreated, the pressure from an abscess will build, pushing the pus into new tissues along the

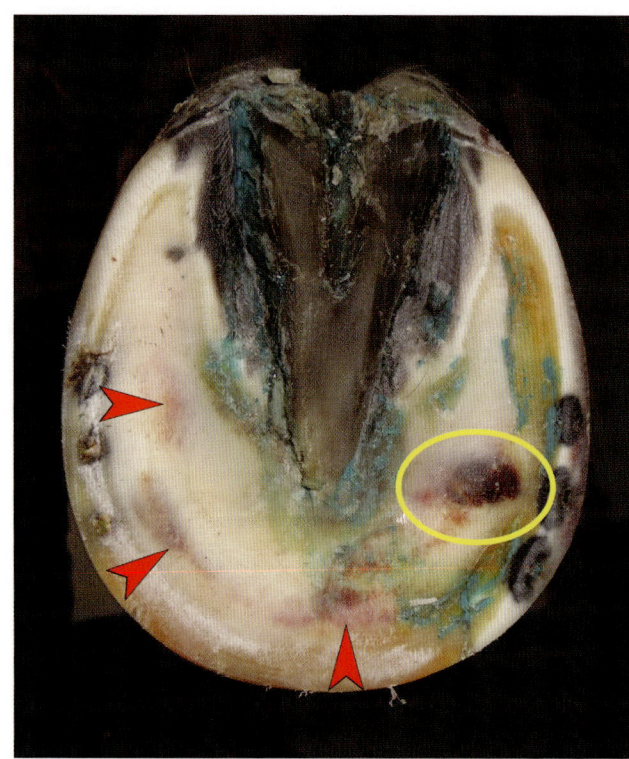

10.23 Sterile abscesses, like the one circled here, are a common consequence of the compromised circulation and bone displacement often seen in laminitis. Notice the bruising of the sole (red arrows), occurring for the same reasons. (Note: Green areas on the bottom of the foot are residue of a packing material that has been removed.)

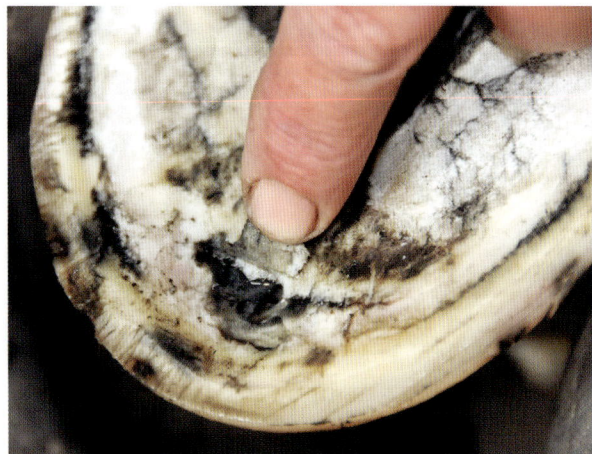

10.22 Like most abscesses, this one was caused by bacteria entering the foot, probably through a fissure in the sole.

path of least resistance until it finds a way out of the foot. If it is not treated, it will eventually rupture, and the pus will then drain out, which usually provides an immediate reduction of pain. Though abscesses typically start at the bottom of the foot, it is quite common for them to erupt through the heel bulbs or the coronet, as these tissues are much softer than the hoof wall and provide an easier exit (fig. 10.24). Sometimes, the pressure and infection can do a fair bit of damage to the laminae or other parts of the hoof along the way, which is why many veterinarians prefer to drain and clean out an abscess, rather than allowing it to mature and break out on its own (fig. 10.25).

The most common point of entry for abscess-forming bacteria is the white line, so anything that weakens or punctures the normally tight connection of the laminae can open the foot up to an increased risk of abscesses. Part of the problem is that a weakened laminar connection will tend to stretch and widen, making it easier for debris and bacteria to get into the hoof. Another issue is that diseased or bruised lamellar tissue creates a welcoming breeding ground for anaerobic bacteria, which can proliferate rapidly in such a warm, moist, protected environment. White line disease, laminitis, and mechanical stresses are therefore all factors that can set the hoof up for the formation of abscesses.

Misplaced shoe nails that go up into or through the sensitive laminae are another common source of introduced bacteria. This is commonly called "quicking," and if your farrier realizes that your horse has been quicked, the nail should be pulled immediately and the wound tract flushed with an antiseptic solution such as Betadine®. Some

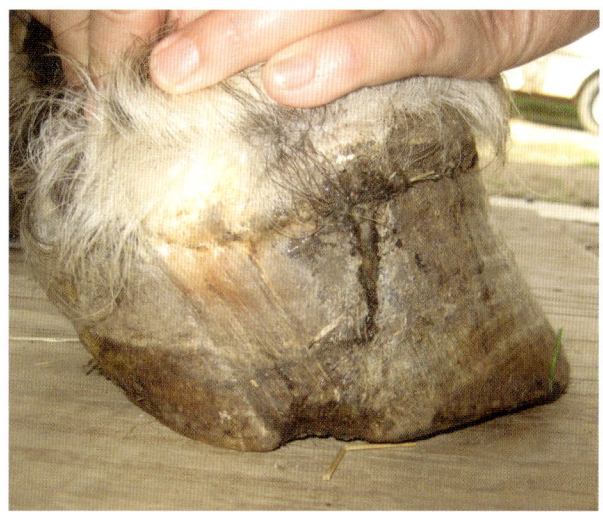

10.24 Many abscesses will migrate upward and break out at the coronet. When they do, pus and exudate will drain from the rupture, as seen here.

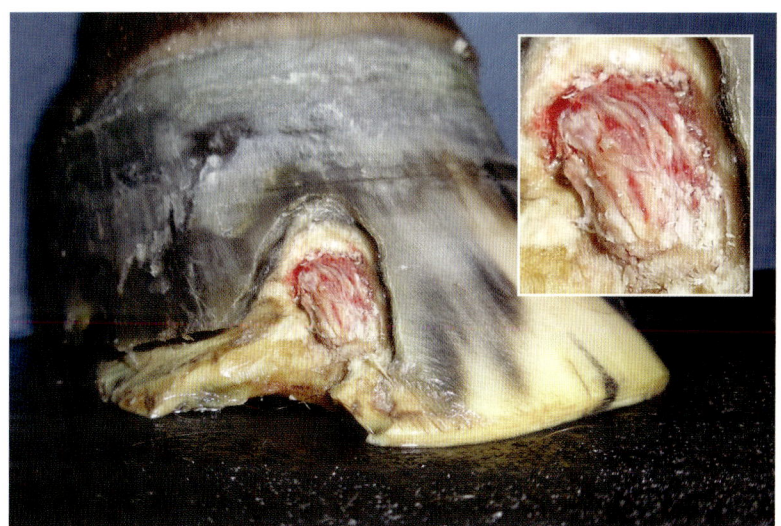

10.25 This migrating abscess had spread out under quite a bit of the hoof wall and caused the dermal laminae (see p. 34) to swell and prolapse (see inset) before the horse was taken to a vet for treatment. In order to access the infection, the separated hoof wall had to be removed, which allowed the vet to use an ultrasonic curette to remove necrotic material without further damaging delicate tissue.

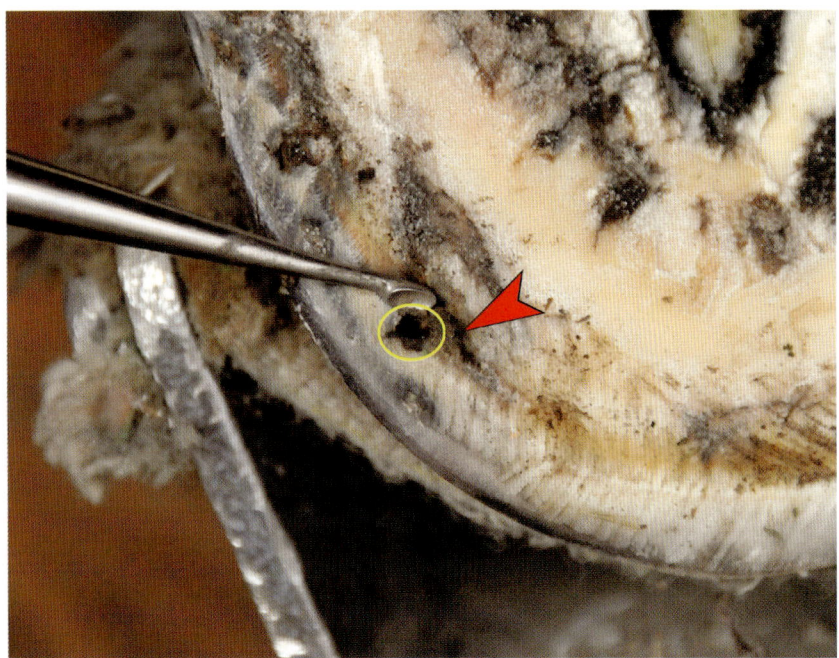

10.26 Shoe nails that get into or too close to the laminae can cause abscesses. The hole in this hoof wall, circled in yellow, is from a nail that went up into the white line (laminae), which caused a small, local abscess (red arrow).

leave the sole more likely to sustain damage if the horse steps on anything hard or sharp. Continual exposure to manure and urine is also damaging to the sole, leaving it weaker and more likely to develop cracks and fissures. Couple this with the fact that these substances create a hotbed of bacteria, and you can see why horses forced to stand in their own waste have a significantly higher risk of developing abscesses.

The sole area under the bars can also end up with both bruising and abscesses when the bars are overgrown and pushing on them (fig. 10.27). Thinning the sole through excessive trimming is another factor that pushes the risk of both bruises

veterinarians additionally advise putting the horse on a short course of broad-spectrum antibiotics as a preventive measure. It is also a good idea to wrap the foot and keep it protected for several days to prevent dirt and bacteria from entering the hole left by the nail. A so-called "close" nail, which means that the nail has not gone into the sensitive laminae but is very close to it, can lead to abscesses, as well. Abscesses caused by close nails tend to develop slowly, taking up to two weeks for symptoms to show (fig. 10.26).

Another common avenue of entry for bacteria is a crack or fissure in the sole. These can develop at any time for a variety of reasons, but are especially likely to occur during prolonged wet weather, or repeated cycles of wet and dry weather. Sole horn is much more porous than wall horn and it becomes relatively soft when wet, so soaking up water can

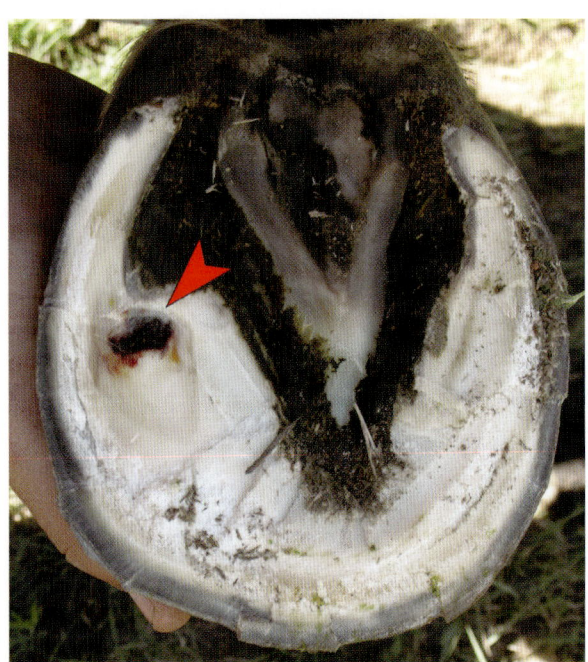

10.27 The abscess on this foot likely started as a bruise, and was caused from an overgrown, laid-over bar that put excessive pressure on the sole. The root cause was likely manmade mediolateral imbalance, as the foot was left too tall on that side.

and abscesses into the stratosphere, and puncture wounds anywhere on the foot are invitations for bacterial invasion and the formation of abscesses (see p. 156).

Abscesses that get into the sole will sometimes build up and fan out between the sensitive and insensitive sole, forming what is called a *subsolar abscess.* This can sometimes cause large portions of the outer layer of the sole to peel away. When this happens, the foot will be very tender, similar to what a person might feel if the outer skin of a large blister peels off. There will also be only the

A Note on
Aggressive Trimming of the Sole and Abscesses

As we have mentioned, some hoof-care professionals have the mistaken idea that paring the sole is the best way to "create" concavity, increase flexibility, and improve hoof mechanism. Whatever their reasoning, aggressive thinning of the sole is seldom appropriate and can be extremely damaging to the foot. Countless horses have suffered bruising, repeated abscesses, and even prolapsed coffin bones due to some well-meaning but badly trained person swiping away with a hoof knife.

Certain barefoot trimmers who were trained to use such methods may even tell their clients that repeated abscessing is a necessary part of the healing process when transitioning a horse out of shoes, and that it is the hoof's way of ridding itself of the toxins that build up in the foot due to shoeing. Please be aware that there is no truth to such statements. An abscess is a bacterial infection, and while the hoof is indeed trying to get rid of the pus that results from the infection, this has nothing

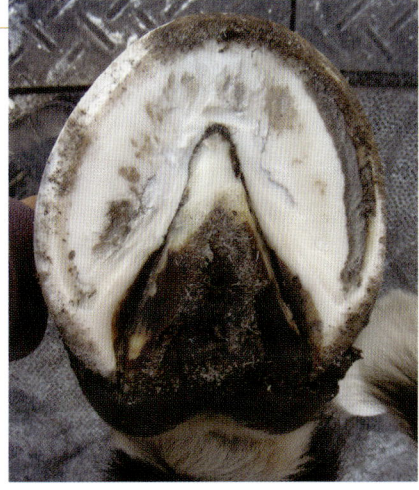

10.28 Paring of the sole (whitish area), for any reason, should be done with caution and expertise, as it can easily lead to a host of problems, including making a horse more vulnerable to abscesses.

whatsoever to do with any buildup of toxins. There is also zero evidence that these alleged toxins even exist, let alone build up as a result of shoeing.

Care should be taken even when merely "cleaning up" the sole, a common practice where hoof-care providers scrape away a thin layer of sole to create a smooth surface or sometimes to gauge the level of the live sole (fig. 10.28). While this practice can be necessary and even beneficial at times, it can be detrimental to horses whose soles are already thin. Many horses are kept unnecessarily "ouchy" due to having that little bit of sole pared away every six weeks.

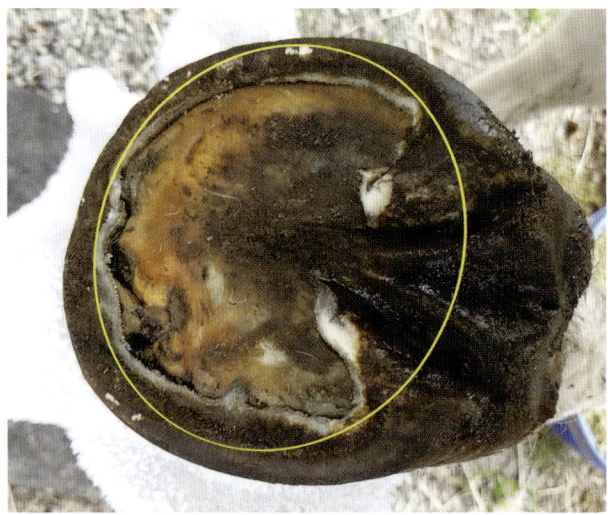

10.29 A broom's bristle that got under the hoof wall of this foot led to a large subsolar abscess, which caused most of the insensitive (outer) sole to peel away in the circled area. What you see here is the new sole beginning to grow in. While the horse was very tender and had to be managed carefully, the prognosis for his recovery was good.

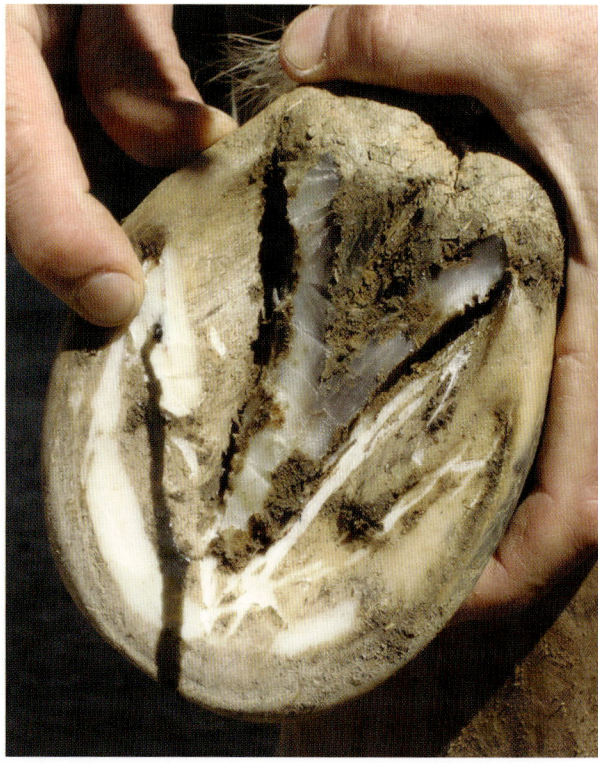

10.30 When an abscess ruptures or is still draining, the gunk that comes out will often be black or grey.

thinnest layer of material between the coffin bone and the rough, dirty world, so to avoid further injury and infection, it is critically important for the hoof be kept clean and protected while the new sole is growing in (fig. 10.29).

Signs, Diagnosis, and Treatment of Abscesses

The most common sign of an abscess is pain, but abscesses can vary in how much pain they cause. Some result in only mild soreness that can easily be missed or taken for something else, but most will cause obvious, and often extreme, pain. When the pain from an abscess is minimal or the animal is particularly stoic (often the case with donkeys), you may not discover the abscess at all until you see evidence that it has broken out. This usually involves

sighting black or grey exudate draining from the rupture (fig. 10.30), but if the drainage stops quickly or gets rubbed or washed off, you may not even see that. In such cases, the only evidence is most often a small horizontal crack or hole growing down in the hoof wall or heel when the eruption occurred in one of these areas.

More often, though, pain from an abscess will be of the "he was perfectly fine yesterday and now he's dead lame" variety. The pain can be so severe that the horse tries to avoid even touching the affected foot to the ground. There may also be heat or swelling, particularly around the coronary band, which may be sensitive to the touch. With more severe abscesses, the swelling can go all the way up to the hock or knee.

In addition to pain, abscesses are often accompanied by an increased digital pulse, which may be stronger on the side of the foot where the abscess is located (see sidebar, p. 175). The increase in the strength of the digital pulse is caused by the disruption of the normal pattern of blood flow within the foot. If you feel a bounding digital pulse and are also observing sudden, dramatic lameness, you might think that your horse has laminitis. However, if you remember that laminitis usually affects both front feet, while an abscess will affect only one, this will point you in the direction of what might be going on.

Still, if your horse is markedly lame, you should get your vet to take a look, as you need to rule out other problems that can have the same presentation. Once it is confirmed that you are dealing with an abscess, your vet will try to pinpoint its location to determine the best course of action. This usually involves a visual examination to find the point of origin as well as the use of hoof testers (see fig. 11.14, p. 177), but X-rays may be necessary in some cases.

Treatment of an abscess is initially aimed at getting it to drain, which is usually fairly easy for vets to accomplish if they have located the spot where the abscess got started. When the tract is in the white line, the vet can open it using a tool such as a thin, narrow loop knife, or a surgical bone curette. Once the tool gets up into the pocket of the abscess, drainage will start and the horse usually feels quite a bit better right away. When the opening is in the sole, your vet or hoof-care professional will pare out a small hole to allow the abscess to drain. It is not necessary to make a large hole, as the continual

pressure and release of the horse walking on the foot will help to expel the exudate. Keeping the hole as small as possible is the best way to preserve sole integrity and minimize the chance of further damage. Flushing of the wound, a process known as *lavage,* can help remove pus and speed healing in some cases, but where damage is more extensive, surgery may be required to remove infected or necrotic tissue (fig. 10.31).

Once drainage is established, it is important to keep the opening clean, so wrapping the foot in a medicated poultice is recommended. There are commercially available poultice products such as Animalintex®, which is moistened in hot water, applied, and left on for approximately 48 hours. Poultices can also be made at home out of cotton bandage materials saturated with a "drawing agent"

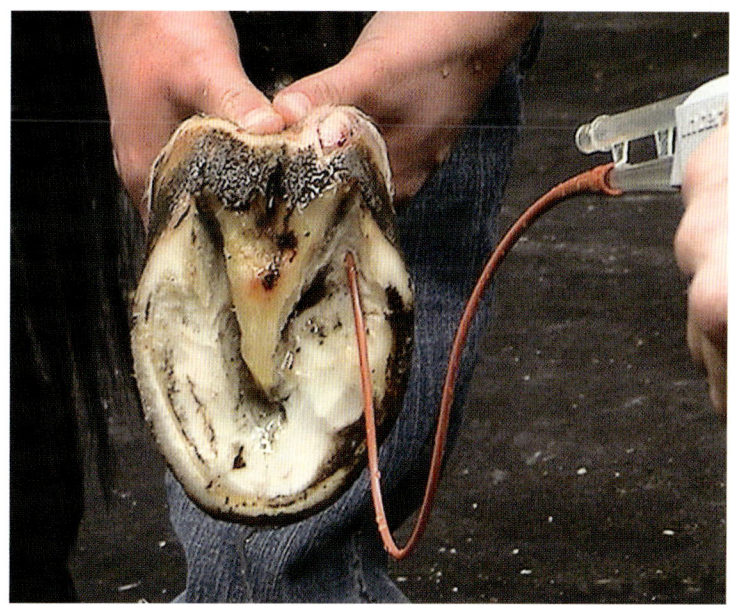

10.31 This abscess, located in the bar area, is being flushed out to remove infected material in the wound track. The fluid is exiting in the heel area.

such as a combination of Epsom salts and Betadine®. Any poultice will need to be covered and held in place with a bandage.

As for soaking of the foot, this time-honored practice has fallen out of favor with many hoof experts. The traditional soak of warm water and Epsom salts was supposed to be done for at least 15 minutes, two to three times a day, for as many days as it took for the abscess to rupture. The purpose of the Epsom soaks was to soften the hoof and "draw out" the abscess, which would supposedly allow the abscess to mature and break out faster. Unfortunately, there is no evidence that abscesses resolve any faster than they would have otherwise as a result of soaking, and in fact, some equine podiatry experts say it can actually slow the healing process and prolong the horse's pain. What happens is that horn material expands as it absorbs water, which can choke off the draining tract of an abscess, trapping the exudate inside the abscess. As an abscess needs to drain and dry out to heal, anything that

keeps it wet and prevents drainage is detrimental. In addition, repeated soaking is known to be damaging to both hoof and sole horn, and may cause widening of the white line, allowing more harmful organisms to invade the sole-wall juncture.

Critics of repeated soaking only recommend it as a short-term application to soften a very hard foot in order to make it possible to pare the sole or frog to create a drainage channel. They also emphasize that the fastest way to relieve the often excruciating pain caused by an abscess is to open it up and drain it, which can usually be accomplished very quickly by a skilled veterinarian or hoof-care professional (fig. 10.32). Leaving the horse in pain for days and doing nothing but soaking the foot is, in their opinion, allowing unnecessary suffering.

Finally, they argue that abscesses not drained therapeutically are more likely to migrate up under the hoof wall and exit at the coronary band, which can potentially cause a permanent disorganization of the horn tubules that grow from that area. While most abscesses that pop out at the coronet don't cause a permanent problem, it does happen, and it can leave the horse with a weakened hoof wall more vulnerable to cracking or splitting in the future. Even worse, a migrating abscess can move deep into the foot where it may damage the internal structures, possibly leading to permanent lameness.

Of course, there will always be people telling you that they soaked their horse's foot and the abscess popped out the very same day without issues, but as they have no way of knowing whether or not the abscess would have ruptured that day on its own, they cannot say that the maturing of the abscess was the result of the soaking. Every horse owner has to decide who to listen to when it comes to treating

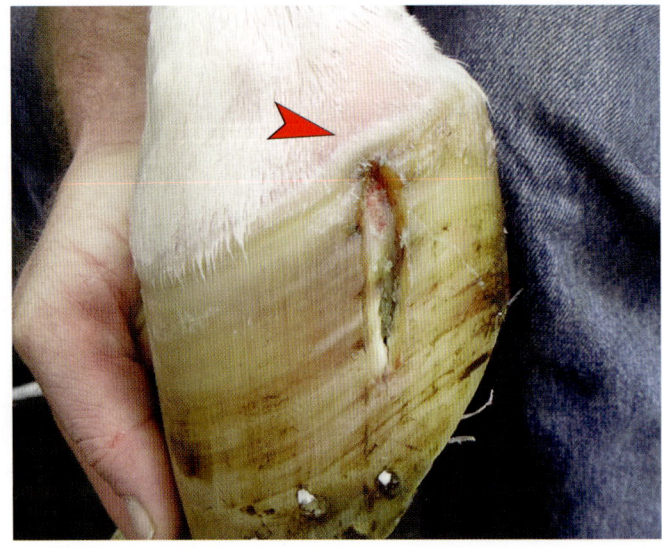

10.32 Before being opened to drain by a veterinarian, this abscess was very painful, as you can imagine from the swelling, redness, and distortion of the coronet.

10.33 When an abscess causes the loss of a large portion of hoof wall, as seen here, it is worth getting your hoof-care provider or vet to take a look at it to see if it needs any special treatment or support.

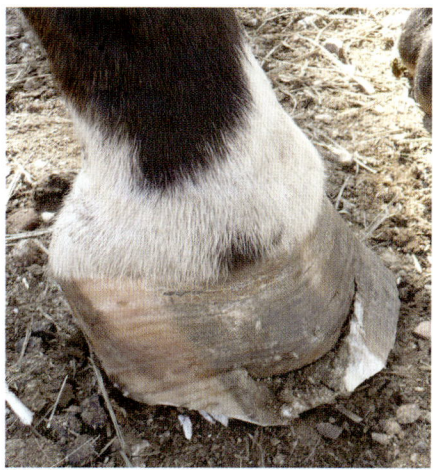

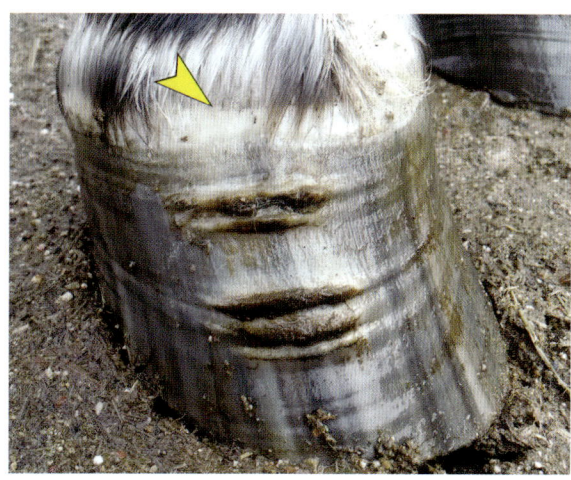

their horse's ailments, but it is always wise to at least consider the science—or lack thereof—before choosing a course of action.

One adjunct to treatment that almost everyone agrees on is giving a horse with an abscess a tetanus shot. Even if your horse has had a regular tetanus shot within the past year or so, your vet will likely recommend a booster to maximize your horse's resistance to the potentially fatal *Clostridium tetanii* bacteria, which is widespread in the soil of just about every environment your horse is likely to be in. Secondary tetanus infection is a real risk when your horse has an opening in the foot, so best not to take any chances with this easily pre-ventable problem.

Once an abscess has drained and healed, the hoof may be left with a crack or hole in the wall, sole, or heel. Most of the time, these will simply grow out and disappear, leaving no lasting damage. However, it is true that in some instances, abscesses that rupture at the coronet will change the way the tubules grow at that point, in which case you will need to keep an eye on the wall and be proactive about managing any tendency it has to crack. The good news is that not all disrupted tubules will cause cracking—some are really just a blemish that will not affect the foot at all. Another possible aftereffect of an abscess, as we mentioned in the

10.34 This horse suffered from chronic white line disease, which led to repeated bouts of abscessing. It is likely that there is permanent damage to the area of the coronet (yellow arrow) where the abscesses keep breaking out, making that the path of least resistance every time another abscess gets started. This is why the blow-out cracks you see in the wall are all lined up. As for the pronounced growth rings, each one is a sign that the foot was experiencing inflammation at the time, so it is not surprising that the blowouts correspond with the rings, as abscesses can cause tremendous inflammation in the foot.

cracks section, is that the wall below the blowout may chunk off. While usually not a problem, this can be pretty dramatic in some cases and may require some attention from your hoof-care provider or veterinarian (fig. 10.33).

If your horse is having repeated abscessing, especially in the same foot, it is time to have a dis-cussion with your veterinarian. Random abscesses can happen to any horse, but frequent abscessing is abnormal. If the abscessing is affecting different feet, there may be a metabolic problem or systemic infection afflicting your horse, or if the abscessing keeps occurring in the same foot, there may be a foreign object lodged in there or an infection that is not healing. White line disease can also lead to repeated abscessing, in one or more feet (fig. 10.34). Frequent abscessing can lead to permanent damage

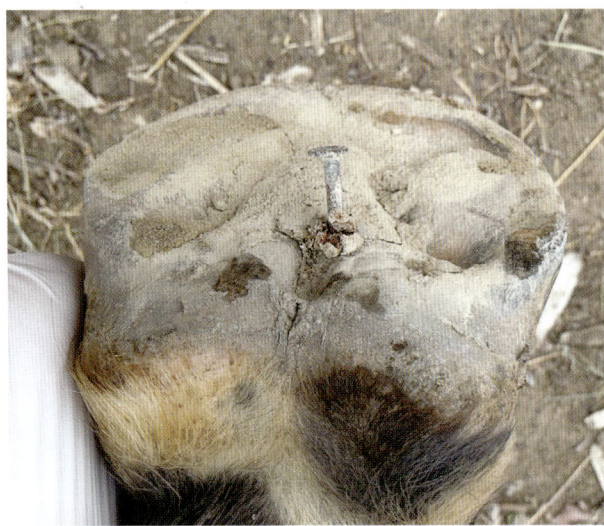

10.35 Finding a penetrating object in the foot is definitely alarming, but at least it gives you the chance to take appropriate measures right away. When a "stealth" puncture occurs without there being any way to really know it happened, it can sometimes end up being worse.

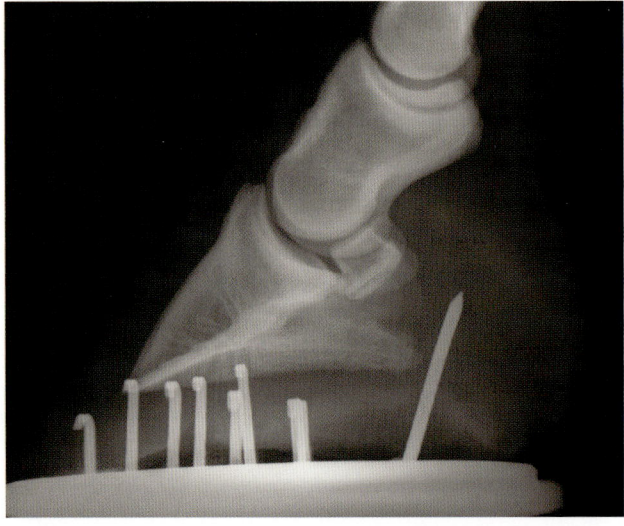

10.36 Deep puncture wounds in the heel or frog area can cause serious problems, as there are so many sensitive structures in this area of the foot. This horse was extremely lucky, as the deeply embedded nail managed to miss all of the critical structures.

of the coffin bone, so it is in your horse's best interest for you and your veterinarian to determine the cause of repeated abscessing and eradicate it.

Puncture Wounds

When it comes to puncture wounds of the hoof, some are obvious and easy to find, with the horse suddenly coming up lame and an examination of the foot turning up something sharp poking into the solar surface (fig. 10.35). Unfortunately, we sometimes don't know a horse has had a puncture in the foot until well after the fact. There may be no visible object to find, and the tract where penetration occurred often closes up quickly once the horse steps off or shakes loose whatever caused the injury. The problem with such "stealth" punctures is

that any object that has penetrated into the foot can cause infection, and depending on what structures are involved, these infections can quickly become dangerous and very difficult to treat.

Deep puncture wounds are divided into three categories depending on where in the foot they are and what structures are affected. Type I wounds are located in the sole and may have caused damage to the solar corium and coffin bone. Type II wounds are found in the frog or heels, and because so many important structures are located just above the frog, these injuries can be extremely serious (fig. 10.36). Structures affected by Type II puncture wounds may include the navicular bursa, the DDFT, the sheath of the digital flexor tendon, the impar ligament, the navicular bone, the coffin bone, the coffin joint, and the digital cushion. Type III injuries are less common and involve punctures of the coronary band. Damage from Type III wounds may involve the coffin bone, lateral cartilages, or the coffin joint. All three types of wounds can easily become septic and cause catastrophic damage to the internal structures of the foot.

If the infection walls off and forms an abscess, it is often very painful but not always a big problem. However, if the object has penetrated into any of the synovial structures located under the frog (such as the navicular bursa, coffin joint, or DDFT sheath) or into the bones of the foot, you have an extremely serious situation on your hands, as sepsis is a very real possibility. Infection in the interior structures of the foot can cause permanent damage that may result in irreversible lameness, and in some cases, the horse's pain is so bad that euthanasia is the only humane option.

The best way to try to prevent a puncture wound from becoming a dire problem is to get your vet involved immediately. Even if the puncture looks minor, you should still call your vet, as infection can develop without any signs until the problem is well established. People often make the mistake of pulling out a penetrating object and thinking all is well because the horse seems better right away, then a few days later the horse goes lame and the foot is already septic. It is always better to be safe rather than sorry with puncture wounds, so get the vet on the phone as soon as possible and describe what you are seeing. If you can take pictures and send them to the vet right away, that will be helpful and will provide your vet with important information so that he or she can advise you how to proceed.

When you find the horse with the penetrating object still in place, most vets will recommend that you *not* remove it, as they want a chance to examine it and possibly X-ray it while it is still in the foot. In some instances, they may want to perform an MRI to get a better look. Whether your vet wants to do X-rays or an MRI, diagnostic imaging is truly worthwhile when it comes to puncture wounds, as it allows the vet to see exactly where and how deep the object has penetrated, and whether or not any underlying structures are involved.

If you are leaving a penetrating object in place until the vet comes, you should try to stabilize the object to prevent it from being pushed farther into the foot. This can often be accomplished by wrapping the foot with some sort of bandaging but maintaining a space around the object. If the object is on the bottom of the foot, taping a roll of duct tape—or something similar—to the foot so that the object is in the center of the roll can work in some instances, though you may have to come up with some other creative solution (fig. 10.37).

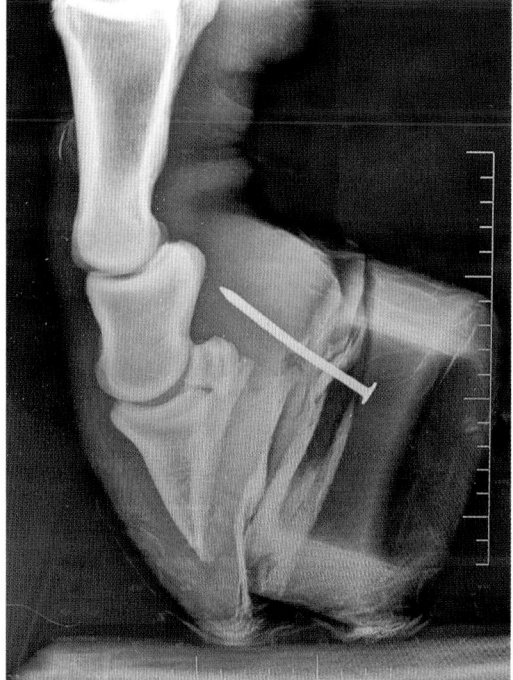

10.37 The owner of this horse taped a roll of duct tape to the bottom of the foot, preventing the nail from being driven in deeper. The vet left the roll on during the X-ray process, so it is visible in the radiograph. While the nail did some damage to the sheath of the deep digital flexor tendon, the horse was treated with antibiotics and anti-inflammatories and recovered completely.

Keep the horse in a clean, dry area, and encourage him to remain as quiet as possible until help arrives. If the vet cannot get to you within an hour or so, or you think the object will get pushed in deeper if you leave it in place, it might be necessary to remove it. Again, getting photos to your vet would be the best way to get advice in this circumstance. If you do remove the object, draw a circle around the spot where it penetrated before you pull the thing out, as the tract may close up and be hard to find afterward, especially if it is in the soft, elastic tissues of the frog. Try to make note of the angle of penetration (take pictures if possible), and make sure to keep the object to show the vet.

Should you see something that you suspect could be a puncture but there is no visible object in the wound, you should still call the vet and mark the spot you are seeing. As long as the vet can find the spot, it is often possible to use a sterile probe or contrast dye in conjunction with X-rays to figure out the depth and direction of the tract the object left

behind. Keep in mind that punctures don't always look like a hole; they may appear to be a crack or fissure, often black in color.

Oftentimes, however, there will be nothing to see on the foot itself, and the puncture will only be discovered through signs of pain and/or infection. These may include:

• Sudden onset of lameness, which can be mild or severe. Sometimes, initial lameness does not last very long, but returns within a few days and likely continue to get worse. Wounds that have punctured through the corium or deeper are usually quite painful soon after the foot is injured.

• Gradual onset of lameness that gets progressively worse over several days, which in the case of a puncture wound is a sign that infection is developing.

• An increased digital pulse that may be stronger on the side of the leg where the wound is.

• Heat in the foot or around the coronet.

• Sensitivity to pressure applied to the sole, often only around the spot of injury early on, but this may spread to the whole sole as infection takes hold.

• Favoring part of the foot.

• Standing with the injured foot forward.

• Swelling in the lower limb above the foot.

Treatment for a puncture wound depends on the scope of the problem. If no critical structures have been damaged, treatment is not particularly complicated and full recovery is highly likely. Your

10.38 Hospital plates are removable covers (right) that fit onto a horse shoe to protect an injured foot but also allow access to the wound for continued treatment. They can be used with a plastic pad (left) cut out as necessary to expose only the area that needs attention.

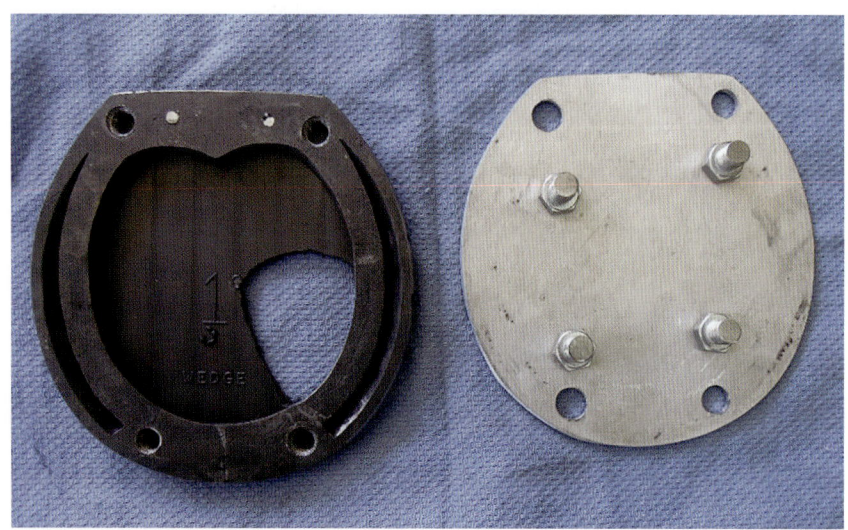

vet will thoroughly clean the surface area of the wound with antiseptic solution, and may perform additional procedures such as *lavage, debridement* (removing damaged or infected tissue), and opening of the wound to allow drainage. A tetanus injection will likely be administered, and the vet may take a sample from the wound to culture, as knowing what types of infectious organisms are present will help in the choice of antibiotics, should they be used.

The foot will then be covered to protect the wound from contact with contaminants. A bandage covered with multiple layers of duct tape on the sole works well as long as you stay on top of it to make sure the duct tape isn't wearing through. Other options include hoof boots over a wrapped foot or removable "hospital plates" added to shoes (fig. 10.38). Bandages will likely need to be changed several times or more, depending on the length of time your vet wants the foot to stay protected.

When internal structures are involved, treatment is likely to be intensive—more so if sepsis has already set in. Surgery may be required to gain access to the area and clean out damaged and infected tissue, and powerful antibiotics will be necessary, likely for a long course (figs. 10.39 A & B). Prognosis will range from good to grim, as some parts of the foot are more likely to recover from

10.39 A & B This Type I puncture wound penetrated into the coffin bone and became terribly infected due to inadequate treatment. The horse was eventually brought to a different veterinarian who opened up the foot and cleaned out all the infected material, then put the horse on a long course of strong antibiotics. The pink area in the inset in A is the coffin bone, and the red dot in the center of that is where the foreign body penetrated the bone. Photo B is an X-ray of the foot, showing how large an area had to be surgically removed (circled) to get to the deep infection inside the foot. Fortunately, damage to the bone was minimal.

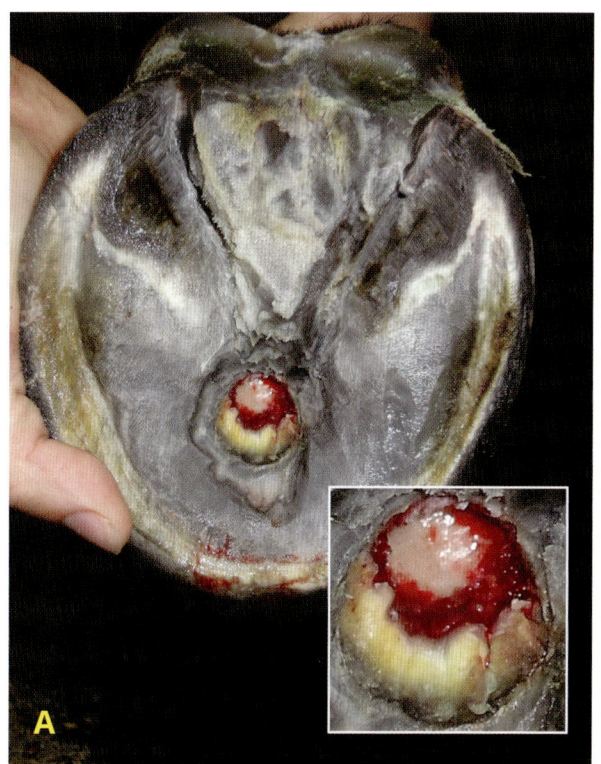

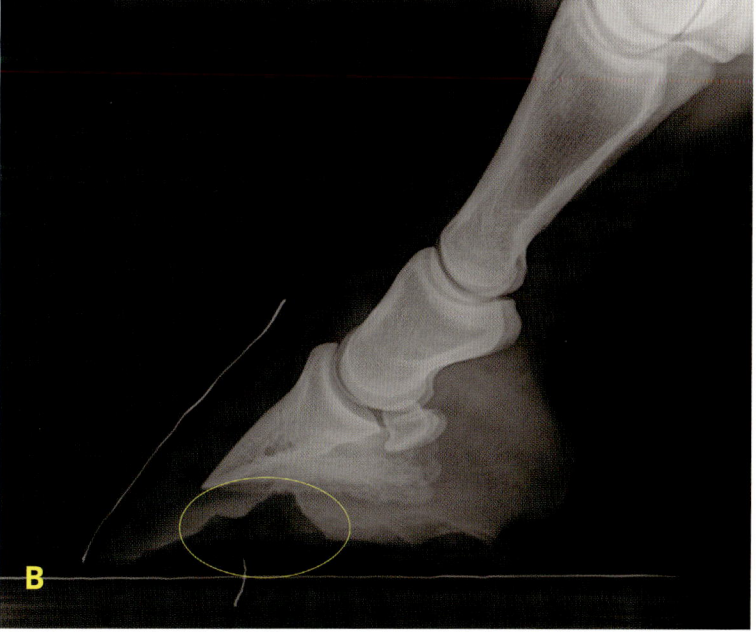

infection than others. If the coffin joint or navicular bursa is involved, the prognosis will be guarded, but the earlier treatment begins, the better the outcome is likely to be.

Wounds that do not appear to be healing need further diagnostic imaging, as problems like *septic pedal osteitis* (infection of the solar margin of the coffin bone) and the formation of *sequestrum* (separated pieces of dead bone) can take weeks to show up (fig. 10.40). When these problems occur, surgery is necessary to remove the necrotic bone tissue, but whether or not this is possible will be determined by what part of the bone has been affected and the extent of damage. If the bone is too far gone in a critical area, the horse may have to be put down.

Truly, any known or possible puncture wound should be evaluated by a veterinarian—not a far-rier—as soon as possible, as only a vet can perform the diagnostic procedures and treatment necessary to keep a deep puncture wound from potentially becoming a disaster. Remember that a very dangerous wound might not look like much at all, so please, play it safe with foot punctures.

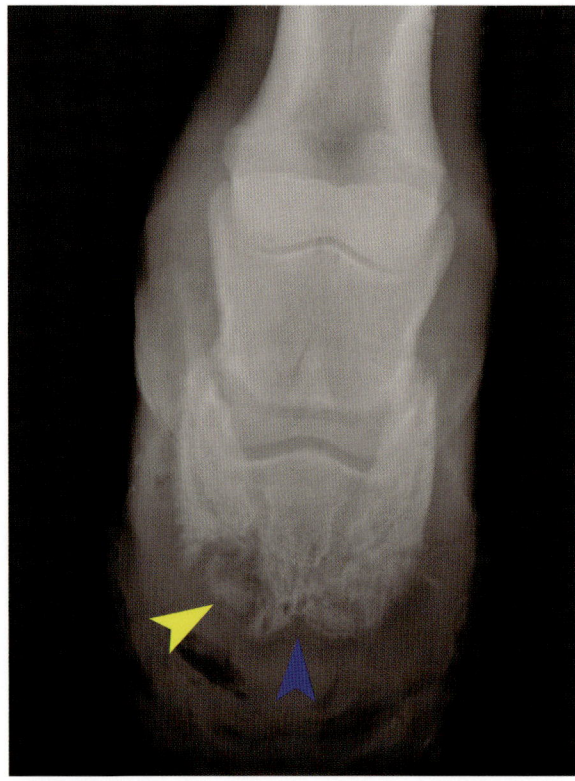

10.40 A puncture wound to this foot caused septic pedal osteitis (see p. 226), which resulted in bone loss that makes the solar margin of this coffin bone appear darker, ragged, and more porous (blue arrow) on an X-ray. The infection eating away at the bone has also caused a piece of bone to break off (yellow arrow). This sequestrum, as dead bone is called, needs to be removed or it will cause chronic problems.

Section Three:

Disease Processes Inside the Foot

Because our eyes can only see the *outside* of the horse's foot, the incredibly complex system of structures and processes *inside* the foot is usually not front-and-center in our minds. However, when disease strikes the interior of the hoof, the consequences can be devastating, and those hidden structures and processes will suddenly demand our attention in a big, bad way. In this section, we'll take a look at the most commonly encountered diseases that affect the inside of the foot so that you can be ahead of the curve when it comes to recognizing and treating these problems, and hopefully preventing them from striking your own horse in the first place.

We'll start off with an in-depth look at the dreaded but frequently preventable disease of laminitis, then examine the collection of palmar foot pain conditions often referred to as "navicular syndrome" or "navicular disease." We'll finish up with an overview of sidebone, ringbone, and pedal osteitis. This material gets a bit deep at times, but the information can be life-saving.

Laminitis/"Founder"

Laminitis is the most serious disease of the equine foot and is considered the second biggest killer of horses after colic. Though it can be excruciatingly painful, it isn't actually the disease itself that kills horses. Rather, because the damage laminitis causes can cause catastrophic lameness, horses often end up having to be euthanized when treatment is unsuccessful. Fortunately, better diagnostics, advances in treatment, and a deeper understanding of the disease itself have brought new hope for horses suffering from laminitis, and it is now possible to rehabilitate many of them that in the past would have been considered beyond hope.

What Happens in Laminitis: A Quick Overview

Laminitis can affect all four feet, but it is much more commonly observed in the front hooves, possibly due to the differences in weight bearing between the front and hind limbs. The disease begins when one or more of many possible trigger factors damage the basement membrane that bonds the dermal and epidermal laminae together, compromising their attachment. If the disruption is bad enough, the basement membrane will be destroyed, along with the capillaries that pass through it and the laminae themselves. The laminae then "unzip," and the bone separates from the hoof capsule (figs. 11.1 A & B).

Laminitis vs. Founder

People often use the terms "laminitis" and "founder" to mean the same thing, but founder actually refers only to chronic cases of laminitis in which the coffin bone has become displaced within the hoof capsule. A horse with a mild case of laminitis may never progress to founder.

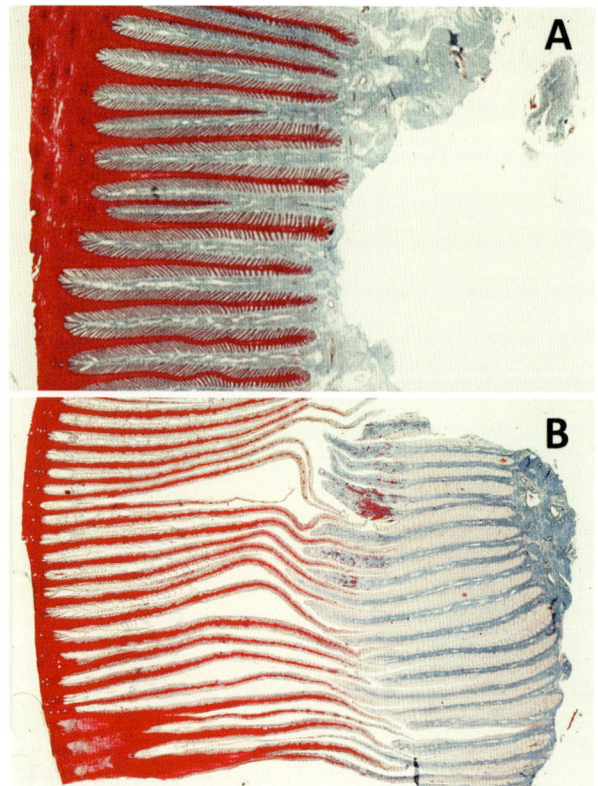

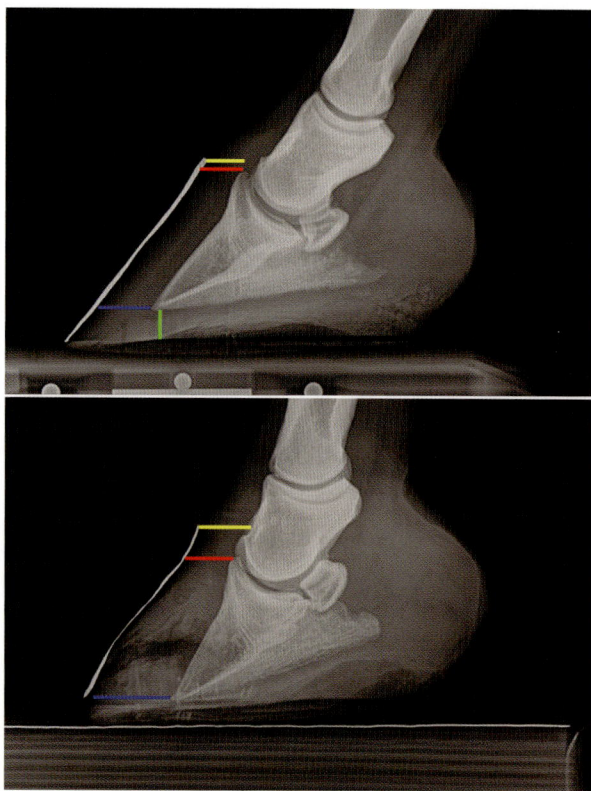

11.1 A & B Healthy laminae are interlocked and tightly bonded (A), but when laminitis strikes, they can become extremely damaged and separate (B). (Note: The blue and red colors seen here are two different stains the researchers used to differentiate the dermal [blue] from the epidermal [red] laminae.)

11.2 There are several difference to note between this normal foot (above) and the foundered foot (below): 1) In the normal foot, the width of the space between the red and blue lines is fairly consistent, as the wall is strongly attached. In the foundered foot, the space is much wider at the bottom due to rotation of the coffin bone. 2) In the normal foot, the distance between the coronet (yellow line), and the top of the extensor process (red line), is very small. When the coffin bone "sinks" in relation to the hoof capsule as it has in this foundered foot, this distance gets greater. 3) The normal foot has a reasonable amount of sole under the tip of the bone (green line), while the foundered foot has none, as the bone is actually penetrating the sole.

Further damage occurs when the coffin bone, no longer anchored to the wall, moves within the hoof capsule. This movement is called *displacement*, and it can take two forms: 1) *rotation*, and 2) *distal descent*, commonly known as "sinking." *Rotation* means that the tip of the coffin bone has moved downward and away relative to the hoof wall. Depending on whom you listen to, rotation is due to either the horse's weight pushing against the ground and displacing the loosened hoof capsule, or the pull of the deep digital flexor tendon, or both, with the latter taking place after the former. *Distal descent* means that the entire bone has moved downward relative to the hoof capsule. Rotation and distal descent are not at all mutually exclusive, as "sinkers" will typically also have rotation (fig. 11.2).

Whatever form of displacement takes place, it wreaks havoc inside the foot. As the coffin bone moves in relation to the hoof capsule, it destroys blood vessels, alters blood flow, wrenches the tissues of the coronary band, pushes on the digital cushion, and crushes into the solar corium. All of this can cause intense pain and lameness, the degree of which will depend on the extent of the damage. Left uncorrected, displacement causes a cascade of problems that can lead to severe and sometimes permanent lameness. Learning to spot early symptoms of laminitis is therefore critical, as early, appropriate intervention is your best chance at minimizing damage inside the foot.

Unfortunately, recognizing laminitis is not always that easy. Most of us think of laminitis appearing quickly and dramatically, a situation called *acute laminitis*. The disease certainly can, and often does, show up this way, but that is not always the case. Horses can also suffer from ongoing or repeated episodes of *subclinical laminitis* in which symptoms may be absent, overlooked, or mistaken for something else. This insidious problem is much more common than people realize and is usually the result of a diet too high in sugars and/or starches, sometimes in combination with an undiagnosed metabolic disorder. Such horses do not present with sudden, obvious lameness, but may instead have intermittent or continual problems such as flaring, white line disease, thin soles, flat soles, tender-footedness, shortness of stride, or a general lack of forwardness that often gets labeled as laziness (fig. 11.3).

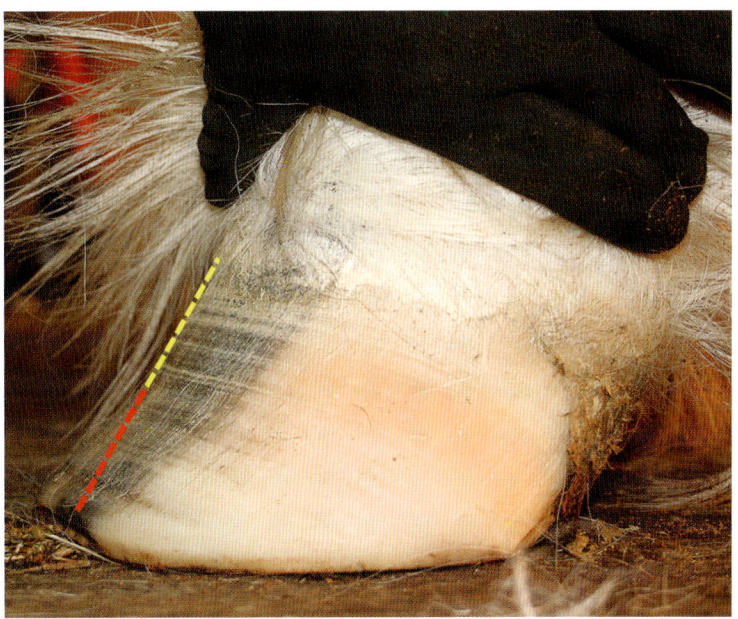

11.3 Flaring can be due to overgrowth and mechanical leverage, but it can also be a sign of subclinical laminitis that often goes unrecognized. In this foot, everything to the left of the dotted line is flare. You can see that the flaring starts at the level where the line turns red.

Whether the onset of laminitis is acute or subclinical, it can have serious consequences for the horse, especially if appropriate steps are not taken to address the needs of the hoof and eliminate the factors that brought on the laminitis in the first place. Too often, treatment of laminitic horses fails because necessary changes to diet and other contributing factors are not implemented. Successful treatment of laminitis requires more than just good hoof care—it requires a thoughtful and thorough examination of management practices, especially diet, as well as a detailed understanding of where your horse is in the recovery process at any given time. The best treatment plan will be a reflection of what is going on, how long it has been going on, and why it happened in the first place.

Delving Deeper:
Phalangeal Rotation vs. Capsular Rotation

When the tip of the coffin bone moves downward and away relative to the hoof wall, most people will say that this is the result of rotation of the bone itself. While this is true in some cases, it is not what is going on in many others. Very commonly, the coffin bone maintains its alignment with the bones above it, meaning it has not rotated downward at all. Instead, it is the hoof capsule that has rotated upward in relation to the bone. This scenario is most correctly referred to as *capsular rotation*.

True rotation of the coffin bone, called *phalangeal rotation* or *digital rotation*, occurs when the coffin bone actually does rotate out of alignment with the bones above it. This is thought to occur from the continual pull of the deep digital flexor tendon, possibly made more intense by muscle contraction in response to pain. The distinction between the two types of rotation is thought to be important by many hoof care experts, as they have found that cases of capsular rotation are often easier to rehabilitate than true phalangeal rotation (fig. 11.4).

It should be noted, however, that because the coffin joint does have some natural mobility, the way the horse is standing or tensing his muscles can change the angle of the bones, so care must be taken when

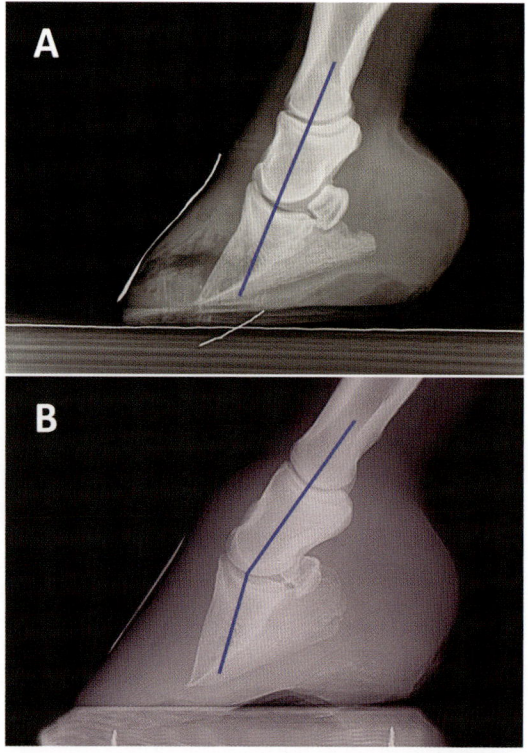

11.4 When a hoof has capsular rotation, the coffin bone maintains alignment with the bones above it (A). When the hoof has phalangeal rotation, the coffin bone has a broken-forward angle in relation to the bones above (B). Notice how straight the blue line that runs down the center of the bones is in X-ray A, and how that line takes on an angle in X-ray B.

taking and interpreting X-rays to get an accurate picture of what is going on inside the foot. If the cannon bone is not upright when the image is taken, for example, the angle of the bones will not read correctly.

Known Triggers of Laminitis

The saddest thing about laminitis is that in the majority of cases, it is a manmade disease caused by management and feeding practices that are not in line with the natural requirements of equine physiology. Unfortunately, many horse owners simply don't have enough information to avoid the practices that can lead to laminitis. Let's make sure you *do* have that information, starting with a look at common triggers that can cause the disease:

• *Diets high in starches and sugars*: The ingestion of significant amounts of non-structural carbohydrates (simple sugars and starch) can cause systemic inflammation in the horse, just as it can in people. Sometimes, that inflammation leads to laminitis. Horses that eat significant amounts of grain, hay that is high in sugars or starch, or pasture high in sugars or starch are therefore at increased risk for laminitis (see *Feeding the Foot*, p. 238) This is especially true for "easy keepers," obese horses, or those who have a metabolic disorder. Breeds that evolved to get by on sparse or poor quality forage should be assumed to be high risk, even if they are not overweight. These include Andalusians, Arabians, Paso Finos, Morgans, Tennessee Walkers, Mustangs, ponies of any breed, and donkeys (figs. 11.5 A & B).

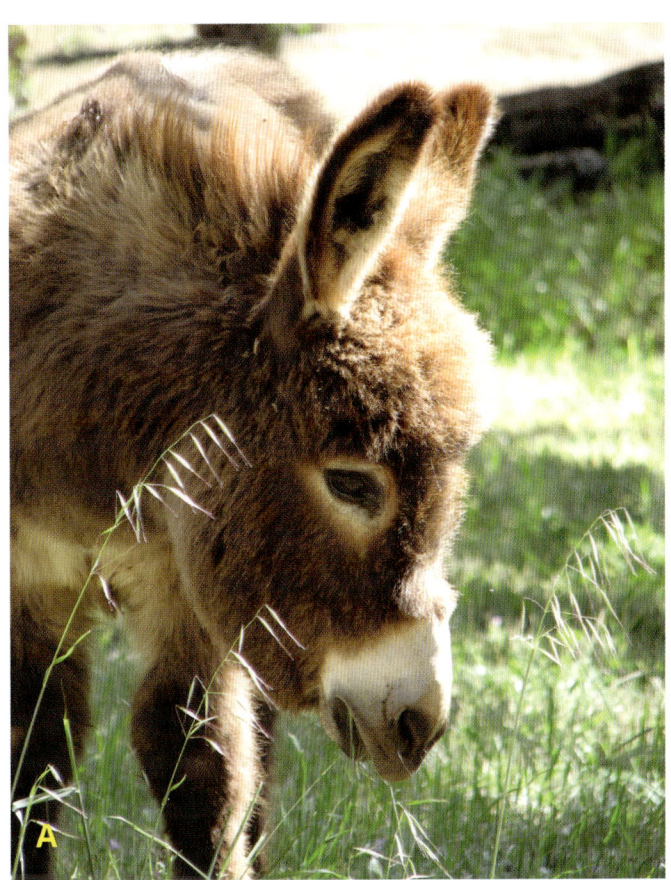

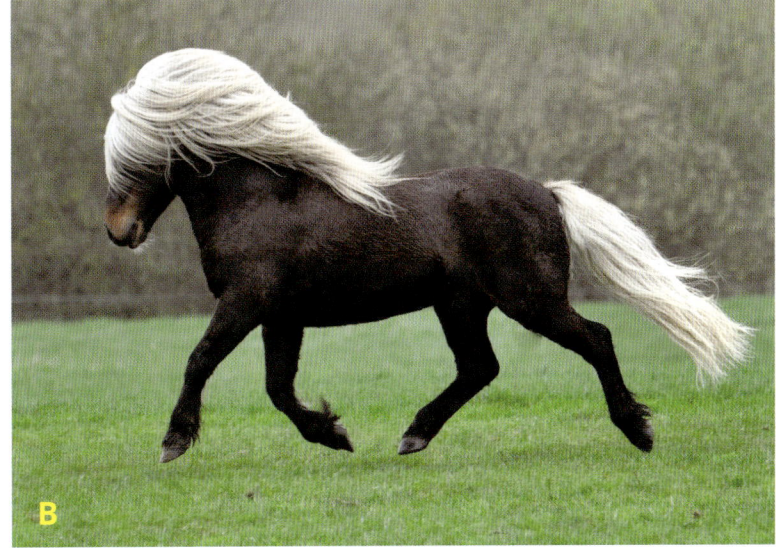

11.5 A & B Easy-keeper equines, including all ponies and donkeys (A), are especially prone to obesity and laminitis, so extra care must be taken with their diets. The handsome Shetland pony stallion Silbersee Luxux (B) is an excellent example of how fit and trim a pony can be when given a proper diet and plenty of exercise.

• *Sudden consumption of a large amount of starch or sugar*: Carbohydrate overload—the classic "horse got into the grain bin" scenario—has long been known to cause laminitis. What happens is that undigested soluble carbohydrates (sugars) reach the horse's hindgut where they rapidly ferment, resulting in a buildup of lactic acid. The horse's hindgut is not designed to handle much lactic acid, so this causes a dramatic decrease in pH. The newly acidic environment promotes an overgrowth of certain exotoxin-producing bacteria, along with the lysis

(bursting) of other bacteria, which releases endotoxins from their cell walls. The lining of the hindgut gets damaged by the lactic acid and becomes "leaky," allowing the bacterial toxins to circulate throughout the body. The exact mechanism by which this causes laminitis is still being studied, but the toxins appear to induce activation of very large amounts of metalloproteinases MMPs—those enzymes that tell the laminae to "let go" (see p. 36)

• *Non-carbohydrate-related gastrointestinal distress*: It is not unusual for problems like colic and colitis to be followed by episodes of laminitis. Different gastrointestinal issues may initiate laminitis through different pathways, but secondary laminitis should be considered a possibility when dealing with any such problems.

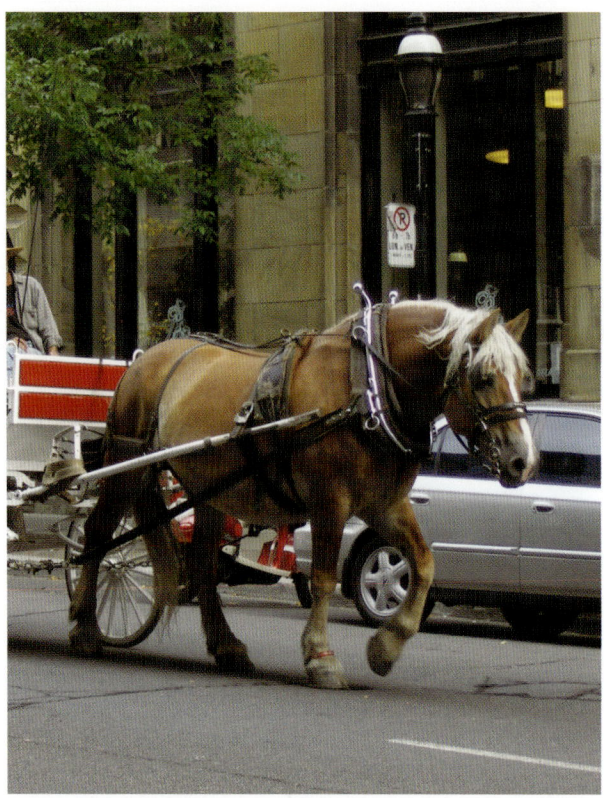

11.6 Healthy hooves can withstand quite a bit of pounding, but working a horse too fast or too long on hard surfaces without protective pads or boots can lead to road founder. Carriage horses like this one often have anti-concussion pads under their shoes to prevent this problem.

• *Mechanical laminitis, aka "road founder"*: Working on hard surfaces exposes the hoof wall and the laminae to tremendous amounts of concussion, which is magnified if the other parts of the foot meant to share in weight bearing are lifted off the ground by peripheral loading or contraction. When the laminae are forced to bear more load than they are designed to handle, inflammation, damage to the blood vessels, and separation can occur. However, a strong, healthy, correctly functioning foot can withstand a fair amount of pounding without ill effects, so if a horse gets road founder, it is possible that some kind of compromise was already in play (fig. 11.6).

• *Insulin related*: Horses with disorders like Equine Metabolic Syndrome, insulin resistance, and Cushing's Syndrome (also called Cushing's Disease or Pituitary Pars Intermediary Dysfunction or PPID) are highly susceptible to laminitis. One reason for this may be that these horses often have unusually high

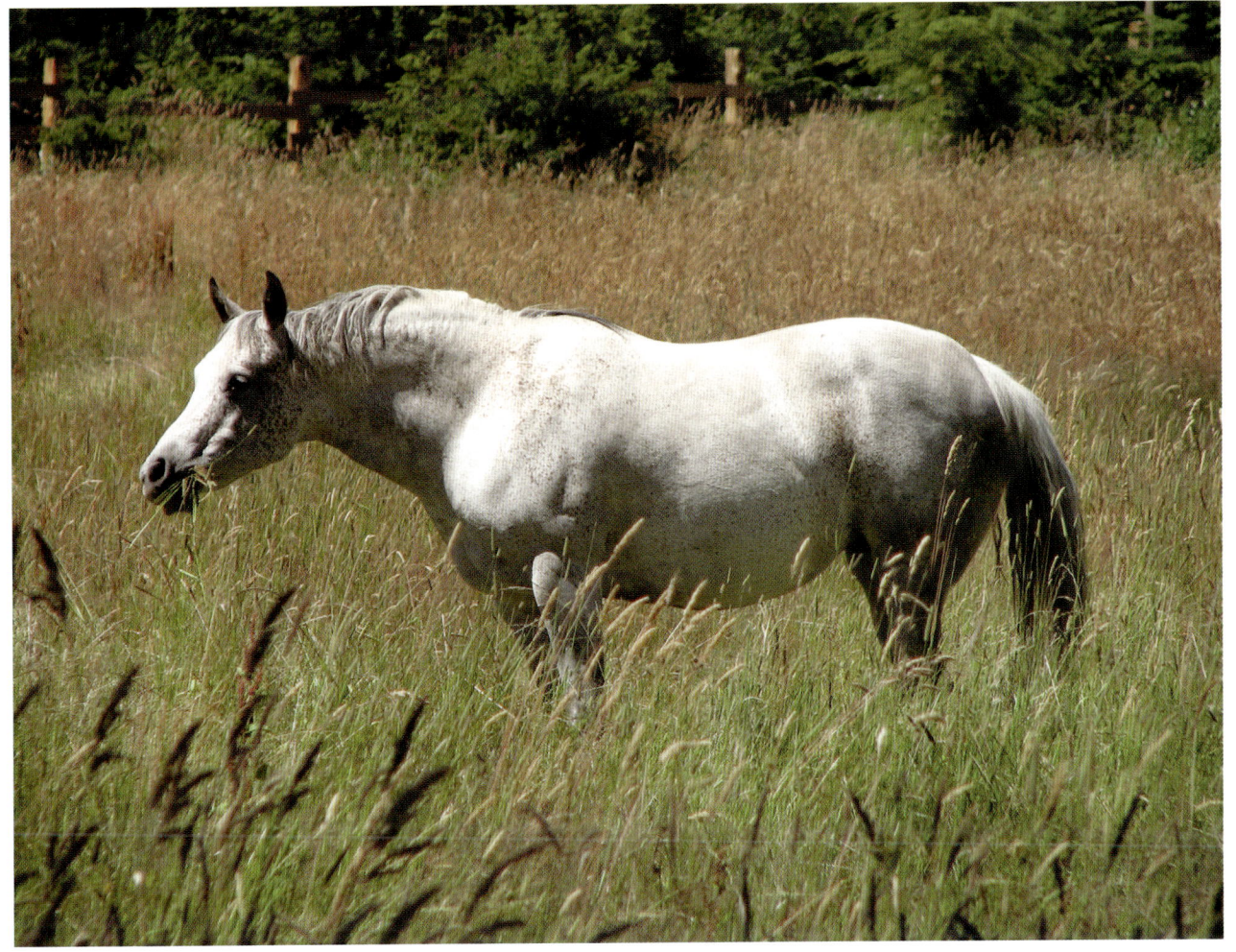

11.7 This obese horse has the classic signs of insulin resistance: a thick, "cresty" neck and patchy pads of fat around the tail head and on other parts of the body. Allowing such a horse to graze freely is almost guaranteed to cause laminitis.

levels of insulin, a condition called *hyperinsulinemia*, which has been shown to induce laminitis, particularly when blood plasma levels of insulin are more than 100 µIU/ml. Normal range is 8 to 30 µIU /ml. These horses may also have trouble regulating cortisol, which can be a factor as well. Horses with metabolic issues should, therefore, be closely monitored and fed a diet low in sugars and starches. Usually, this means keeping them off grass entirely, as grass is too likely to cause a problem for them (fig. 11.7).

• *Seasonal hormonal changes:* Cushing's Syndrome is an endocrine system disorder in which the pituitary gland and adrenal gland can't communicate properly. This causes an overgrowth of cells in the *pars intermedia* area of the pituitary gland. The result is abnormally high production of many pituitary hormones, including adrenocorticotropic hormone (ACTH), which regulates levels of cortisol in the body. Horses with PPID have a problem regulating cortisol, which can cause laminitis at any time of year, but they are especially vulnerable in the fall, when ACTH levels rise in all horses.

• *Corticosteroid use*: Steroidal drugs such as cortisone, dexamethasone, and triamcinolone can bring on laminitis. The stronger the drug, the more likely it is to induce laminitis. The use of such drugs in horses already at risk for laminitis due to other factors should be avoided if at all possible.

• *Stress*: Stress triggers the adrenal gland to release cortisol, a hormonal steroid. Elevated levels of cortisol are associated with an increased risk of laminitis, similar to what happens with the use of steroidal drugs.

• *Other forms of illness*: A wide variety of health issues, including retained placenta, high fever, and pneumonia can all trigger laminitis. Toxaemia and septicaemia, whether related or unrelated to gastrointestinal illness, can also lead to secondary laminitis.

• *Supporting limb laminitis*: Like road founder, supporting limb laminitis is the result of mechanical forces. When a horse has an injury that causes one limb to be non-weight bearing, the limb on the other side has to do double duty, placing it under enormous strain. The constant, intense weight bearing restricts the perfusion of blood into the foot, and after two to three days of this, the foot may develop laminitis. You may recall the wonderful racehorse, Barbaro, who had to be euthanized due to supporting limb laminitis eight months after breaking his leg in the Preakness.

The Three Phases of Laminitis

With so many possibilities, we can't always know what triggered a particular case of laminitis, but whatever the cause, the disease is known to follow a certain progression. Understanding this progression is critical, as it helps you determine what treatment options are best at any given point. Most experts now think of laminitis as having three distinct phases: the developmental, the acute, and the sub-acute/chronic. Here is what happens in each one:

• *Phase 1—Developmental:* Usually, there is a problem in some other part of the body—most commonly the GI tract or the endocrine (hormonal) system—that precipitates the developmental phase of laminitis, which ends when symptoms of lameness appear. During this period, which may last anywhere from 8–48 hours or thereabouts, vasodilation (opening of the blood vessels) leads to increased blood flow in the lamellar region, bringing in trigger factors that damage the basement membrane and capillaries, which later leads to separation of the laminae. Lameness is not yet present. Because horses don't show noticeable symptoms, it is easy to miss the developmental phase altogether, which is unfortunate, as this is the best time to potentially stop or significantly reduce damage inside the foot.

• *Phase 2—Acute:* The acute phase is when the laminae are actually separating (fig. 11.8), causing foot pain and noticeable lameness, and it lasts until displacement of the coffin bone appears or the horse stabilizes. The degree of lameness is proportional to the severity of the separation. Some people put a time frame of no more than three days on the acute phase, but in reality, it can range from a couple of days to six weeks or more. How long the acute phase lasts will depend on the severity of the case, as well as the speed and quality of supportive care the animal receives.

• *Phase 3—Subacute:* If the horse makes it through the acute phase and no bone displacement occurs, the horse is said to be in the subacute phase. With good hoof care and appropriate changes aimed at eliminating precipitating factors, such horses stand an excellent chance of making a full recovery, though they are thought to be more vulnerable to repeat episodes of laminitis in the future.

• *Phase 3—Chronic:* When displacement of the coffin bone does occur, the horse has entered the chronic phase, also called "founder." This is the indefinite phase of laminitis in which displacement shows up on X-rays, and external changes to the foot become evident. Chronic laminitis can cause minor or severe problems depending on how much the coffin bone has rotated and/or descended, the care the horse receives, and how long the condition has been present before treatment is initiated.

Signs of Laminitis

Every horse owner should be familiar with signs of laminitis, as detecting the disease as early as possible is your best shot at minimizing damage to your horse's feet. Signs will vary considerably, depending on what phase of the disease your horse is in.

Developmental Phase Signs

It is a simple and frustrating fact that there are not many clinical signs when laminitis is in the developmental phase, and those that are sometimes

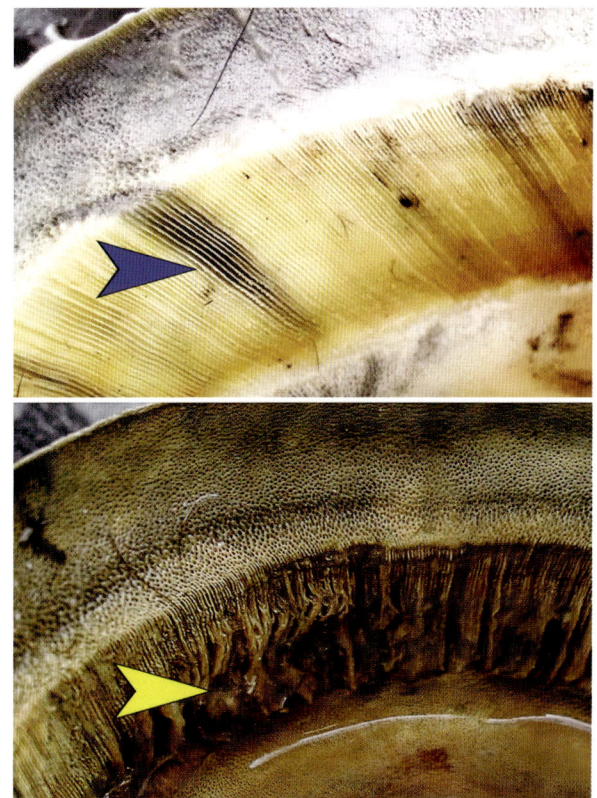

11.8 When the laminae are actually going through the process of separation, the horse experiences terrible pain. Compare the healthy, neatly aligned epidermal laminae in the interior of the hoof capsule (above, blue arrow) to the ones damaged by laminitis (below, yellow arrow), and you can imagine how much this kind of tissue destruction would hurt.

detectible are not always present. In some cases, there will be noticeable warmth in the hoof wall and coronet resulting from vasodilation. However, not all horses with warm feet *have* laminitis and not all horses with cool feet *don't* have it. Hoof temperature has natural variation throughout the day, and it can also be affected by various factors such as fever, exercise, or standing in the sun (warmer), as well as exposure to water, snow, or cold air (cooler).

Delving Deeper:
Enzymes, Blood Flow, and Stopping Laminitis Cold

We don't yet fully understand all the mechanisms by which the different trigger factors cause laminitis, but thanks to the work of Dr. Chris Pollitt and his colleagues, it is now generally accepted that laminitis involves the release of uncontrolled amounts of enzymes called *metalloproteinases* (MMPs). As mentioned on page 36, MMPs are usually released in minute amounts as part of the remodeling process that allows the hoof wall to grow. The MMPs cause tiny sections of laminae to temporarily separate so that the hoof wall can slide down in relation to the coffin bone. Under normal circumstances, this temporary separation is reversed by the release of other enzymes called *tissue inhibitors of metalloproteinase* (TIMPs), which lock the laminae back together. However, various laminitis triggers somehow initiate an overwhelming flood of MMPs, resulting in massive damage to the basement membrane and associated capillaries (fig. 11.9), and causing large portions of the laminae to separate.

Changes in the blood supply also play an important role in the development and progression of laminitis. Fortunately, Pollitt also made important discoveries about what

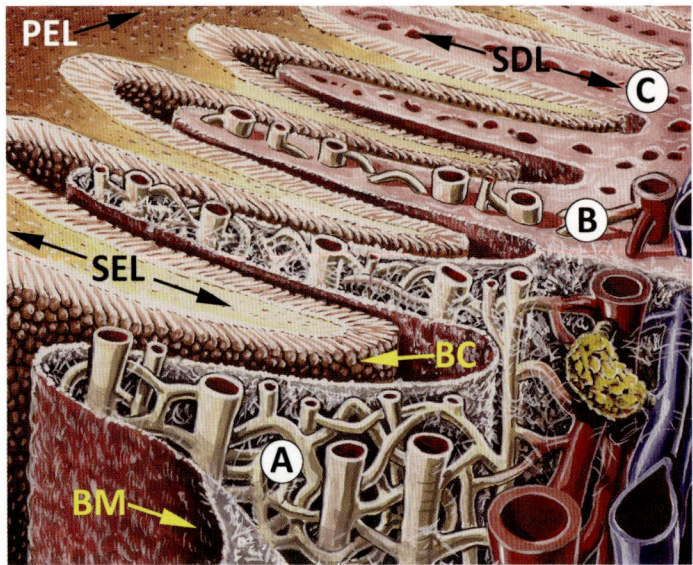

11.9 The basement membrane is the continuous sheet of material that binds the dermal and epidermal laminae together. When the epidermal laminar basal cells and the basement membrane are damaged, the laminae may separate. This diagram illustrates the basement membrane (BM) and the associated complex of blood vessels (tube-like structures). The foreground (A) shows the blood capillaries in a secondary dermal lamina (SDL) as they would look stripped of other tissue. Area B shows an SDL in a non-stripped state. Forward of C, the diagram shows the BM teased apart from the basal cells (BC) of the secondary epidermal laminae (SEL), for illustrative purposes. Note that secondary epidermal laminae branch off from a primary epidermal lamina (PEL). (Review fig. 4.22 on p. 36 if you need a reminder about the anatomy of the laminae.)

laminitis does to the vasculature and blood flow within the foot and how this may tie in with the damage caused by MMPs. These discoveries have led to invaluable changes in treatment approaches, sometimes allowing us to halt the development of the disease altogether.

For example, one longstanding and widely believed theory about laminitis is that the damage to the laminae is caused by *vasoconstriction,* which means constriction of the blood vessels. Vasoconstriction in the laminae would result in ischemia (inadequate blood flow), which would starve the tissues of oxygen and nutrients, leading to separation. For this reason, drugs that increase blood flow, called *vasodilators,* were often administered in the early stages of laminitis in hopes of minimizing damage. Rather than employing vasodilators, what is really needed is cryotherapy.

Cryotherapy involves submerging the limb in extremely cold iced water for an extended period of time. Cryotherapy is an effective vasoconstrictor, but the main benefit comes from the inhibition

of the enzymatic processes that dissolve the bonds between the laminae. It is the only therapy that has been proven to be able to stop the development of the disease and prevent damage to the laminae when applied early enough (see *Cryotherapy,* p. 187). While some believe that the use of vasodilators is appropriate in cases of acute laminitis, others disagree and are choosing to go the cryotherapy route instead.

What everyone agrees on is that once the pathology of laminitis destroys laminar anatomy, there are radical changes in blood flow all over the foot and even part way up the limb. These changes start when the basement membrane and its capillaries are destroyed, causing the blood that would normally flow into the laminae to bypass them entirely by diverting through vascular

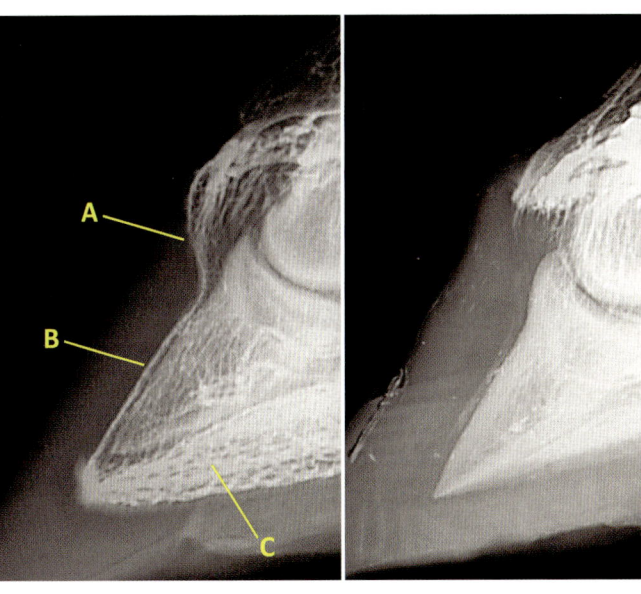

11.10 These venographic images show some of the changes in blood flow that happen in the foot during acute laminitis. Note the flow in the healthy foot (left) in the cascade of blood vessels known as the "lamellar waterfall" (A), the laminae (B), and into the solar corium (C). Then look at those areas in the foot on the right and you'll see that blood flow is almost nonexistent.

shunts (fig. 11.10). Resistance to blood flow increases, and in many cases, you can actually feel this as a bounding digital pulse. Damage to the coronary and solar coria also produces changes in circulation and may result in abnormal and/or slow growth of the hoof wall and sole, and even necrosis (tissue death).

What you need to look for is a hoof that feels warmer than normal and stays that way for an extended period of time, well after a hot horse or a sun-warmed foot would have cooled down. When that happens, you may be dealing with laminitis. It is a very good idea to get familiar with what is normal for the temperature of your horse's feet at different times of day and in different conditions, as knowing this will allow you to determine if they are hotter than usual. You can use your hand to get a general sense of hoof temperature, or you can buy an inexpensive handheld infrared thermometer and keep it on hand in your barn (fig. 11.11).

Another indicator of laminitis you might find in the developmental phase is a bounding digital pulse. This can be so strong in some instances that you can actually see it pulsing, but more commonly, you would have to feel for it (see sidebar, p. 175). If it is present at all, the bounding pulse can come and go during the developmental phase. But, like heat in the feet, a bounding pulse does not necessarily mean laminitis. Increased pressure in the digital arteries can be associated with other kinds of pain or inflammation in the foot, such as can result from an abscess.

And, the lack of a bounding pulse does not rule out laminitis. While this symptom is quite common, it does not always show up in the developmental phase, and sometimes you won't find one even during the acute phase, when it is very common. It can also be difficult to find the digital pulse, bounding or not, if there is significant edema (accumulation of fluid) in the leg. Still, getting to know what a normal digital pulse feels like for your horse is an important tool in your laminitis detection kit, as this will allow you to feel when the pulse is abnormal.

The third possible early warning sign is an increase in resting heart rate. Increases in this phase will be small, possibly as little as 6 beats per minute (bpm), but researchers have found this rise to be quite common a day or two before lameness appears. Normal resting heart rates for adult horses generally range between 30 and 40 bpm, and tend to be quite consistent for an individual horse. Of course, factors such as exercise, excitement, stress, and ambient temperature can raise a horse's heart rate, so it is important to try to get the horse quiet and comfortable before taking his pulse (see sidebar, p. 176). If the horse is in a resting mode and his heart rate is elevated, especially for any length of time, laminitis could be brewing.

Unfortunately, even when early signs are

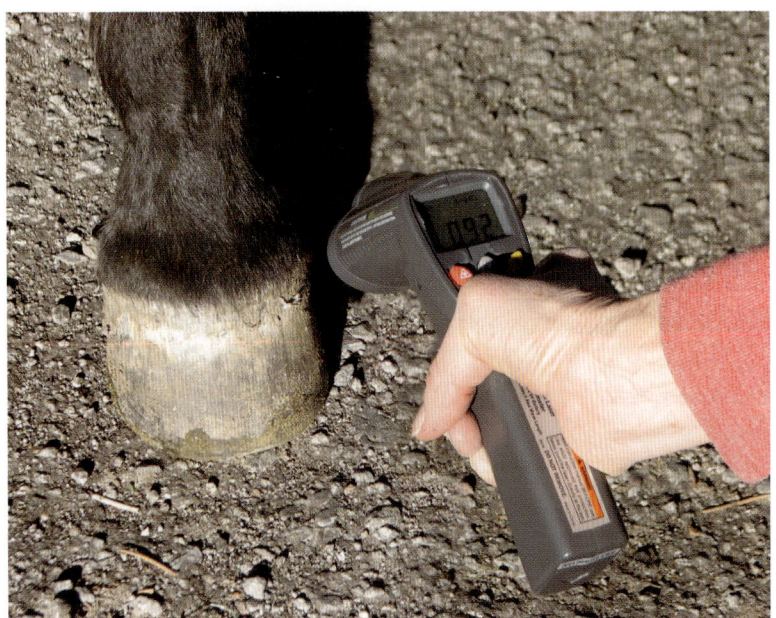

11.11 An infrared thermometer is an easy and quick way to take a hoof's temperature, and more accurate than trying to gauge it with your hand.

Hands-On Activity:
Checking Your Horse's Digital Pulse

There are a number of places where you can feel a horse's pulse, but the *digital pulse,* found in several spots low down on the limb, is a particularly useful one. When blood pressure in the vessels of the hoof and the digital arteries is normal, the horse's digital pulse feels quite faint—if you can find it at all. However, when there is laminitis or other problems causing inflammation in the foot, blood pressure may increase, causing the pulse to become far more palpable.

The easiest place to find the digital pulse is just below the fetlock joint, pretty much lining up with the back of the outer heel bulb. You want to use your first two fingers to try to find the pulse—not your thumb, as pressing with your thumb may cause you to feel your own pulse in the thumb, which could be mistaken for the horse's pulse.

With your horse safely restrained and standing reasonably square, place your two fingers below the fetlock and roll them sideways in a back and forth motion until you find what feels like a ¼-inch–½-inch cord under your fingers. This cord is formed by the lateral VAN (vein, artery, nerve) bundle running into the hoof (fig. 11.12). Once you find it, press down a little and see if you can feel a pulse. If you don't, try pressing a little harder, but note: if

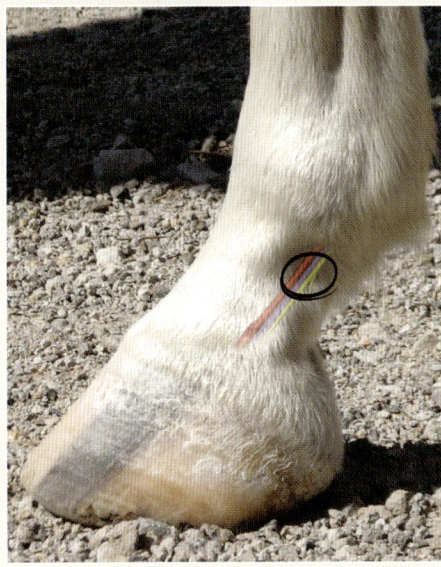

11.12 The VAN (vein, artery, nerve) bundle just below the fetlock is easy to feel, although you may not always feel a pulse in it, which is perfectly fine (see circle).

you press too hard, you will cut off the blood flow and also feel nothing as a result. Play with different pressures and take your time.

If you have found the bundle but can't feel a pulse, this is okay—your horse is not a zombie! What this tells you is that blood is flowing well. If the pulse is there but faint, it is also okay. Get to know what "normal" feels like in your horse in different situations—after exercise, and at different times of day. Then, if you ever feel a significantly stronger "bounding" pulse, you will know something is going on. Last word of advice: check all four legs when looking for increased pulses. Laminitis usually shows up in both front feet, but it can affect the hind feet too. If only one foot is affected, the bounding pulse may be due to something other than laminitis.

present, they are usually missed due to the fact that they are simply not noticeable unless you are actively looking for them. It is, therefore, a good idea to make a quick check for bounding pulses, elevated heart rate, and hot feet part of your daily routine, especially if you have any reason to suspect that your horse is at increased risk of laminitis. Once you are used to checking these things, they won't take more than a minute or two, and they could save your horse's life.

Acute Phase Signs

The acute phase has started when signs of pain become readily observable. The appearance and

Hands-On Activity:
Assessing Your Horse's Heart Rate

Being able to assess your horse's heart rate is an important skill that is helpful in many situations, not just the onset of laminitis.

The average resting heart rate for an adult horse is 30–40 beats per minute (bpm). Some individual horses, especially those that are very fit, can have a slightly lower resting pulse rate. Young horses, on the other hand, have a higher pulse rate than adult horses, with the rate for foals ranging from 70–120 bpm, yearlings from 45–60 bpm, and two-year-olds from 40–50 bpm.

Taking a horse's pulse manually is not hard to do, though it may take practice to locate the arteries and count the beats. Some "pulse points" that are generally easy to find are inside the front part of the jowl, just below the chestnuts on the inside of the front legs, and along the inside of the cannon bones just below the knee. Feel around in these areas for what feels like a thin rope under the skin—this is an artery. Most people like the one inside the jowl, as you don't have to bend over to get to it (fig. 11.13).

Once you locate the artery, use your forefinger to press firmly enough to feel the beats distinctly, and use a watch to count the beats for 30 seconds. Multiply this by two and you have your beats per minute.

If using a stethoscope to take your horse's pulse, place the instrument on the horse's barrel behind the left elbow, which should allow you to hear the heart beat clearly. Remember to count each "lub-dub" as one beat, not two.

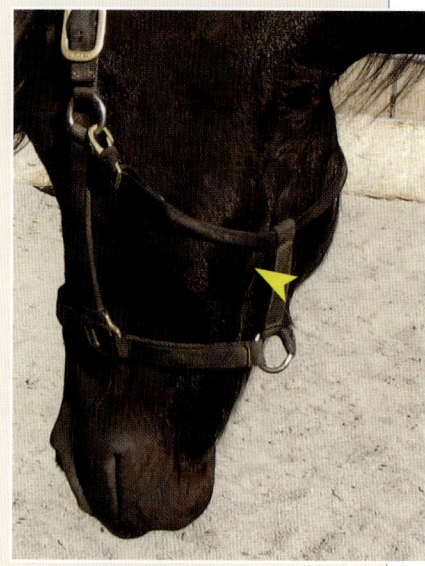

11.13 Finding the mandibular artery under the jowl is usually fairly easy and is a good place to take your horse's pulse (see yellow arrow). Remember to use your fingers, not your thumb, so that you don't feel your own pulse and confuse it with your horse's heartbeat.

intensity of these signs correlate with the severity of the changes going on inside the foot. Signs most commonly observed include:

• *Shifting weight from foot to foot*: This is often the earliest observable sign of acute laminitis. It is most often seen in the front feet, but can occur in the hind feet as well. Under normal circumstances, horses shift their feet up to 5 times a minute, but when the pain of laminitis hits them, this will increase dramatically, up to 25 times a minute, or more. If one foot is more painful than the other, it may be rested more often.

• *Bounding digital pulse*: A bounding digital pulse is extremely common, though not universal, in the acute phase.

• *Elevated hoof temperature*: Hoof temperature increases can happen in both the developmental and the acute phases. Remember, though, that laminitis can be occurring, even in the absence of warm feet.

• *Trembling, sweating, elevated pulse rate and respiration*: The pain of laminitis can be relatively minor in low-grade cases, or absolutely excruciating in more serious cases. When the pain is significant, horses may react by trembling and sweating, and both their heart rate and respiration rate can be quite elevated. This is much more dramatic than the slight increase in heart rate you might note in the developmental phase.

• *Pain response to percussion*: Tapping the front of the hoof wall will often elicit a marked pain response in horses with acute laminitis.

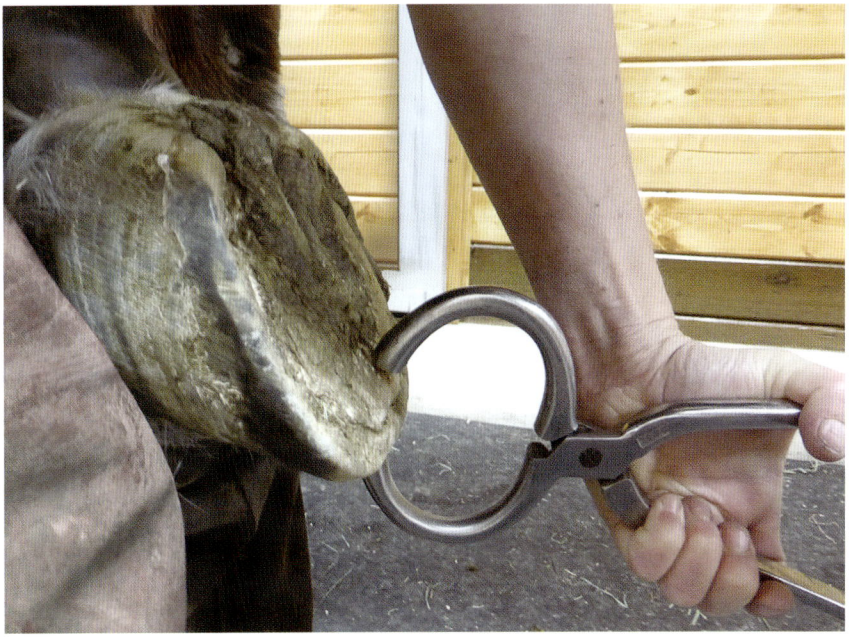

11.14 Vets and hoof-care providers will sometimes use hoof testers to see if the horse is sensitive to pressure in the toe area. Training and experience in the correct use of hoof testers is key in getting an accurate response, as it is easy for a novice to produce false negatives and false positives by applying too little or too much pressure.

• *Pain response to toe pressure*: Pressure applied to the sole in the toe area usually elicits a positive pain response during the acute phase (fig. 11.14).

• *Stiff gait, reluctance to move*: Pain often causes laminitic horses to move stiffly or be hesitant to move, with symptoms worse on harder surfaces. Turning in tight circles may be especially painful, and they may hunch their back when they try to move in an attempt to take the weight off their painful feet. Abnormal heel-first landing may also be observed as the horse attempts to relieve pressure on the toes.

• *Abnormal stance*: Because the toe area is so painful, standing laminitic horses often take on a variety of abnormal postures. Many try to shift their weight to the heels of the affected feet, and because the front feet are usually where the problem is, they try to shift their weight off the front feet as much

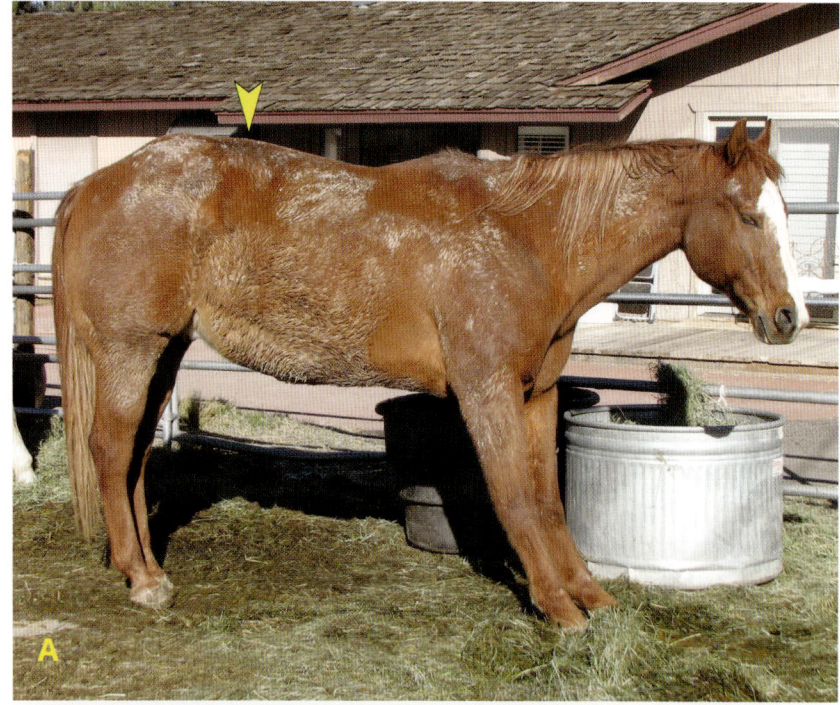

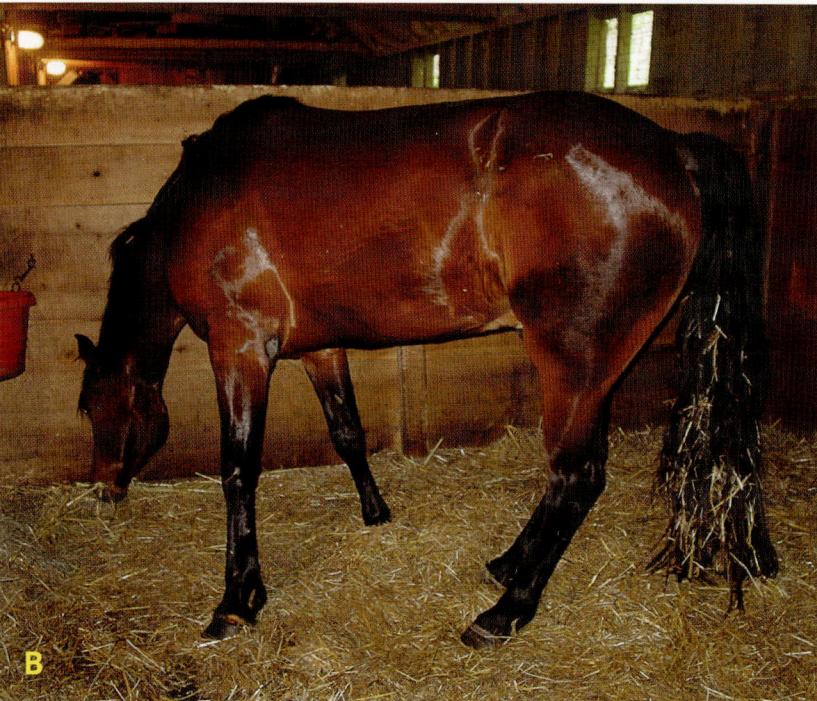

11.15 A & B The horse in A is exhibiting the "sawhorse stance" often seen in laminitic horses. His weight is shifted to his hind end and his front legs appear farther forward than normal, both of which are an attempt to relieve pressure and pain in his front toes. Note the abnormal hump in his lower back (yellow arrow), which is a sign of the strain his hind end is under due to this stance. Some horses will have their hind feet farther forward than seen here. The horse in B is attempting to eat without putting his weight on his front toes, so he has his weight shifted back onto his hindquarters as much as possible, and has spread his front feet apart—a modified version of the classic "sawhorse stance."

as possible. In such instances, horses often stand with their front feet farther ahead than normal, and their hind feet moved forward toward the belly, what is called a "sawhorse stance" (figs. 11.15 A & B). Some horses will do a **"standing-on-a-dime"** stance, with the front feet moved back, the hind feet moved forward, and the limbs flexed (fig. 11.16). This position relieves tension on the deep digital flexor tendons and may provide some pain relief in these cases. Other unusual postures or simply increased muscle tension may also occur, depending on which feet are affected and the severity of the case.

• *Increased recumbency:* Laminitic horses will sometimes lie down more than usual and may be reluctant or find it difficult to get back up. While remaining recumbent may provide some relief to the feet, it can cause other health issues if it goes on for more than a few hours. For one thing, the weight of a recumbent horse's body puts a lot of pressure on the parts touching the ground, which can damage the skin, muscles, nerves, and blood vessels. Other risks include fluid accumulation in the lungs and reperfusion injury, which is when blood that has been squeezed out of an area suddenly returns and overwhelms the tissues in the area.

Chronic Phase Signs

There is a tremendous amount of variability in chronic laminitis. In low-grade cases, the feet will have changes, but because they are relatively subtle and extremely common, many people don't recognize them as problems at all, or chalk them up to the horse simply not having the greatest feet. These changes may include slow growth, mild lameness that comes and goes for no apparent reason, general tenderness on gravel or rough ground, shortened stride, a preference for soft footing, seasonal tenderness associated with grazing on spring or fall pastures, prominent growth rings on the hoof, a stretched white line, toe flare, toe cracks, a dished (concave) dorsal wall, thin and flattish soles, and white line disease (fig. 11.17). Of course, many of these signs can be associated with other problems as well, which makes it even more difficult to determine exactly what the issue is with the feet.

Horses with greater degrees of internal damage will have increasingly obvious external changes to the foot and lameness that is more severe. Any of the low-grade symptoms may be present, but the degree will be worse. They may also have multiple, prominent growth rings giving the hoof wall a rippled appearance. In addition, these horses are likely to have divergent growth rings in which the rings are wider at the heel than at the toe (fig. 11.18). This is generally attributed to damage in the toe region causing growth to slow, and separation causing the toe to flare forward, while growth at

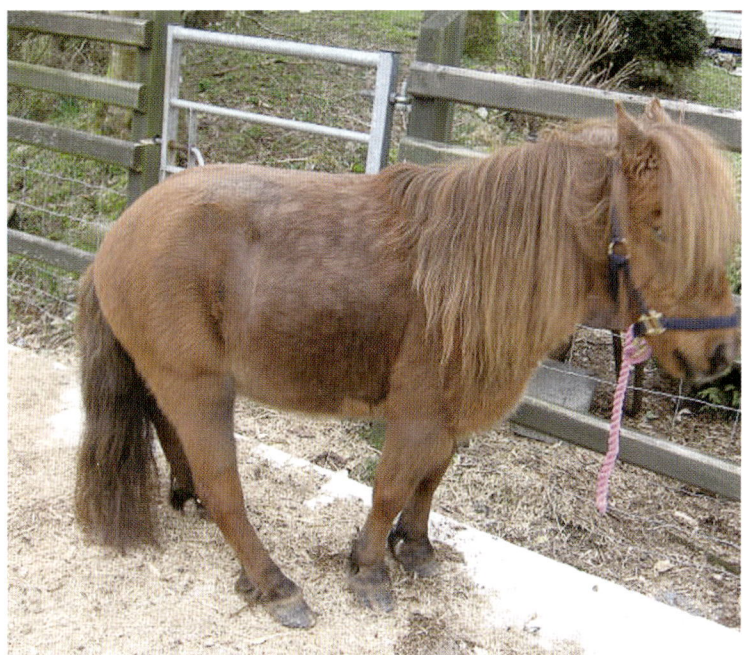

11.16 The "standing-on-a-dime" stance, where the hind feet are forward and the front feet are back is another posture you might see when a horse has laminitis.

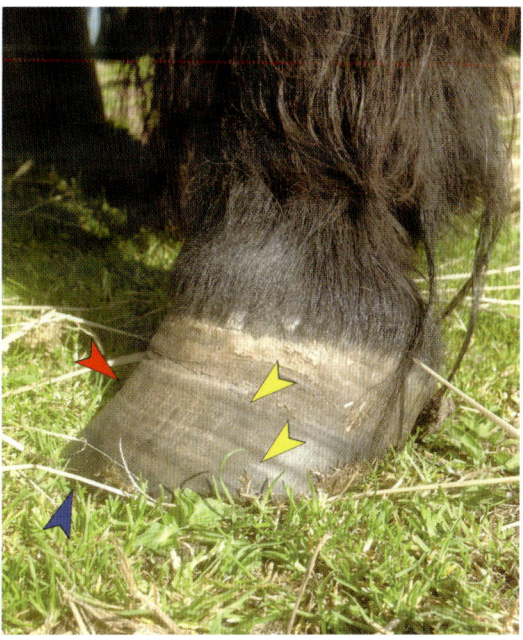

11.17 Many people would look at this foot and simply think the toe is too long, but the dished wall (red arrow), toe flare (blue arrow), and prominent growth rings (yellow arrows) all suggest low-grade laminitis.

11.18 The dished hoof wall, prominent growth rings that are wider at the heel, and toe flaring forward on this hoof capsule are all classic signs of severe, chronic laminitis. Milder cases may have similar features, just not to this degree.

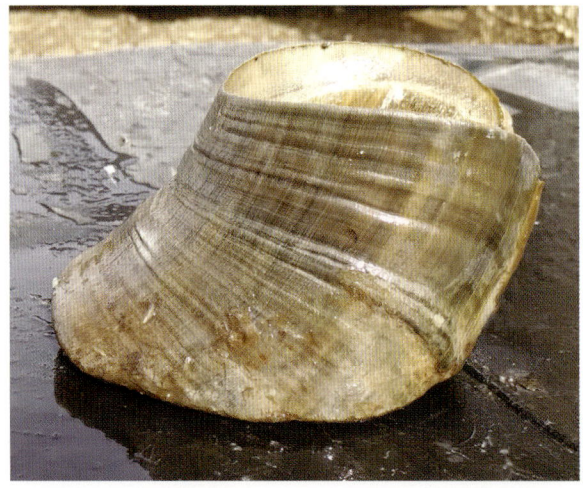

the heel continues more normally. If feet in this state are neglected, they can develop extremely elongated and upwardly curved toes, often called "Aladdin's slippers" (fig. 11.19).

Other problems seen in such horses may include "dropped" (flat) or bulging (convex) soles, which result from abnormal pressure of the coffin bone pushing down on the solar corium. This pressure may also cause bruising under the front edge of the coffin bone that often appears as a reddish, crescent shaped discoloration (fig. 11.20). Bruising may occur prior to the sole bulging. Dropped and/or bulging

11.19 Neglected laminitic horses can end up with severely overgrown and distorted hooves known as "Aladdin's slippers."

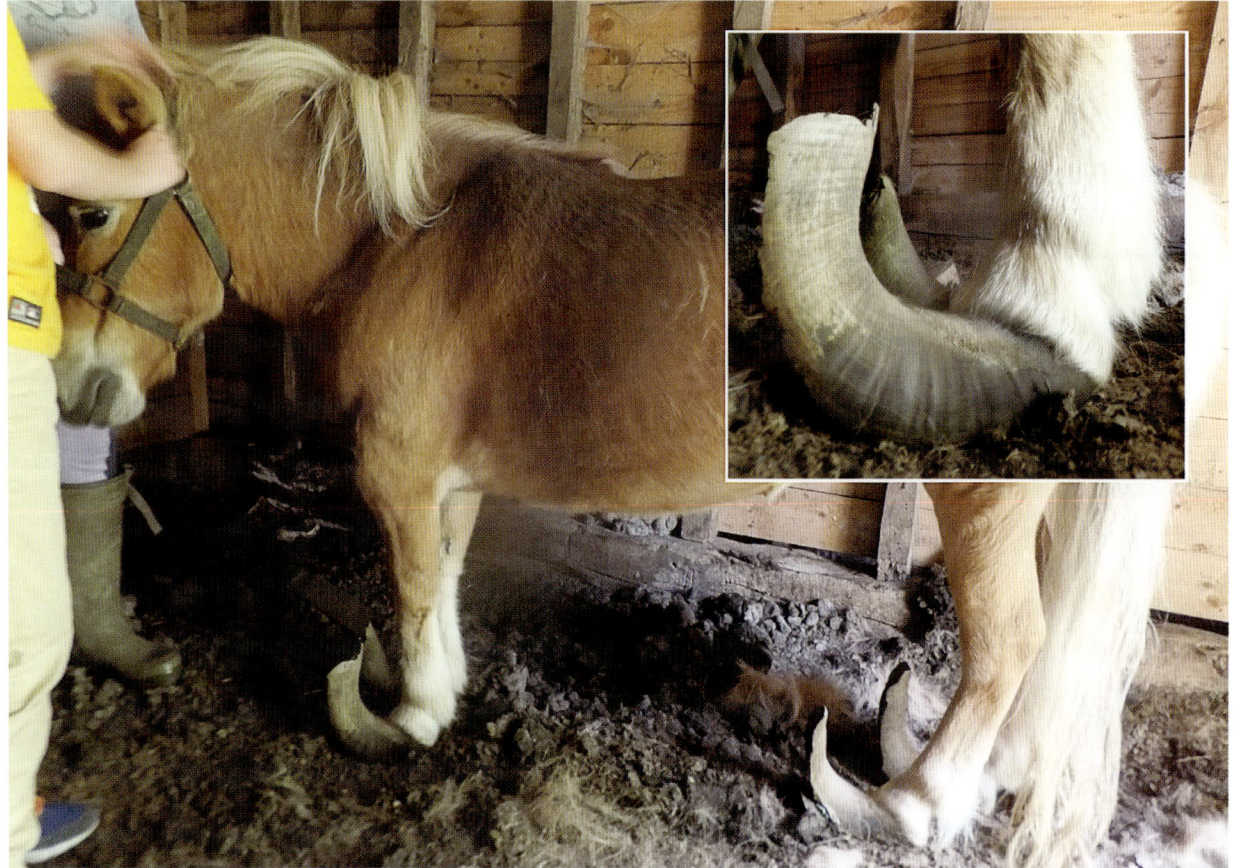

soles are a serious issue, as they indicate a substantial degree of displacement of the coffin bone, which causes a host of problems. Compression of the solar corium impedes growth, resulting in a thin, sensitive sole and a coffin bone that is dangerously close to the ground. Internal structures like the digital cushion are also displaced and rendered less functional by the altered position of the bone, leaving the bone even more vulnerable to impact forces. The flat or convex sole is also unable to flex, adding to the dysfunction of blood flow within the foot.

In some cases, you will see a dip, groove, or shelf form in the front of the coronet area, which is caused by the coronary corium being dragged downward along with the coffin bone (fig. 11.21). In very serious cases, the entire coronet will prolapse as the coffin bone detaches and descends within the hoof capsule. In such cases, the skin may separate at the hairline and exude serum or bleed (fig. 11.22).

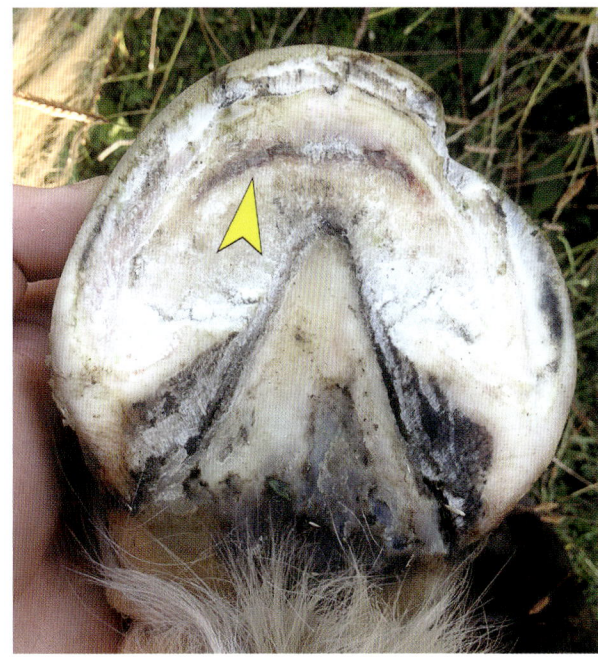

11.20 This crescent-shaped bruise is very worrisome, as it indicates that the coffin bone is pressing down into the solar corium.

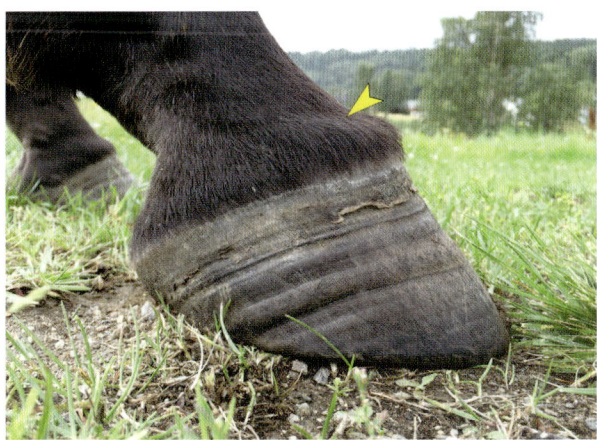

11.21 A shelf has formed in the front of the coronet area of this hoof. While this could be related to low ringbone, the prominent growth rings are strongly suggestive of chronic laminitis. This would be a situation where X-rays would definitely be in order to determine exactly what is going on inside the foot.

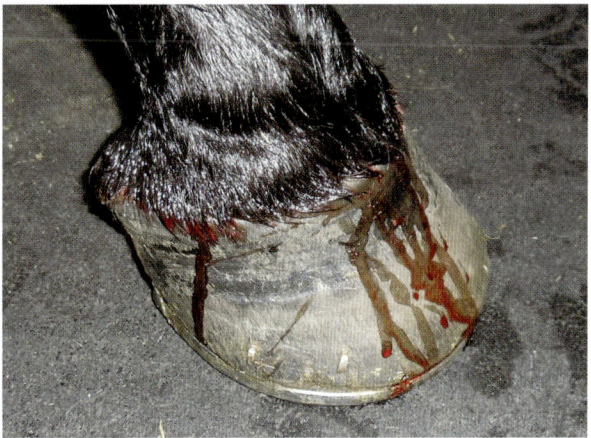

11.22 When the coffin bone detaches and moves within the hoof capsule, it pulls the coronet downward as well. Severe cases will experience tearing at the coronet/hoof wall junction, which may result in blood or serum seeping from the damaged areas.

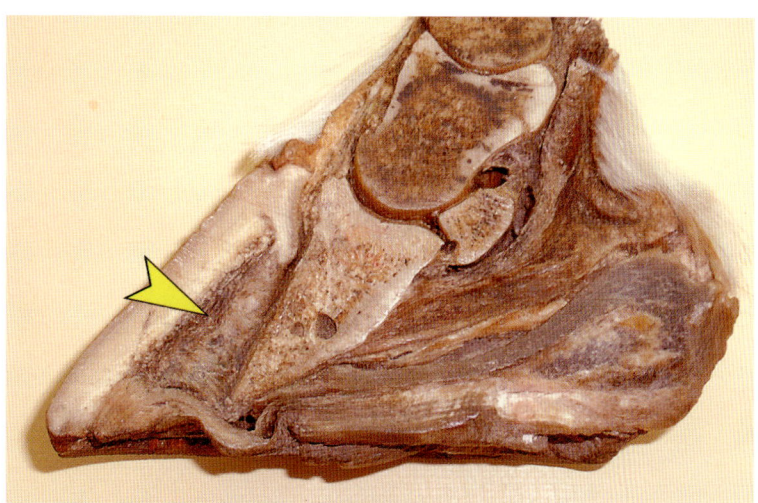

11.23 This cross-section of a foundered foot clearly shows how lamellar wedge material fills in the area between the hoof wall and the displaced coffin bone.

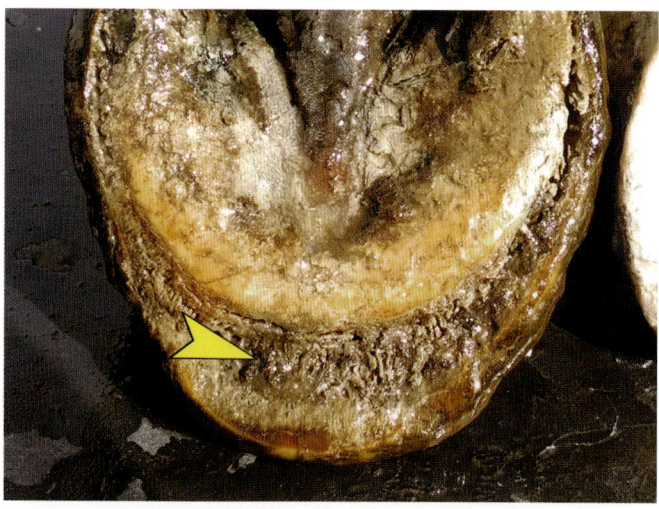

11.24 On the bottom of the foot, lamellar wedge material will be soft and somewhat porous looking when it is first being laid down, but it hardens over time.

The most catastrophic cases may see the entire hoof capsule detach and slough off.

Additional symptoms may be changes in the angle of the hoof wall, creasing of the hoof wall, frequent hoof infections, bruising of the sole and/or wall most noticeable when the foot is freshly trimmed, blood or bruising in the white line, and the development of a *lamellar wedge*, which is when the space between the sole and the separated wall gets filled in with structurally disorganized horn material (fig. 11.23). This wedge will look like a very stretched white line when viewed from the bottom of the foot, sometimes up to an inch wide or even more (fig. 11.24). When the inflammation is active, the lamellar wedge will be soft and spongy, but when the inflammation has subsided, the disorganized wedge horn will harden over. The lamellar wedge can impede the regrowth of healthy, well-attached wall by increasing leverage on the wall.

In the most serious cases, the coffin bone may continue to rotate and/or sink. Many of the previously mentioned signs will undoubtedly be present, but they will likely continue to worsen as time goes on if steps are not taken to stabilize and support the foot. Without such support—and sometimes despite every effort being made—the coffin bone may penetrate completely through the sole (fig. 11.25). Even without sole penetration, repeated abscessing and infection are likely, and pain will be constant and extreme. Over time, pressure on the front edge of the coffin bone will cause it to deform, a process called *remodeling*, and it may eventually lose bone mass and dissolve, which is referred to as *osteolysis* (fig. 11.26).

However, as horrible as all of that sounds, it cannot be overemphasized that the care the horse receives, and when he receives it, will dictate, to a very great extent, how bad things get and what

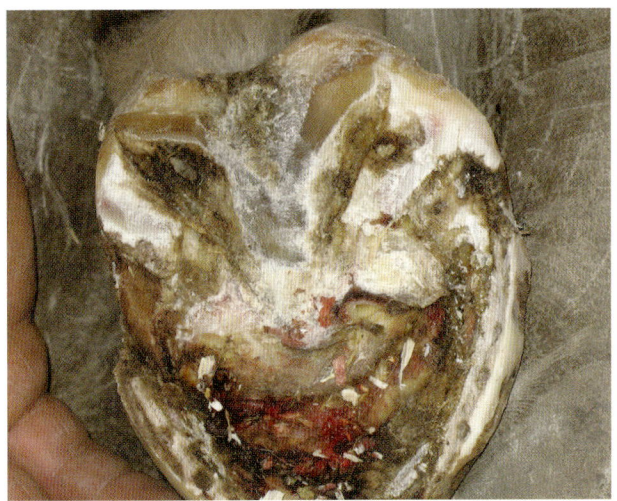

11.25 Penetration of the sole by the coffin bone results from catastrophic failure of the laminar connection.

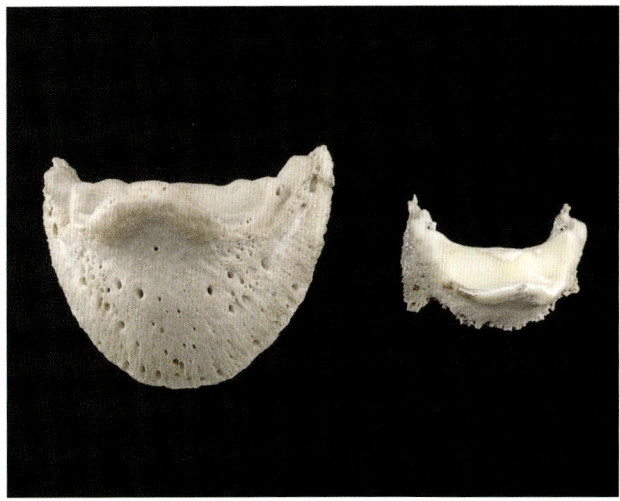

11.26 Compare the healthy coffin bone on the left from a full-sized horse to the one on the right, which came from a pony with long-term, chronic laminitis that caused enormous damage and bone loss.

the horse's chances are for recovery. Even if the situation appears dire, that doesn't always mean that euthanasia is the only option, though it often gets presented that way. The sad fact is that many professionals simply don't know how to help a horse that is in a very bad way, but a significant percentage of these horses can be saved in the right hands. For example, while many veterinarians will tell you that a horse with sole penetration is too far gone to recover, that is not always the case at all. Barefoot specialist Pete Ramey and many others regularly rehabilitate such horses, so it is definitely possible with the right approach, especially if it is done early enough, before serious damage to the bone occurs.

Doing the "Impossible": Recovering from Sole Penetration and Reversing Distal Descent

When the coffin bone penetrates through the sole of the hoof, there is no doubt it is a terrible situation. However, veterinarians and hoof-care professionals who say that such a horse is a hopeless case and should be put down may simply not have the understanding of how to bring such a horse back from the brink. Fortunately, thanks to Pete Ramey and other pioneering hoof-care educators, there are an increasing number of professionals who do have that understanding and are out there saving the lives of horses many others have written off. One such professional is hoof-care provider Paige Poss, who first found that it can be done with the case of a Connemara pony named Druid.

Druid's founder was so bad that he had solar penetration on all four feet. However, no one

Pete Ramey on
Rehabilitation Following Sole Penetration

"There is no doubt that rehabilitating horses with sole penetration can be done," says Pete Ramey. "Here is one of many examples: In May of 2004, I went to see a horse that had 14-degree rotation and the coffin bones penetrating the soles of both front feet (fig. 11.27). The owner stood up to countless people telling her this horse couldn't be helped. The 'after' picture, from December 2005, was taken on the day this horse was awarded the Speed Event Championship Buckle for the year in our local saddle club. This horse and rider have dominated in competition—so when I say, 'It can be done,' I don't mean survive, I mean *perform*!"

Part of what needs to happen for such horses to recover is a reversal of the distal descent that allowed the bone to get too close to the sole in the first place. While such reversal has long been considered by many to be impossible, there are now many examples of horses whose coffin bones have defied gravity and moved back up within the hoof capsule, effectively achieving the "impossible." Here is how Pete Ramey explains how he reverses distal descent, using another laminitis case as an example:

"The first time I saw this foot was after four years of lameness and numerous shoeing protocols. The horse was a very nice school horse that had a fortune spent on her trying to restore some soundness. The previous owner tried everything, then finally gave her to one of my customers.

"When I saw the horse she was very lame, with a huge amount of distal descent. The coffin bone was lower than any part of the hoof wall and almost exposed. The collateral groove at the apex of the frog was only ⅛ inch deep. This should immediately tell you that you will not be able to shorten this long toe from the bottom. In order to build adequate sole depth under

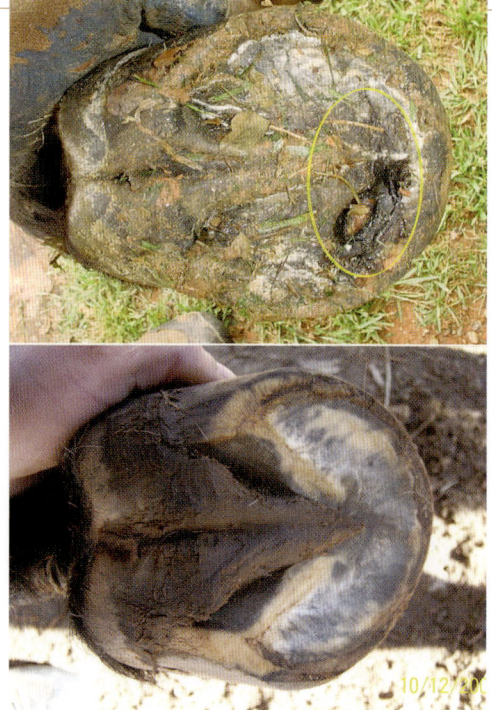

11.27 With severe rotation and the coffin bones coming out of both front feet (above—yellow circle shows area of penetration), this horse was considered a "goner" by just about everyone. While some would say such a thing isn't possible, the feet fully recovered (below), and the horse was not only sound, but competing and winning.

P3, thus lifting the collateral grooves off the ground, almost a half-inch of sole needed to be built up! In fact, you can clearly see the imprint of P3 on the sole in figure 11.28. I traced its 'footprint' with my hoof pick so it shows up white in the photo (fig. 11.28).

"It also should be clear that the walls are no longer attached to P3 either, and lamellar wedge (keratin proliferation by the laminae, between the dermal and epidermal laminae) has filled in the void between P3 and the wall. Many professionals think this area in front of P3's callus ridge is sole, when in fact it is intertubular hoof horn produced from cells migrating down from the coronet with the epidermal laminae. The sole only grows from the bottom of P3.

"The bone position is so low, cutting this long hoof to a 'natural length' would actually cause you to rasp away part of P3! At the same time, the walls should be rolled or beveled out of a 'lifting role,' and P3 should be loaded through the sole so the coronet can migrate toward a more natural position relative to P3. You might think that if you add a half-inch of sole to a hoof this long, the hoof capsule will end up even longer. The opposite is true. With the walls rolled and the sole unmolested and callusing, the hoof capsule actually becomes much shorter as the coronet moves down to its normal position relative to P3 and the lateral cartilages.

"After six months of rehabilitation using these techniques, the horse had excellent hooves and was gloriously sound. The coffin bone moved up into a natural position in the hoof capsule,

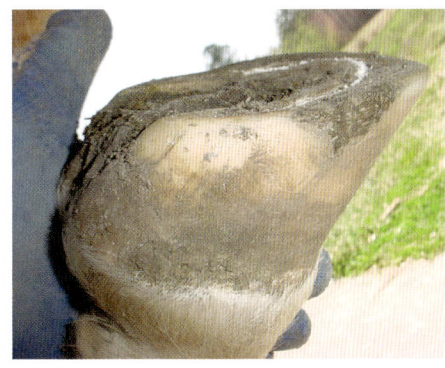

11.28 "When I first saw this foot, it had marked distal descent indicated by the long hoof capsule, flat sole, and bulge under the coffin bone (marked with white scrape mark) and the coffin bone was dangerously close to penetrating the sole."

shortening the hoof, while building the necessary sole (fig. 11.29). It is very important to understand that the sole was never trimmed throughout this whole process. It was too thin to start with, so it needed to build. You have to keep this in the front of your mind if you are trying to rehabilitate a horse with thin soles.

"I also want to stress that you should use foam padded hoof boots when a laminitic horse is in any discomfort, if the soles are thin, or if the terrain is rocky. Running around in rocks on a thinned sole is dangerous. You need to build a thick callused sole *before* you do this. Pressure to an unnaturally thinned sole can cause bruising and can even restrict

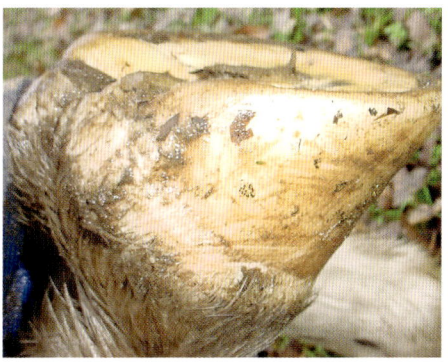

11.29 "This is the same hoof eight months later, before the mare's six-week maintenance trim. Note that the hoof has now reached a more natural length, but the collateral groove at the apex of the frog is now recessed within a ⅝ inch deep bowl of solar concavity. This healthier toe length that would have 'quicked' the horse eight months ago exists with much more armor underneath, at the same time. P3 has moved upward (relative to the coronet) significantly. At no time was the sole of this horse cut. This concavity was built by adding adequate sole thickness under P3."

blood supply to the sole by restricting flow through and from the circumflex artery that follows the perimeter of the distal border of P3. This can 'starve' the sole and reduce its ability to thicken and callus.

"Keep the horse on yielding terrain at first, and/or use the foam insoles in boots to avoid this pitfall. *It is critical that any means of sole support provide a total release of pressure to the solar corium during hoof flight.* This is why I prefer boots over fixed shoeing systems for laminitic horses."

11.30 When Druid's feet collapsed about a month after he first came down with laminitis, he ended up with solar penetration in all four feet.

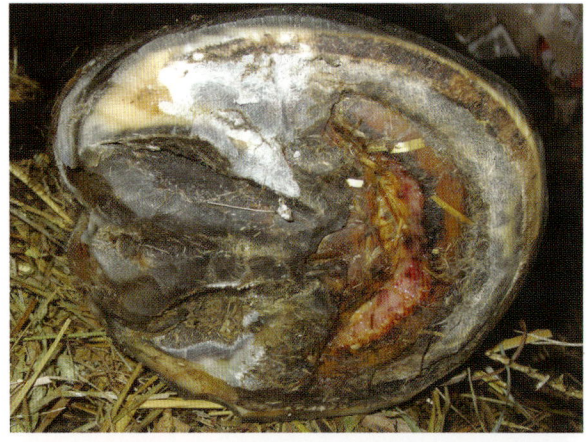

11.31 This photo was taken only 18 days after figure 11.27. "This new sole was very soft and felt like skin," says hoof-care provider Paige Poss.

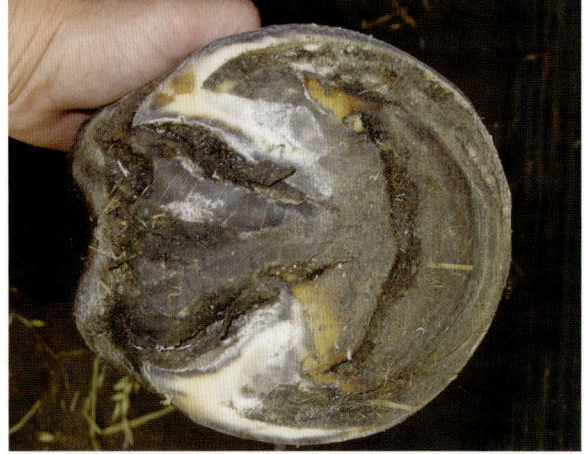

11.32 Looking at Druid's feet after his recovery from quadrilateral solar penetration, you would never know he had suffered from laminitis at all.

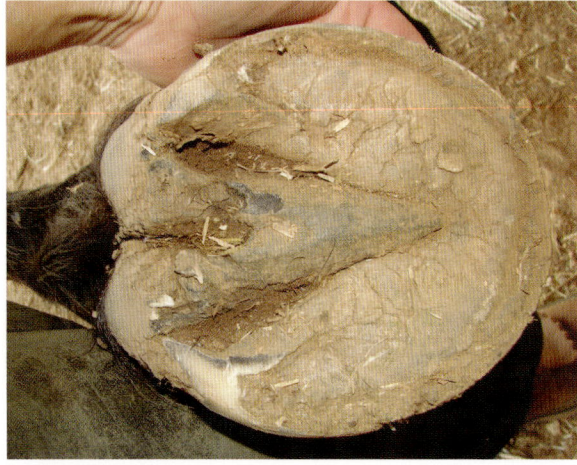

wanted to give up on this lovely boy, so Poss and the pony's owners and supporters went to work trying to save him (fig. 11.30). No one was more amazed than Poss to see how quickly the feet began to repair themselves. Within a few weeks, the coffin bone was growing a new covering (fig. 11.31). Ten months later, Druid was well enough to start riding again. It was not an easy road at times, especially given that everyone involved was learning as they went, but the end result is a happy, healthy horse whose feet bear no visible trace of the catastrophic damage they suffered (fig. 11.32). While Druid remains sensitive when walking on gravel and requires boots for riding on rocky trails, that is true of many domestic horses that have never had laminitis at all.

Poss emphasizes that close attention to diet was a huge factor in Druid's rehabilitation, clarifying for her that laminitis is a whole-horse issue, not just a foot issue. Druid continues to be on a diet appropriate for laminitic horses in order to prevent another episode, and exercise has also been important in keeping him healthy since he has been able to move comfortably. Having now worked with many badly foundered horses, Poss also stresses that every case of laminitis is unique, and some horses will do well with certain methods, while others will not. As she puts it, "The horse has the final say. If it isn't working, it isn't 'right.'"

Ultimately, the decision of whether or not to try to save a horse with such severely damaged feet must be considered very carefully. The horse could be in a substantial amount of pain for some time (though this may be manageable with medication), and there can be setbacks, even when the horse appears to be making good progress. In some cases, the rehabilitation process may just be too hard on the animal—and it is likely to be emotionally difficult for those who care for the horse, as well. Still, for those who feel that attempting to save the horse is the right thing to do and who have the level of commitment to see it through, the rewards can be worth it. Some supposedly hopeless horses have even returned to active competition—proof positive that it can be done.

Emergency Treatment for the Laminitic Horse

Recognizing laminitis in the earliest stage possible gives your horse the best chance of recovery. If you have any suspicion that your horse is suffering from

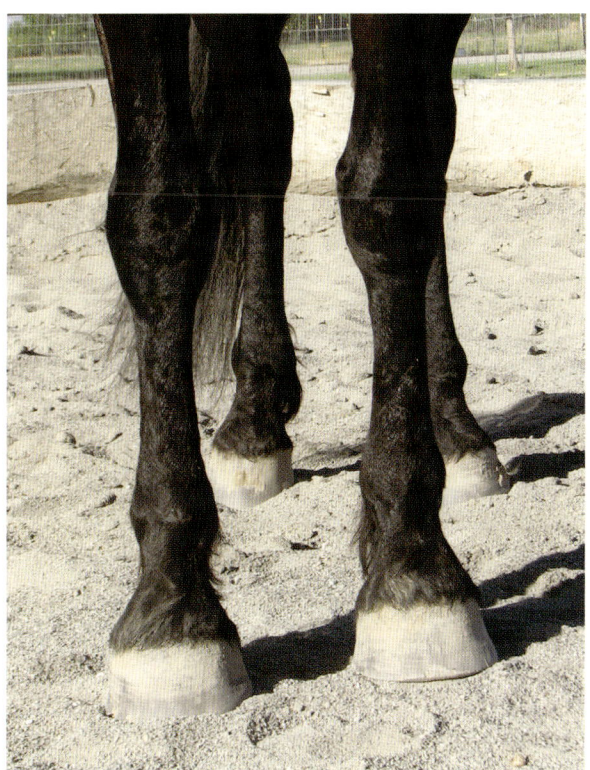

laminitis, or experiencing any other health issue that could precipitate laminitis, do not hesitate to contact your veterinarian and hoof-care provider immediately. Laminitis should be treated as the potentially life-threatening emergency that it is, and early diagnosis and intervention is critical in order to minimize the damage.

While you are waiting for the vet or farrier to arrive, there are immediate steps you can take to help your horse. First, you want to remove any grain, avoid feeding anything sweet (including carrots and apples), and take the horse off grass if he is grazing. The carbohydrates in any of these feed sources may be causing the crisis. The horse should be put in a contained area that will limit movement (or kept haltered and restrained), and the footing should be supportive but conformable. Loose sand is ideal for this purpose, as it will allow the foot to sink in but still provide support for the coffin bone (fig. 11.33). If you don't have any loose sand, a thick layer of shavings is better than a flat, hard surface.

When the horse is extremely reluctant to move, it may be best to just halter him and wait for help, rather than forcing the horse to move to another area, as movement may increase damage if separation is already underway.

Cryotherapy

Horses with laminitis will often choose to stand in cold water or snow if they have the opportunity, likely because the cold relieves some of their discomfort (fig. 11.34). However, if you want to really harness the benefits of cold temperatures on

11.33 Standing a horse in loose sand is a good way to provide immediate, emergency support for laminitic feet.

11.34 Laminitic horses will often seek out natural ways to cool their feet, but they will not be able to get them as cold as they need for as long as they need to halt the progression of laminitis.

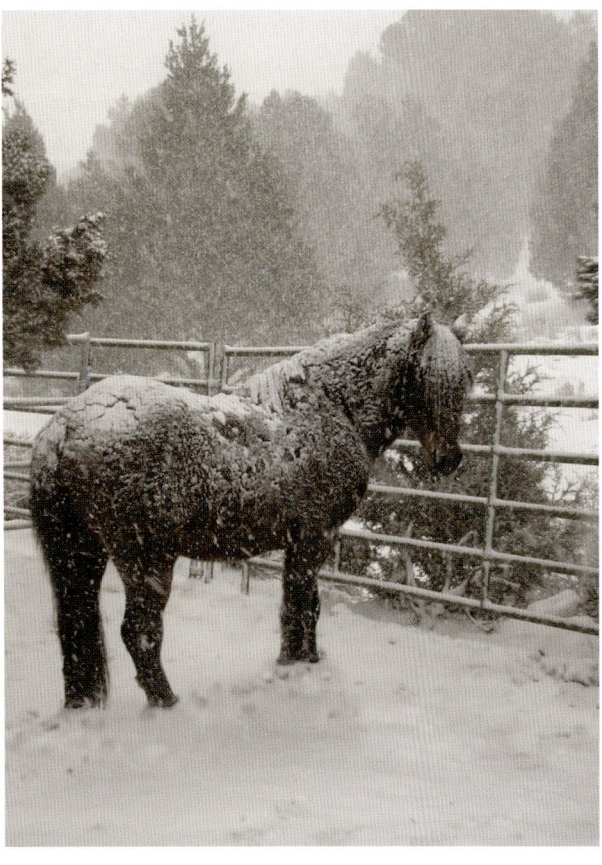

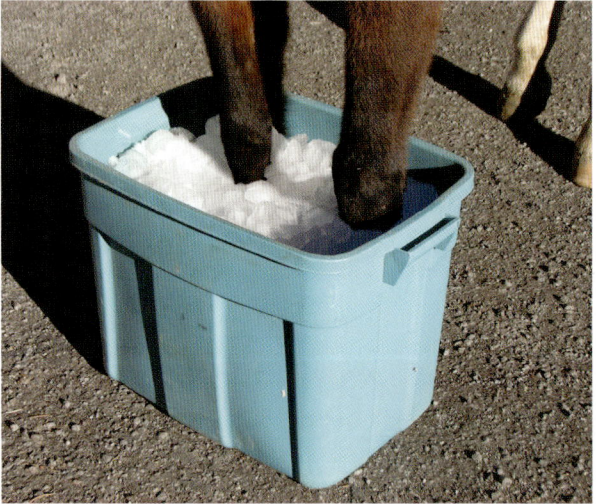

11.36 A storage bin like this one can work well for cryotherapy, and is deep enough to get the water/ice mixture up to the knees. Some people may find it easier to use one bin for each foot.

11.35 There are two things wrong with this picture, from a cryotherapy-for-laminitis perspective: First, only the foot is submerged in ice, when it should be the entire limb up to the knee. Second, there is far too little ice to keep the temperature as low as it needs to be.

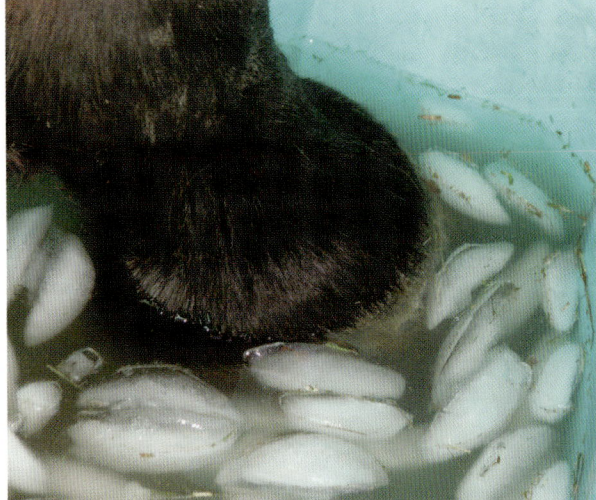

laminitic feet, you have to employ serious cryotherapy, which is the only method we currently know of that can halt or reduce the progression of laminitis.

Cryotherapy can be implemented by standing the affected feet (or feet you suspect might become affected) in tubs of ice water that is as cold as possible—*lots* of ice! Get the level of the water as close to the knee as you can (higher is okay), as it is necessary to cool the blood coming into the foot, not just the foot itself, in order to have the desired effect (fig. 11.35). There are cryotherapy boots and "spas" on the market now, but as these are costly and unlikely to be available in a pinch, a Rubbermaid® type storage container or small water trough can work well for emergency purposes (fig. 11.36). As cryotherapy also has benefits beyond the treatment of laminitis, equine clinics and larger barns may want to invest in or build a more substantial cryotherapy setup, some of which can be designed to be portable and will be able to treat all four feet (figs. 11.37 A–C).

If you are utilizing cryotherapy, it is critical to keep adding ice and sluicing out water as needed to maintain the water at close to freezing temperature, no higher than 40 degrees Fahrenheit. You will need a lot of ice and another person or two to help with this, as you have to keep it up for a minimum of 24–48 hours, or until your vet tells you otherwise. Be aware that cooling wraps and other devices meant to lower hoof or limb temperature have not been shown to get the limb cold enough, reach high enough, or stay cold for a long enough time to make a difference in acute laminitis.

One thing you don't have to worry about is the cold being uncomfortable for the horse or damaging to the limb. Horses are well adapted to withstand extremely cold temperatures, and cryotherapy, even when applied for up to a week, has been shown to cause no discomfort or harm. Its biggest drawback is that it is labor intensive, as someone has to keep the water icy cold continually. However, since cryotherapy is the only method proven to be able to prevent or minimize damage inside the foot, it is definitely worth doing if the horse is in early enough stages to benefit from it.

If the horse is already in the acute phase when you find it, cryotherapy will not reverse damage that has already occurred, but it will provide some pain relief and may help to stabilize the foot. It was previously thought that cryotherapy was only of benefit if applied during the developmental phase, before symptoms of lameness occurred. However, a groundbreaking study conducted at the University of Queensland showed that the benefits can be significant beyond the developmental phase. After

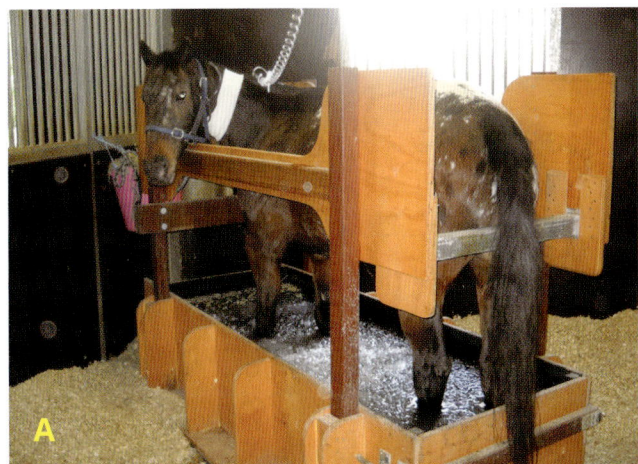

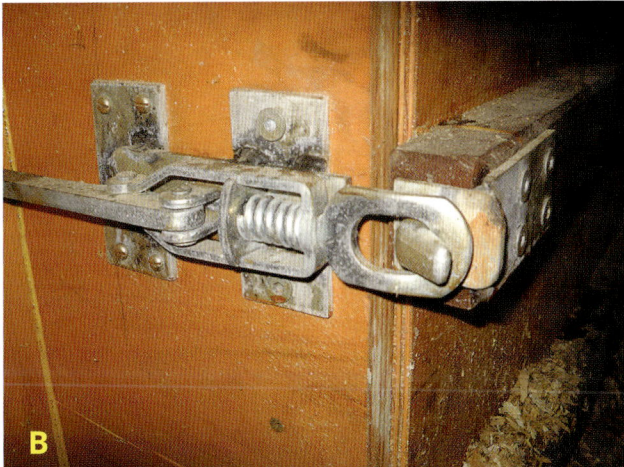

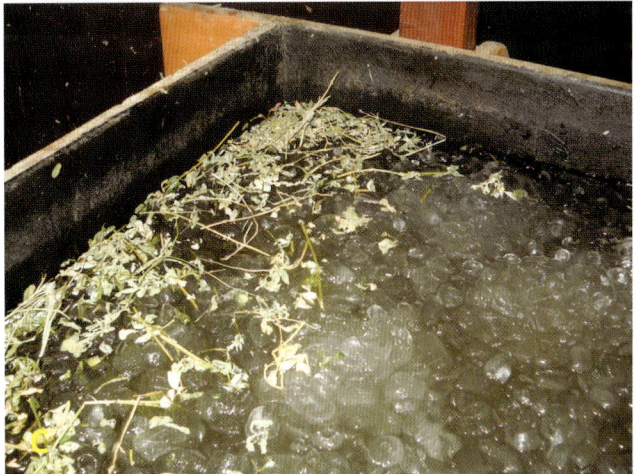

11.37 A–C This portable cryotherapy setup at Anstead Veterinary Hospital in Queensland, Australia, was designed by Dr. Chris Pollitt (A). It can be taken apart for easy transportation. The compression latch on the back door of the box holds everything tight (B). The ½-inch thick, rubber liner compresses when the back door is latched, keeping the water in (C).

11.38 Taped-on polystyrene pads can help support the sole while relieving pressure on the toe. The photo on the left shows how to apply a cross of duct tape to the pad to easily start the process of putting it on the foot. The photo on the right shows the pad in place before it was fully covered with more layers of tape to protect the pad and secure it.

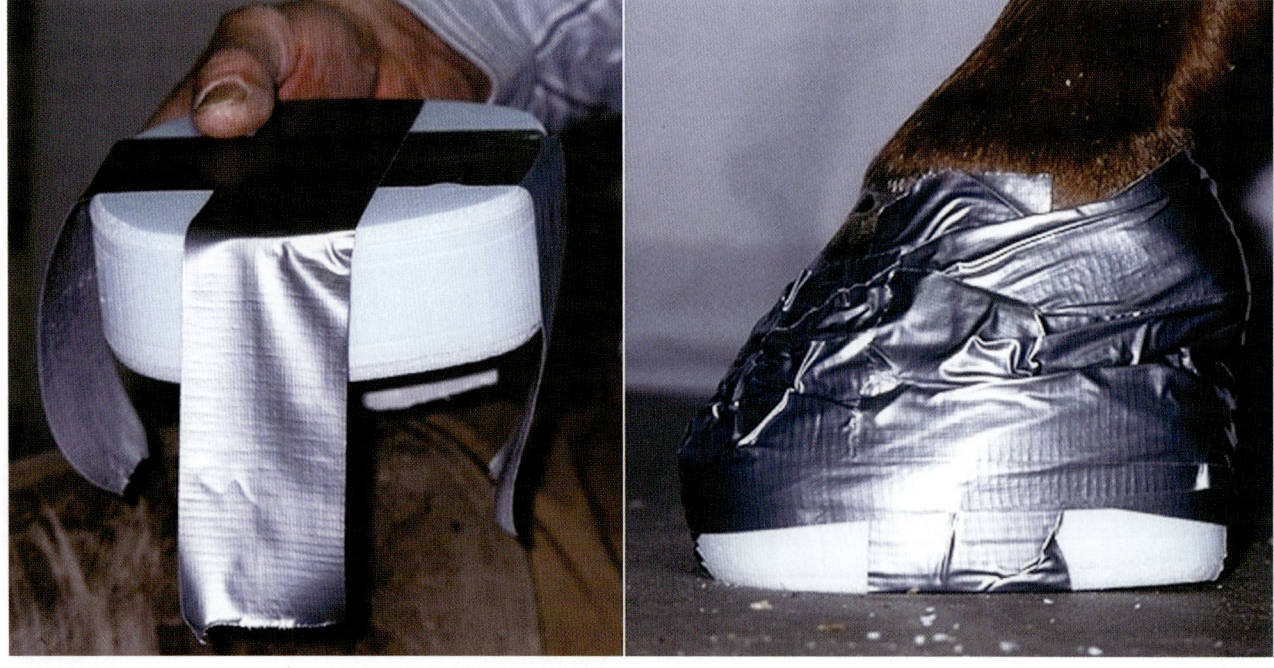

inducing bilateral laminitis in the test subjects, the researchers waited until lameness was evident, then applied cryotherapy for 36 hours to one limb only on each horse. Results showed that disease progression was much lower in limbs that had undergone cryotherapy than those that hadn't. On a scale of 1–4, with 4 being the most severe, the cryotherapy feet scored an average of one, while the untreated hooves had progressed to an average of 3.5. They also found that four out of eight untreated hooves experienced total separation of the laminae, but among the treated feet on the same horses, three had a score of only 1, and one had a score of 2.

This data means that even if your horse is already showing visible signs of lameness, you may still be able to halt or reduce the progression of the disease with cryotherapy. It is certainly a "the earlier, the better" scenario, but the results of the Queensland study bring new hope for untold numbers of suffering horses and their owners.

Supporting the Foot

In situations where cryotherapy is not an option, there are other things that can be done that may be helpful when a horse is showing signs of lameness from laminitis. One is to find a way to support the coffin bone via the sole, while relieving pressure and levering forces on the toe. As previously mentioned, providing conformable footing (such as sand or deep shavings) for the horse to stand in is an easy way to achieve this, but you can also apply supportive padding to the foot itself to relieve pain and assist in the stabilization of the coffin bone.

There are a number of different ways to do this, and because each case of laminitis is different, what works for one horse might not work for another. It is equally important to realize that laminitis is a process, and thus a technique that works for your horse today might need to be changed for something else tomorrow or next week. This is something you simply have to experiment with, paying close attention to whether your attempts to support the sole are making the horse feel better or worse. If the horse is more comfortable, you are on the right track, but if discomfort seems to increase at all at any point after application, remove whatever you have done immediately and get the horse onto some conformable footing.

One commonly used method of sole support is the application of taped-on polystyrene (Styrofoam®) pads, which conform to the horse's foot and weight-bearing pattern, providing custom support (fig. 11.38). Research has shown that that such pads increase surface contact area, decrease contact pressure and peak contact pressure, and move the center of pressure toward the back of the foot—all helpful for a majority of horses with acute laminitis.

Of course, as with everything else, there are different opinions on how best to apply support pads, but Master Farrier Gene Ovnicek's technique is simple and effective. What he recommends is first applying a pad shaped to fit the entire foot, including the toe, and duct taping it onto the hoof. After 24–48 hours, that layer will crush down, at which time it is necessary to add a second layer cut to fit behind the sore area around the toe. You can get more detail and see him demonstrating his method in this video: www.youtube.com/watch?v=DzUeYjYe5yE.

There are pre-made pads made specifically for temporary sole support, which are a good thing to keep in your equine emergency kit, especially if you have a horse at increased risk for laminitis. However, you can also make pads yourself using 2-inch-thick, high-density insulation polystyrene, sold in large sheets at most home improvement stores. If your local store only carries thinner sheets, you can double them up.

Other approaches to first-aid supportive padding include packing the foot with dental impression material, taping a roll of gauze under the frog, or putting the horse in padded hoof boots. Any of these, when used correctly, may provide relief and help to minimize further damage for some horses, but once again, it must be emphasized that if whatever you are using causes greater discomfort, you need to modify your approach or you may do more harm than good. If you are not sure about putting something on the bottom of the foot, you can keep the horse standing in sand, soft dirt, or a thick layer of shavings until help arrives.

Diagnostic Imaging for Laminitis

The visible signs of laminitis can only give you very limited information about what is happening to your horse. In order to get a real understanding of how bad things are—and how bad they are likely to become—you need to get a look inside. Diagnostic imaging is absolutely essential, as it is the only way to assess the disease, chart its progress, and formulate treatment options most likely to minimize the damage and maximize the chances for your horse to recover.

11.39 While this is a good X-ray in many ways, the radiopaque marker used on the hoof wall goes far above the coronet, making it impossible to use the coronet as a reference to accurately gauge distal descent. The coronet might be somewhere around the yellow arrow, but without a good marker, you can only guess.

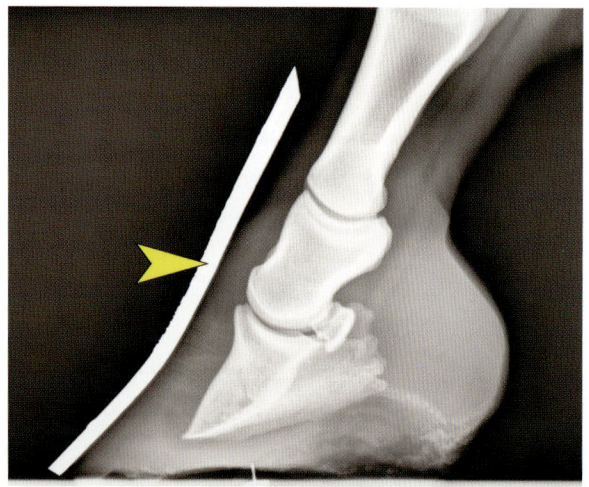

11.40 Both of these images show a hoof with flexion in the coffin joint. However, the foot in top photo is perfectly healthy, with no rotation at all. The joint is flexed because the foot is flexed, which looks somewhat similar to phalangeal rotation, except that the hoof wall is still well attached, as you can see by the uniform distance between the front of the coffin bone and the marker on the outer hoof wall. The foot in the photo below has actual phalangeal rotation due to laminitis. The space between the coffin bone and the hoof wall marker is much greater at the solar margin than at the top, indicating rotation.

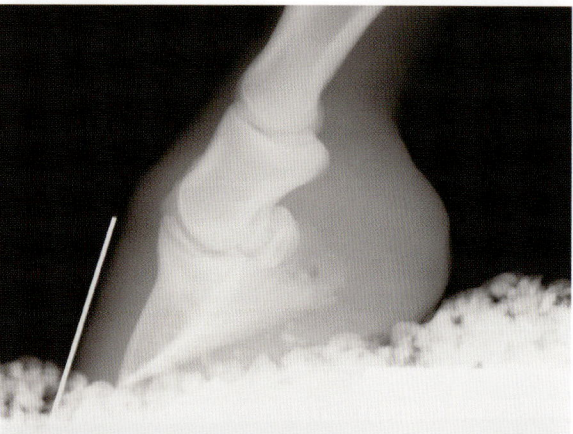

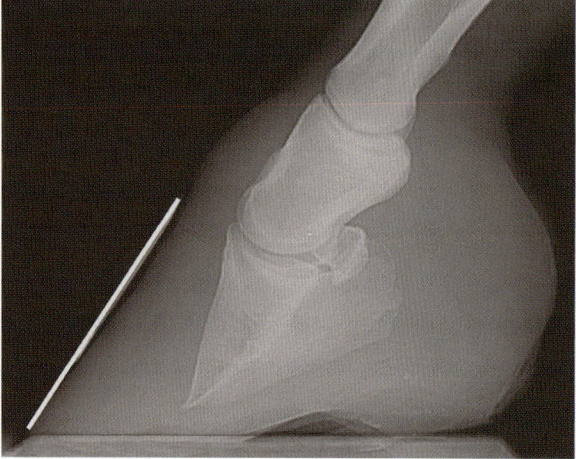

Radiography (X-Rays)

If your horse has laminitis, it is extremely beneficial to get X-rays of the feet as soon as possible as they will show you exactly how much, if any, rotation/distal descent has happened in the foot. Your vet will also likely want to take additional X-rays at various points in the following weeks to keep abreast of any changes. Without this knowledge, your vet and hoof-care professional will be guessing at what needs to be done, which can greatly impede your horse's recovery. Good X-rays not only show what changes have occurred inside the foot, they also provide a guideline for treatment and trimming to realign the foot if rotation has taken place.

However, it is very important for you to understand that not all X-rays are good ones. Some vets do not correctly position the leg or the beam, or they fail to mark the ground angle or the hoof itself, leaving you without reference points that would allow you to gauge things like how great the distance is between the coronet and the top of the coffin bone's extensor process—an important indicator for distal descent (fig. 11.39). It is worth asking if your vet has specific education in this area, and if not, you may want to get a referral to someone who does. Key points in taking good X-rays include:

• Marking the dorsal wall with something metal or radiopaque to indicate both the coronet (important for gauging distal descent) and the hoof wall (to gauge rotation). Barium paste is ideal for this purpose.

• Standing the leg so that the cannon bone is upright and the foot is flat—necessary for getting a correct reading of the angles of the bones. When the foot is flexed, the joints will reflect that, making it trickier to see whether or not there is any phalangeal rotation (true rotation of the coffin bone—fig. 11.40).

• Positioning the beam to get a true lateral image, not skewed forward or back, up or down.

• Marking the true apex of the frog, an important reference for trimming and gauging hoof-capsule distortion. A shortened-off thumb tack is often used for this purpose—a full-length one may be too long and poke into sensitive tissue.

When viewing X-rays, a veterinarian is looking for a number of possible changes, but you can also learn what to look for. Here are some questions to ask yourself when viewing X-rays of laminitic horses:

• Is the space between the outer surface of the hoof wall and the front surface of the coffin bone larger at the bottom than at the top? If so, that foot has rotation. You can determine the degree of rotation, also called the "dorsal angle," by drawing a line along the surface of the hoof wall, then another along the coffin bone, and measuring to see how many degrees that angle is (fig. 11.41). You can also determine whether the rotation is phalangeal or capsular by checking to see if the coffin bone lines up with the bones above it (see figs. 11.4 A & B, p. 166).

• What is the palmar/plantar angle of the coffin bone? It will often get very high in cases of rotation—far above the 2–5 degrees of a healthy foot (fig. 11.42). This is a critical factor to consider when undertaking rehabilitative trimming to realign the coffin bone.

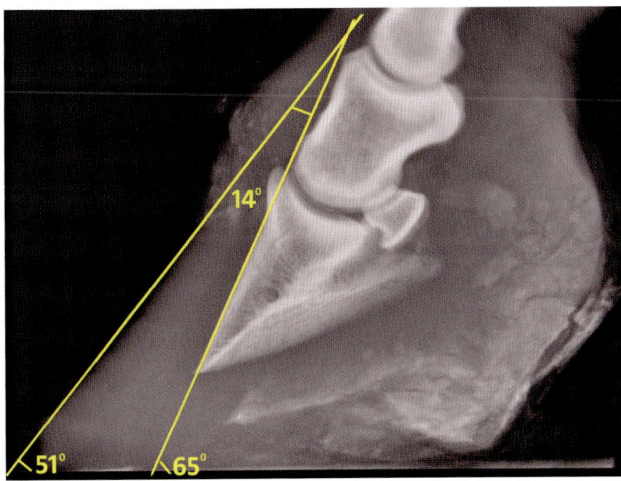

11.41 Dorsal-angle rotation is one of the most important pieces of information you can get from an X-ray in cases of laminitis. In this foot, the angle of the front surface of the coffin bone is 65 degrees, while the angle of the dorsal hoof wall is 51 degrees, which means there is 14 degrees of rotation. Remember that in a healthy foot, the angles of the coffin bone and the dorsal wall would be the same.

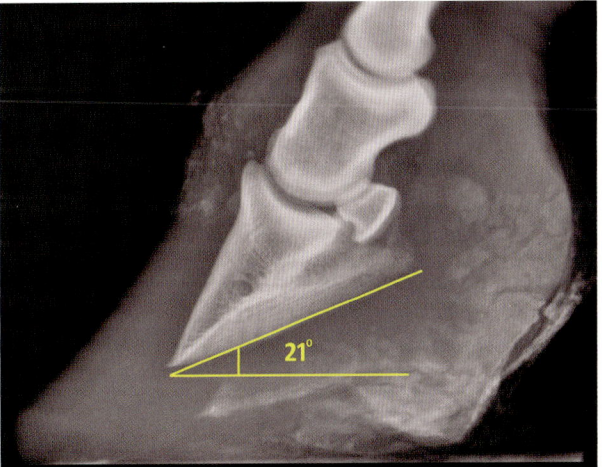

11.42 Being able to visualize the palmar/plantar angle allows hoof-care providers and veterinarians to plan for rehabilitative trimming. This foot has a 21-degree palmar/plantar angle, while healthy feet generally have a 2–5-degree angle.

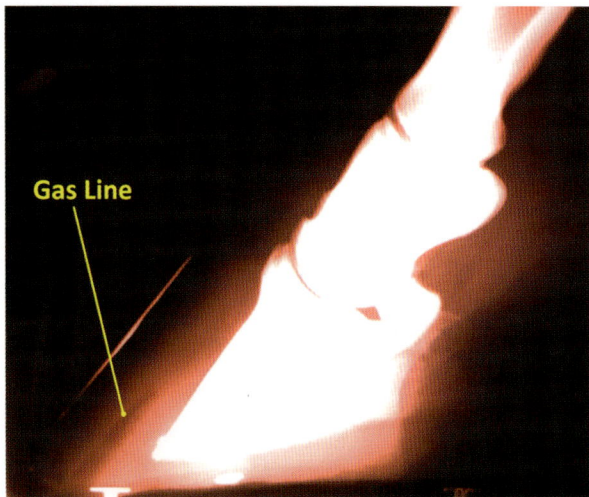

11.43 A "gas line," which is a pocket of disintegrated tissue, shows up in an X-ray as a dark area under the hoof wall. Seeing a gas line is visual confirmation of separation, even if rotation is minimal or absent.

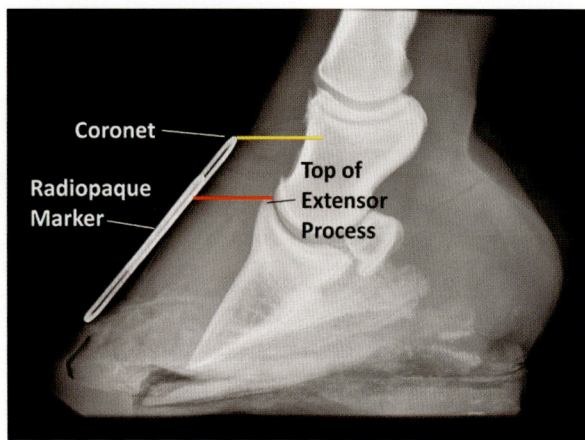

11.44 Distal descent, where the coffin bone "sinks" in relation to the hoof capsule, is a very serious problem. An X-ray with a radiopaque marker placed to show the location of the coronet allows you to see how much descent is present. In a healthy foot, the top of the extensor process lines up with the coronet, or close to it. In this foot, however, there is a large gap between the yellow line marking the level of the coronet, and the red line marking the level of the top of the extensor process, showing a significant degree of distal descent. Being able to see this will help your vet and hoof-care provider to make the best decisions for treatment.

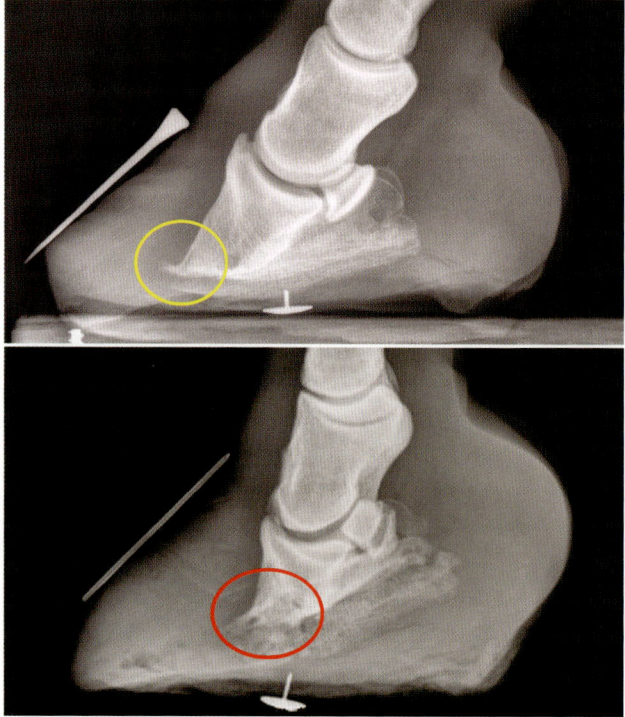

11.45 A "ski tip," also called "lipping" (above, circled in yellow), is usually the first change noticeable when rotation has gone uncorrected for some time. As more time passes, the damage may become more extensive, with the bone dissolving away (below, circled in red). Bone loss of any significant degree makes rehabilitation more difficult or sometimes impossible.

• Is there a visible "gas line"? What the vets call a gas line is a pocket of disorganized, separated material that shows up on an X-ray as a dark area along the inside of the hoof wall (fig. 11.43).

• Does the top of the extensor process line up with the coronet, or is it lower, indicating distal descent (fig. 11.44)?

• If the condition has been present for a while, are there any changes/damage to the coffin bone? Remodeling of the bone often starts with the front of the bottom edge deforming forward from the unnatural pressure it is enduring, often referred to as a "ski tip" or "lipping." As deterioration continues, the tip of the bone may dissolve altogether (fig. 11.45).

A New Tool: The Venogram

A new tool in the fight against laminitis is the *venogram*. A venogram is a vascular study in which contrast dye is injected into the blood vessels of the foot, which is then X-rayed (fig. 11.46). In a normal foot, the vessels show up in a certain pattern, but that pattern changes with laminitis as blood vessels in the laminae are destroyed and others get compressed by an unstable coffin bone.

One of the advantages of a venogram over an X-ray is that it can detect subtle changes before there is measurable displacement of the coffin bone (fig. 11.47). Therefore, to provide the greatest benefit, the first venograms should be performed as early as possible, ideally within the first 48 hours of the horse showing lameness. This will help determine the severity of the case and assist in the selection of a treatment plan. A follow-up venogram anywhere from four days to three weeks later is also helpful in monitoring the horse's response to treatment.

Some experts now feel that proceeding with treatment without a series of venograms can be misleading. Their reasoning is that many cases of laminitis appear to respond to initial treatment because the comfort level of the horse has improved, but despite that apparent improvement, the foot may not be healing adequately. The horse is assumed to be stable, but the lack of improvement eventually leads to the structural collapse of the foot. Such horses usually "crash" four to six weeks

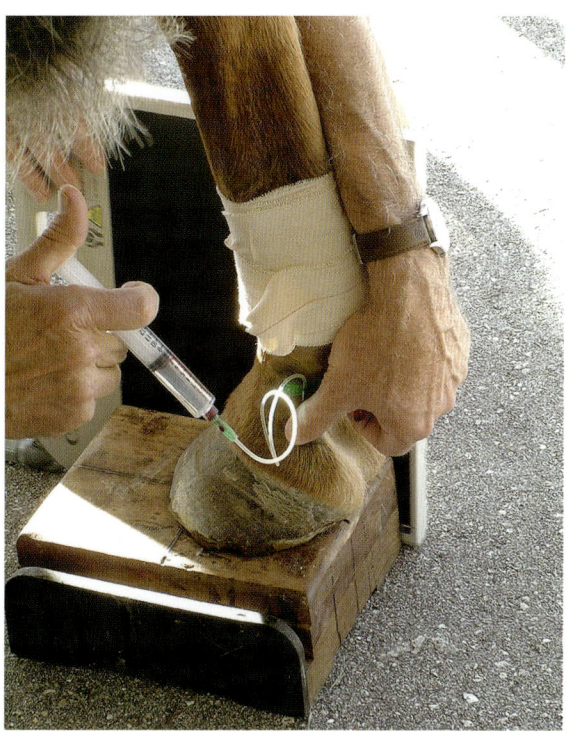

11.46 Blood vessels are not normally visible on X-rays, but the contrast dye injected into the blood vessels for a venogram makes them show up very well.

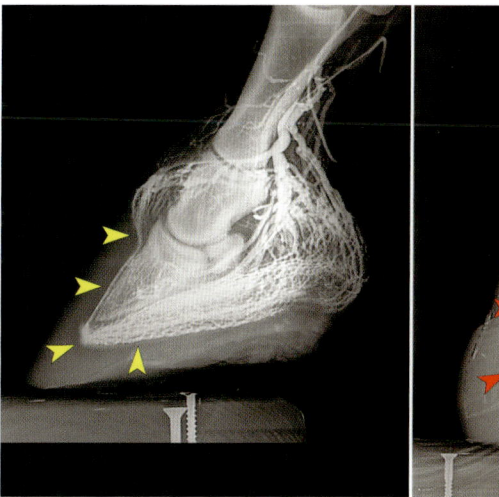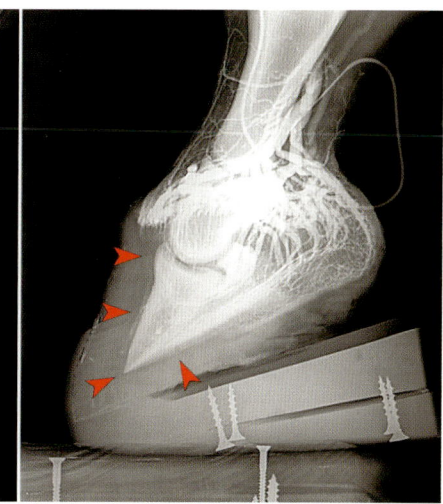

11.47 The changes in blood flow that occur in acute laminitis are visible long before any displacement of the bone. The foot on the left is a normal foot, and the one on the right has laminitis. Although there is no rotation at this stage, you can see that the blood flow to the lamina has effectively ceased, and blood flow under the coffin bone is also greatly diminished. Compare the blood flow in the areas pointed out by the yellow arrows in the healthy foot to the same areas pointed out by the red arrows in the laminitic foot.

Dr. Ric Redden on
The Value of the Venogram

"I developed this clinical protocol out of the need to better understand the degree of vascular damage during different stages of the laminitis syndrome. Working with Dr. Chris Pollitt at my clinic, we used his in-vitro (not within a living organism) study to perform the first in-vivo (within a living organism) venogram procedure in 1992. Since that time, I have modified the procedure to meet the requirements of specific breeds, as well as a variety of foot problems that involve the circulatory system (fig. 11.48).

"Having performed a few thousand venograms over the years, I have discovered a pattern that appears to be repeatable as laminitis progresses from a mild onset to high-scale cases, whether it is acute or chronic. Likewise, the venogram offers a reliable means of monitoring the progress of reperfusion (restoration of blood flow) in compromised areas. It also helps explain why some cases fail to progress in a favorable fashion. Being able to correlate the altered vascular pattern with the clinical picture, growth pattern, and tissue response greatly enhances your insight for the planning and treatment stage.

"A venogram is a discovery experience, as it offers a means to track the disease syndrome as it alters the vascular supply. Therefore, it offers unlimited options concerning the medical, surgical, and therapeutic regimes necessary to revive the compromised areas. Being able to visualize the vascular tree (branching blood vessels):

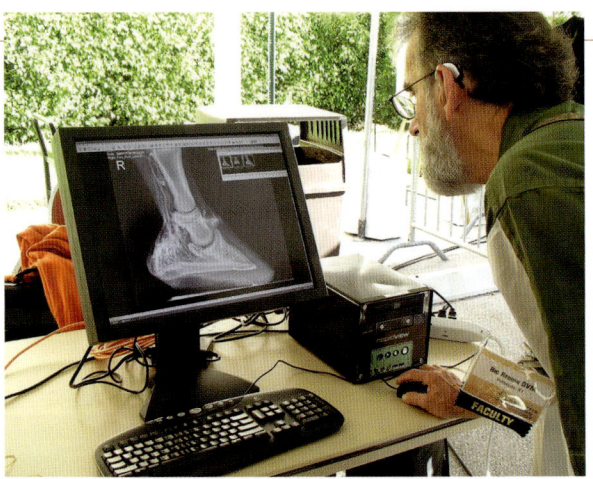

11.48 Dr. Ric Redden pioneered the use of the venogram and developed it to the point where it is now an incredibly powerful tool for the diagnostic imaging of laminitis.

• Helps you better understand the relationship of load (weight bearing) and vascular patency (degree to which the blood vessels are blocked).

• Allows you to see healthy blood supply versus pathology (disease or damage).

• Helps you predict tissue response relative to degree of compromise (how well the foot is likely to heal based on the damage seen).

• Allows you to monitor efficiency of treatment regime.

• Defines various levels of damage and precise location.

• Helps you better understand the requirements of horn growth and maturation.

• Alludes to the timing for the DDF tenotomy (surgical severing of the deep digital flexor tendon) when a tenotomy is appropriate (see p. 203).

- Alludes to prognosis in advanced or high-scale damage cases.

- Ultimately helps save horses' careers and lives.

  "When should you perform a venogram?

- Acute case: Day one or on the very first exam, set the baseline values.

- Repeat venogram in 3–5 days, depending on history.

- Third venogram: 5–10 days later. This one will allude to the prognosis and will also indicate if more aggressive treatment is needed—for example, de-rotation strategies and DDF tenotomy.

  "The venogram is basically reserved for the acute case as an aid to access vascular damage, and it has predictive values in the hands of those with exceptional experience in this procedure. It can also be used as a diagnostic aid and allude to prognosis in advanced or high-scale cases.

  "Caution is due: Technique failure or even slight difficulties can be very deceptive, giving false negative as well as false positive results. Positioning of the limb (loaded versus unloaded) and beam orientation can greatly influence the information obtained. Therefore, the person performing the venogram must be clear of mind concerning precisely the information he or she is seeking and have skills to obtain optimum information with every venogram."

after the initial onset of laminitis. At that point, you can still do a venogram to determine the case severity, but you will have missed the best window of time in which to make effective changes in treatment.

Ongoing Care for the Laminitic Horse

Caring for a horse that has foundered or even one who has had sub-acute laminitis requires dedication, patience, and the help of knowledgeable and experienced professionals. Among those professionals, however, you will find that there are many very different ideas on how to deal with the feet of a foundered horse. Most equine podiatrists do agree that in the early stages at least, it is best to pull a horse's shoes and keep him barefoot until stabilized, as it is both difficult and expensive to keep up with the changes a laminitic foot undergoes when the horse is wearing shoes. The needs of laminitic horses can change quite quickly in the early days and weeks, and being able to respond to those changes by making adjustments in hoof support can mean the difference between successful treatment and catastrophe.

As for the longer term, there are a plethora of options that can be more than a little overwhelming. Not surprisingly, most farriers who apply shoes believe that the best way to help a foundered horse is to use some form of therapeutic shoeing, while barefoot specialists believe that barefoot trimming, often with the temporary addition of padded hoof boots or casting, is the way to go. Vets may take either position, but as most have little experience with good barefoot protocols and the success these can bring in cases of founder, they tend to lean toward shoeing.

It would be wonderful if there was one method that worked for every horse, but the fact is that every case of founder is unique, and ultimately, you, as the horse owner, have to decide which approach you want to take.

That said, there is universal agreement that the main objectives when working on a foundered foot are to return the coffin bone to as normal a position as possible, and to encourage the growth of healthy, well-connected walls and robust soles—but that is pretty much where agreement ends. It would take an entire book (or perhaps several volumes) to go over the myriad options employed to help the feet of laminitic horses, but here are some of the most frequently encountered approaches.

Shoes

Shoeing is the traditional method for helping horses recover from laminitis and is the most common go-to for vets and farriers. There is an abundance of types of shoes that have been used to treat the laminitic foot including reverse shoes, wide web shoes, egg bar shoes, heart bar shoes, rocker shoes, wedge shoes, rail shoes, banana shoes, and plain old keg shoes (fig. 11.49). Every farrier has their favorites, but good farriers understand that each case is individual and must be handled with consideration of each foot's unique needs.

Like any other treatment for laminitis, correct identification of what is going on in the horse is critical, as is correct placement of the shoe. Generally, the idea is to support the heels and relieve pressure at the toe. Setting breakover close to the tip of P3 is normally called for, and then finding optimal heel height and padding/packing options are factored in. Shoeing at all can be problematic for some foundered horses, as driving the nails can cause pain, and standing on a foundered foot while the other one is being shod can be almost impossible.

It is important to be aware that shoeing may worsen the effects of laminitis and promote distal descent if the foot is left peripherally loaded.

Clogs

The Steward Clog, developed by Oklahoma veterinarian Dr. Michael Steward, has become more popular with veterinarians and farriers over the last few years (fig. 11.50). Developed about three decades ago, the Steward Clog started out as a low cost treatment for laminitis. Dr. Steward made plywood stacks up to 3 inches in height, heavily beveled the ground surface, and attached the clog to the hoof with screws, often with soft impression material underneath the sole and frog. The softer and more shock-absorbing platform of wood seemed to make many laminitic horses more comfortable than steel, and the heavily beveled ground surface allowed the horse to easily adjust his hoof angles. Breakover

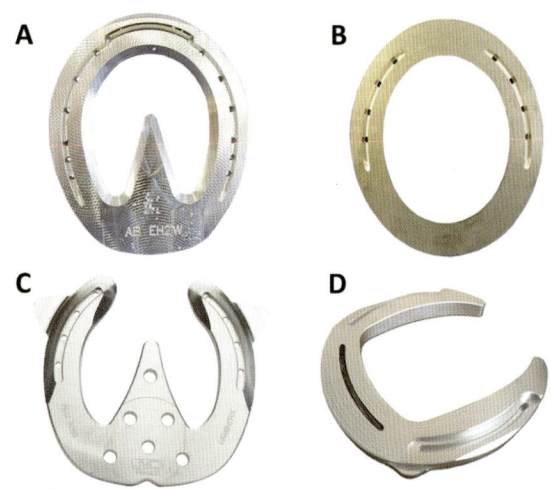

11.49 There are many different kinds of shoes that can be used in the treatment of laminits. The four shown here are: heart bar by Anvil Brand (A), egg bar by RGM (B), JMD Laminitix, which is applied open at the toe (C), and rocker shoe by NANRIC (D).

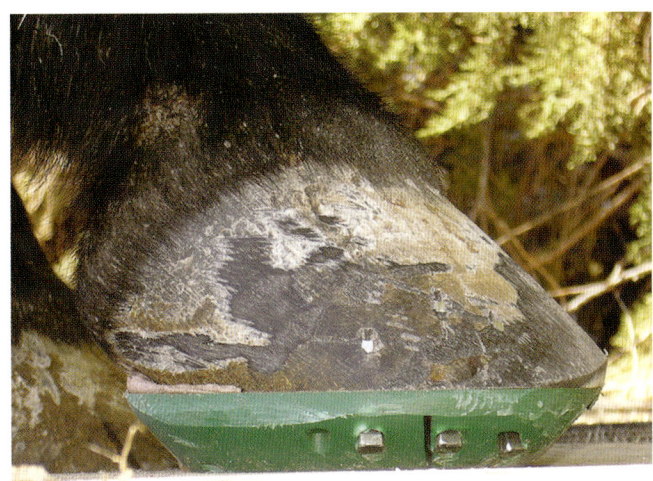

11.50 The Steward Clog can increase comfort and provide good support for many laminitic horses.

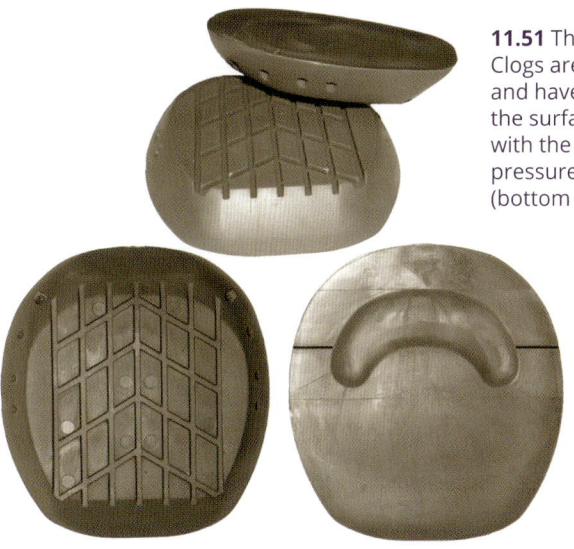

11.51 The new EVA Steward Clogs are softer than wood, and have a recessed area on the surface that interfaces with the hoof to relieve pressure on the coffin bone (bottom right).

could also be set back under the tip of the coffin bone with a Steward Clog, easing mechanical forces on the damaged laminae.

Since their initial introduction, some tinkering has gone on with the clogs to improve them. They can still be solid wood, but they are now sometimes made of EVA (ethylene-vinyl acetate) for an even softer feel, or a combination of wood/EVA or EVA/ leather (fig. 11.51). They are still often screwed onto the horse's foot, but can also be nailed, glued, or casted on. Like any procedure on a foundered horse, the proper application of the clog is impera- tive to good performance.

Hoof Casts

Casts have been used for a long time to set bro- ken bones, and lately their use has become more prevalent in treating hoof issues. Hoof casts reduce the flexion of the hoof, stabilizing it without pound- ing nails into the hoof to affix a shoe (fig. 11.52). This reduced flexion can bring relief to damaged

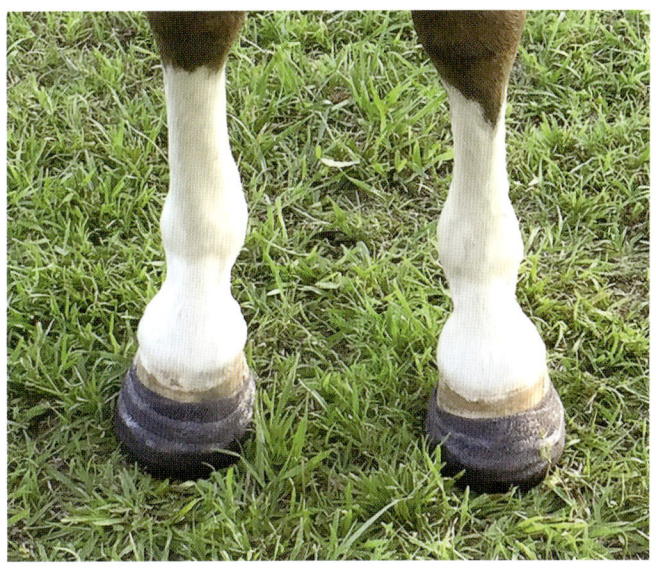

11.52 A hoof cast offers a great way to reduce flexion of the foot without having to use nails. Similar to casting materials used on people, most hoof casting is made of fiberglass that comes in rolls of various widths. Strips are cut as needed, then moistened either before or after application, depend- ing on the ambient temperature. When it is hot out, you generally wrap the foot before wetting the casting material to prevent it from setting up (hardening) too fast. In cold temperatures, strips are typically soaked before application.

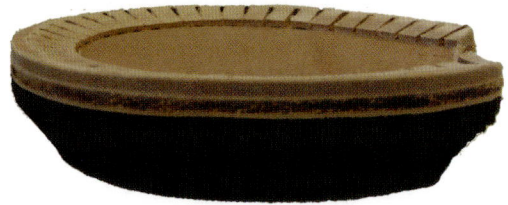

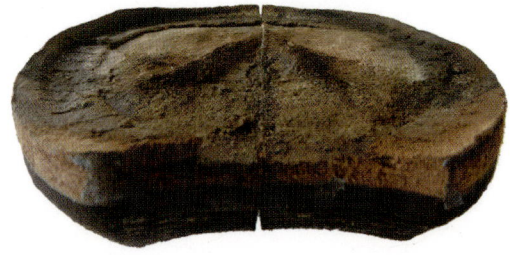

11.53 The EVA (ethylene-vinyl acectate) and leather "shoes" made by Equicast® are specifically designed to be used with hoof-casting materials. The side view (above) shows a profile similar to a Steward Clog, while the used pad (below) shows how the leather takes on the shape of the foot. Other kinds of pads can also work nicely—it just depends on what a horse's particular needs are.

increased discomfort. They are, therefore, best applied by veterinarians or hoof-care providers with experience in their proper use. Casting is often used in situations where shoes are not considered optimal but hoof boots will present difficulties for the owner in terms of day-to-day maintenance.

Hoof Boots

There has been a huge explosion in the number of hoof boots on the market, with new ones coming out seemingly every month. Most hoof boots are meant for riding purposes, but more are becoming available for therapeutic uses, and some are designed to be left on for up to 24 hours at a time (fig. 11.54). Boots can be particularly helpful in many laminitis cases, especially where frequent trimming and adjustments are necessary. The boot is simply removed, the foot tended to, and the boot put back on, all without the use of glues, screws, nails, or

and malfunctioning laminae, giving them a break so they can heal. Casting material comes in widths of 2, 3, and 4 inches. The size used depends on how big the foot is, and if a full sole coverage cast is wanted, or just a rim cast that leaves the sole open. Pads and packing material can be used under a cast if the horse is comfortable with that. One kind of pad, made by Equicast® out of leather and EVA, is specifically made to be used with hoof casting and conforms to the foot very precisely (fig. 11.53). If pads are not used and the center of the sole is left uncovered, disinfectant soaks can still be effectively administered.

One important consideration with casting is that casts can be applied too tight, which might cause

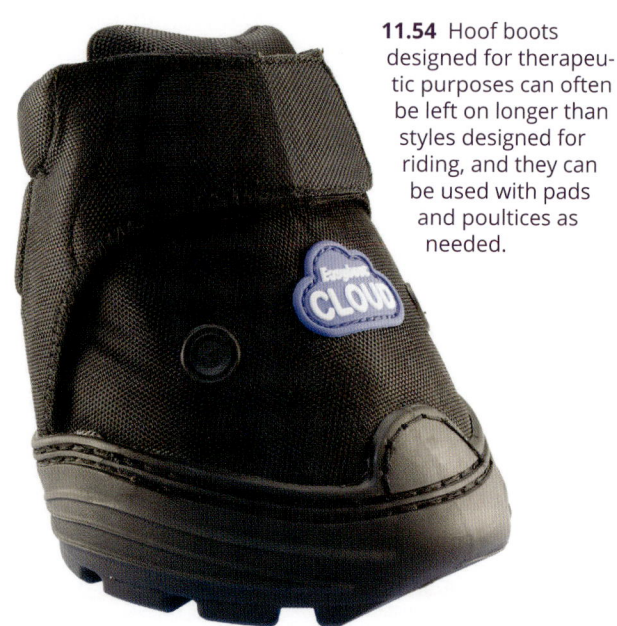

11.54 Hoof boots designed for therapeutic purposes can often be left on longer than styles designed for riding, and they can be used with pads and poultices as needed.

whatnot that might affect the hoof wall. Different padding and packing material can also be used with boots and adjusted as the hoof's needs require. Even without pads, the rubber soles of hoof boots are rather cushy and seem to make many horses more comfortable than steel shoes.

There are many brands of boots available, and every veterinarian or hoof-care provider has his or her favorites to work with. It is hoped they recognize that the best boot for one horse might not be optimal for another, and that the same horse might benefit more from one type than another at different times during his recovery. Ease of use is a further consideration with hoof boots, as some can be safely left on for longer periods, while others require more frequent removal, which can be a strain for some horse owners.

One of the main concerns with the use of boots is rubbing, which can cause sores. Even boots designed for around-the-clock use can still rub certain horses, but usually there is a way to circumvent this. Applying vet wrap or an old sock under the boot is often quite effective, but not always. In addition, because hooves do perspire a bit, boots often need to be cleaned and sometimes dusted with a medicated foot powder to prevent the boot and foot from getting soggy, which can increase the risk of thrush infection.

Pads and Packing Material

If you thought the options available for shoes, therapeutics boots, and casting were overwhelming, you might need to sit down to consider the astronomical number of alternatives in padding and packing material that can be used to support the bottom of a laminitic foot. Packing products come medicated

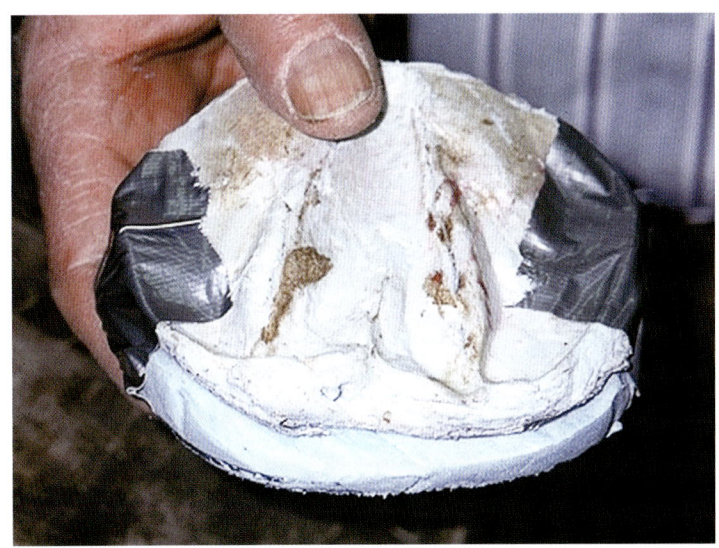

11.55 Impression materials are often used to pack the bottom of a foot under a therapeutic pad. They conform well to the foot but remain flexible. Here, impression material was used under a foam support pad.

and non-medicated, and can be made of many different materials with varying densities (fig. 11.55). Pads can be foam, leather, plastic, rubber, gel; wedge or flat or frog support pads; thin or thick—it really doesn't end. The use of pads and packing is further complicated by the fact that the needs of the laminitic hoof are ever changing. Still, finding the right support materials can make a world of difference in the horse's comfort level, so it is worth trying to figure out what works at any given point in time.

The key principle when using any form of padding or packing is to test the material to ensure the laminitic horse is comfortable in the density of the material being used, and to make sure there isn't any pressure where it will make the horse sore. Often, this means that the padding material needs to be cut away in the toe so it won't put any pressure on the sole under the tip of P3, as this can be a very sensitive area on a foundered horse. In some instances, the horse is most comfortable when the packing material is only applied to the back half of the foot.

There is a lot of trial and error in finding the right material, but if you pay careful attention to the horse's response to the application of pads or packing, and adjust as necessary, it can significantly improve your horse's comfort level, help minimize damage, and assist in the healing process.

Science Goes Barefoot

A few years ago, a group of veterinary researchers led by Dr. Debra Taylor of the Department of Clinical Sciences at Auburn University conducted a study examining the potential benefits of the management protocol for laminitic horses developed by barefoot specialist Pete Ramey. For years, Ramey had been claiming that his methods could routinely rehabilitate many laminitic horses that more traditional experts had deemed hopeless—but could he

prove it under the cold, impartial gaze of scientific inquiry? Turns out he could.

Not wanting to make it easy, the researchers selected a study group consisting of 14 laminitic horses that were seriously compromised. The horses had a mean lameness score of 3.5 on the Obel scale, which ranges from 1–4, with anything above 3 being considered severe. They also had considerable degrees of rotation: the least was 5 degrees; the worst was 29 degrees (fig. 11.56). As the prognosis for return to former athletic function is considered guarded for horses with 5.5 to 11.5 degrees of rotation, and poor for horses with more than 11.5 degrees (six horses in the study had more than 11.5 degrees), this was definitely a group of subjects that would put Ramey's methods to the test.

Taylor's group worked with Ramey to implement his multi-pronged approach, the highlights of which are as follows:

• Very specific barefoot hoof care that involves trimming the foot to unload the toe wall, and supporting the coffin bone through the use of padded boots.

• Diet modification aimed at carbohydrate reduction.

• Exercise introduced and conducted within particular parameters, the aim of which is to develop a healthier foot by encouraging correct, heel-first landing.

The experiment was a resounding success. In a paper published in the *Journal of Equine Veterinary Science,* the team concluded that, "Using the described management protocol, 14 of 14 laminitic horses with rotation greater than 5 degrees and

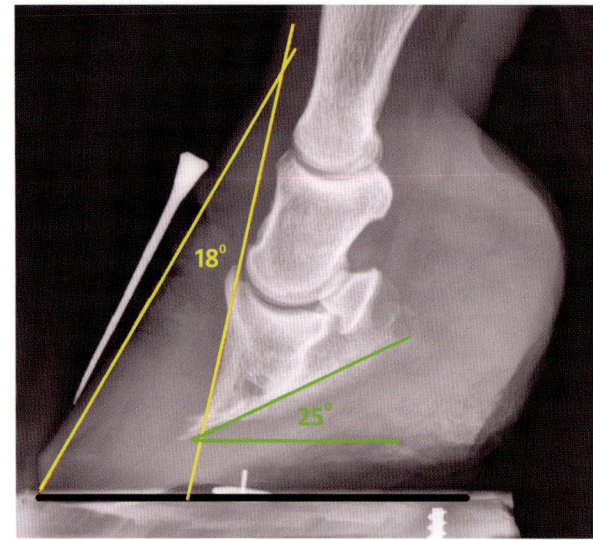

11.56 The horses in the Auburn study had dorsal rotation of up to 29 degrees. The hoof in this X-ray has 18 degrees of dorsal rotation, which should give you a sense of just how badly off the study subjects were. And, imagine what the palmar angles of the study subjects must have been like, when this foot shows a 25-degree palmar angle (healthy being around 2–5 degrees).

a guarded prognosis returned to their pre-laminitis level of soundness by the time of the endpoint radiographic evaluation. A long-term follow-up survey indicated that most of these horses maintained the same level of soundness without incidence of laminitis recurrence or hoof abscess formation. This method of laminitis management is effective and warrants further evaluation."

Ramey's methods have also proven successful with horses even worse off than those in the Auburn study. Ramey and others using his or similar techniques regularly bring around many apparently catastrophic cases—even ones where the coffin bone has penetrated the sole, a situation many traditional experts consider impossible to remedy.

Of course, no method is going to be able to save every horse, and Ramey emphasizes that the greatest likelihood of successful rehabilitation comes when you can start appropriate management before there is significant damage to the coffin bone.

Horses that do already have extensive damage to the coffin bone and other structures may still benefit from a program like Ramey's that emphasizes good barefoot hoof care, attention to diet, and appropriate exercise that encourages healthy development of the feet, but the degree to which they can recover is going to depend on the severity and type of damage, as well as the skill of the hoof-care provider and the level of commitment of the owner.

We hope that if you are ever faced with a laminitic horse and you want to try the barefoot route, you can start taking the right steps before bone damage occurs. (To get the specific details of Ramey's laminitis management protocols, you can read the entire text of the Auburn team's paper with accompanying photos at: http://www.j-evs.com/article/S0737-0806(13)00637-0/fulltext.)

A Surgical Option: Deep Digital Flexor Tenotomy

In cases of laminitis that are not responding to standard treatments, or where rotation is severe early in the disease process, veterinarians will sometimes recommend a procedure called a deep digital flexor tenotomy, which involves cutting the DDFT in the mid-cannon region (fig. 11.57). The purpose of the surgery is to relieve the pull of the DDFT on the back of the cannon bone, which will allow for realignment of the coffin bone through therapeutic trimming and the application of support devices.

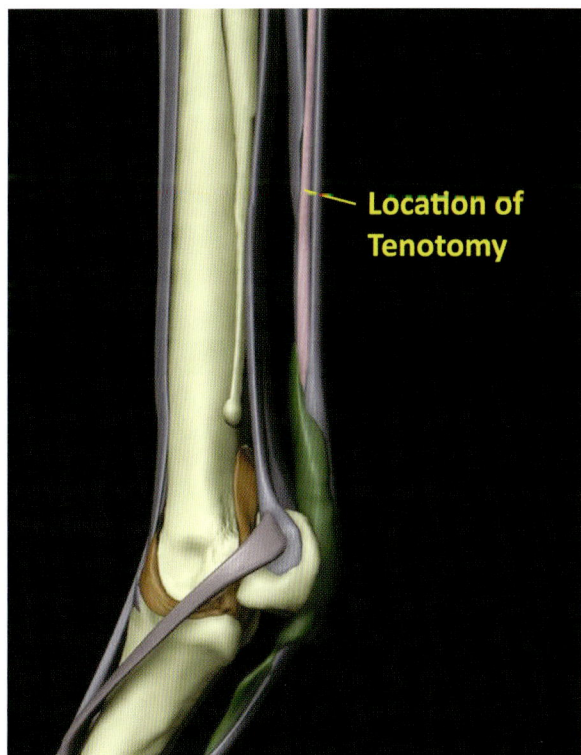

Location of Tenotomy

11.57 When a DDF tenotomy is performed, the DDFT (pink), sandwiched between the superficial digital flexor tendon and the accessory ligament, is severed at the mid-cannon level.

When the surgery and follow-up treatment are successful, the horse is comfortable, blood flow in the foot improves, sole thickness increases, and deterioration of the coffin bone is prevented. Horses are usually only pasture sound after the tenotomy has been performed, but some can be used for light riding. Since this surgery is usually considered a "salvage" operation, meaning that otherwise, the horse would be facing euthanasia, achieving even pasture soundness is a good outcome.

However, studies looking into the effectiveness of the procedure have returned mixed results. Some indicate that it is less effective when performed during the acute phase of the disease, and some concluded that it is not helpful at all in cases where there is distal descent, rather than rotation. One study did find that 73% of owners whose horses were included in the study were satisfied with the outcome and would have the surgery done again if ever faced with a horse in a similar situation.

There are also hoof-care specialists who believe that when laminitis occurs, the primary mechanical force that pulls the laminae apart is the weight of the horse coming down on the foot, not the pull of the DDFT. They have found that while there is a rotational force exerted on the coffin bone by the DDFT, this force can be successfully negated in many cases by unloading the toe wall and supporting the coffin bone through the sole (see Auburn study discussed on p. 203).

If you weigh the pros and cons and do opt for a DDF tenotomy, it is important to understand that the success of the procedure is at least partially dependent on the aftercare the horse receives. The recovery period can be lengthy and requires stall confinement, which may range from one to six months depending on the severity of the case and at what point in the disease process the procedure is performed. Short periods of hand walking may be allowed and recommended, but that will also depend on the severity of the case. Monthly follow-up X-rays are necessary to monitor how things are going in the attempt to realign the coffin bone. Between those and the necessity for intensive farrier care, costs can mount up, even though the surgery itself is relatively inexpensive due to its simplicity and the fact that it can generally be performed with the sedated horse standing.

Feeding the Laminitic Horse

It is a sad reality that the vast majority of cases of laminitis would have been completely preventable had the owners of the horses been aware of how big a role diet plays in most instances of this terrible disease. It truly cannot be emphasized enough that allowing horses to become obese, feeding diets high in non-structural carbohydrates, and allowing at-risk horses to graze on pasture are the primary reasons why laminitis strikes thousands upon thousands of horses each year.

It is equally true that once a horse gets carbohydrate- or pasture-associated laminitis, recovery is far less likely, and prolonged suffering is far more likely if the horse's owner does not take the need for strict dietary changes very seriously. We discuss this in more detail in *Feeding the Foot* on page 238, but the basics for feeding any laminitic horse are:

• Eliminate all sources of grain and grain products, including wheat bran.

• Do not let him graze. Grass, even when it looks dry and dead, can contain surprising amounts of sugar, and as the levels fluctuate all the time, there is no way to know when it might be safe, if it ever is. If you must turn a laminitic horse out on anything other than a dry lot, use a grazing muzzle to restrict his feed intake (fig. 11.58).

• Try to source low-carbohydrate grass hay that has been tested and has sugar (listed on tests as ESC) and starch numbers that add up to less than 10%.

• If low-carb hay is not available, look for somewhat coarse, first-cut hay, as this has a *better* chance of being lower carb, though there is no way to know for sure without testing.

• Soak—meaning completely submerge—any untested hay for approximately one hour just prior to feeding, as this will remove up to 30% of the sugar from the hay. There is no guarantee that this will make it safe, but it will make it *safer*.

• Feed alfalfa cautiously or not at all. Some laminitic horses get an increase in foot soreness on alfalfa, despite it almost always being a low carbohydrate feed. No one is exactly sure why this happens, but it may be that some horses are very efficient at converting protein into glucose, and alfalfa is generally high protein. Be aware that many bagged feeds advertised as low carb contain alfalfa, and so may not be safe for some laminitic horses. Hays containing other legumes, such as clover, can also be problematic.

• Avoid grain hays such as oat or rye unless they test safe, as they are often high in starch.

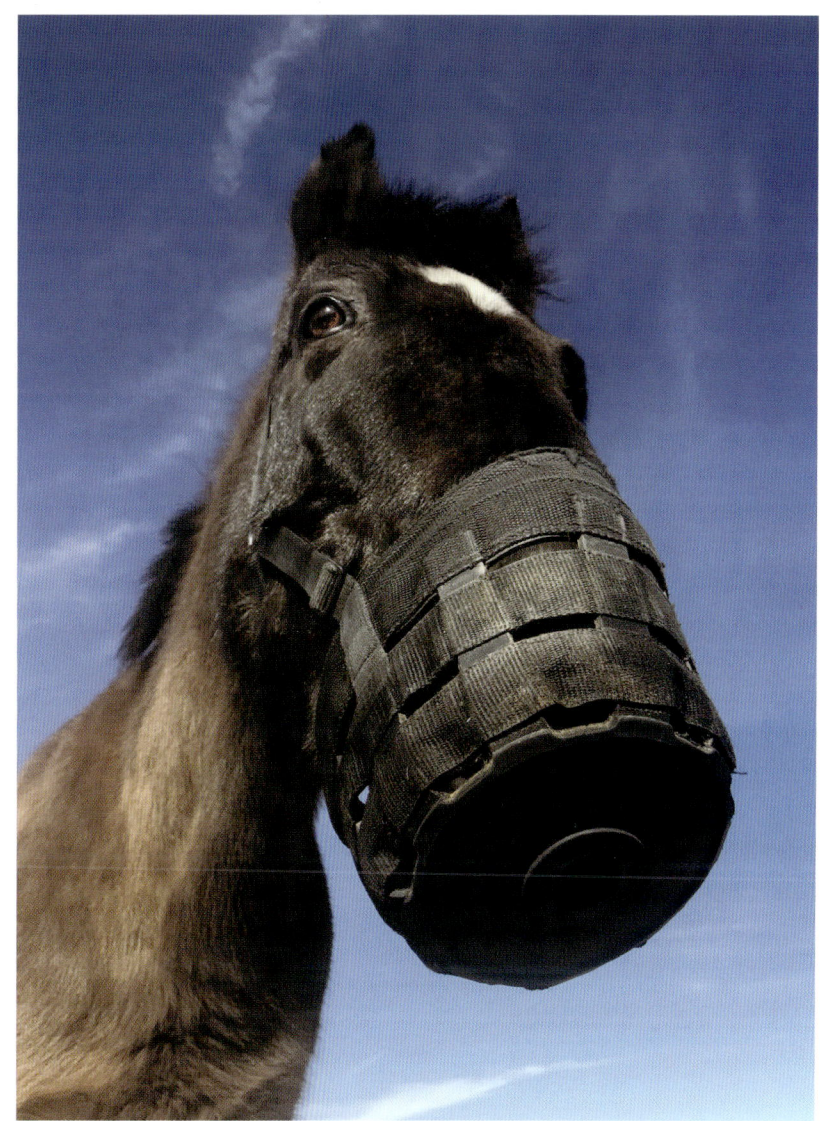

11.58 A grazing muzzle typically has a small opening at the bottom that allows the horse to take in some grass, but not nearly as much as he would consume without the muzzle. Some come with a built-in breakaway halter; others need to be attached to your own halter, which should also be a breakaway model for safety.

• Do not feed sweet treats, fruit, or carrots to laminitic horses. Some will have an increase in soreness with just a bite or two of such treats. A few nuts or a small handful of sunflower seeds are a safer substitute, and most horses absolutely love them.

• Do not feed anything with molasses in it. Molasses is "hidden" in many feeds, some of which don't even list it on the label. If it smells like it could contain molasses, trust that it does, even if it doesn't say so. You can also taste it—if there is any sweetness to it, don't feed it. Some feeds, like beet pulp, are sprayed in molasses that can be removed by soaking and thorough rinsing.

• Do not "starve" a laminitic horse, even if he needs to lose weight. All horses should be fed a minimum of 1.5% of their body weight in forage per day, as their digestive system is designed to have roughage going through it at all times. Instead of going below the 1.5% minimum, opt for a lower calorie (and low carb!) hay. It is always better to feed more low calorie hay than less high calorie hay. Feeding too little can have other health consequences as well, such as the inducement of *hyperlipidemia,* a potentially fatal condition in which the body responds to an energy deficit by increasing blood triglycerides and depositing fat in the liver and other organs. An increased risk of colic is another hazard when feed is too restricted, as is a greatly increased risk of gastric ulcers.

Prevention is at least ten hundred thousand million times better than cure when it comes to laminitis, but whether you are aiming to prevent or treat this disease, what you feed is a major part of the picture. Take that to heart, and your horse's feet will thank you.

12

The Chapter Formerly Known as Navicular Disease

What's in a Name?

The terms *navicular disease* and *navicular syndrome* have both been used to describe lameness attributed to disorders of the navicular bone and surrounding tissues. Whichever term was used, such a diagnosis meant a likelihood of progressive, incurable disability with the specter of euthanasia always looming somewhere down the line. Most often, veterinarians would diagnose navicular disease based on certain signs of lameness, a positive response to a nerve block of the foot, and X-rays showing degenerative changes in the navicular bone, typically in the form of pitting or "lollipop-shaped" lesions (fig. 12.1). Having done the appropriate clinical workup and finding such lesions, it was assumed that the navicular bone was the cause of the horse's pain.

The problem with this method of diagnosis was that horses could have marked changes in the navicular bone yet not be lame at all, while other horses had perfect X-rays but were lame with every "navicular" sign in the book. When presented with such mystery cases, horse owners and veterinarians alike were frequently frustrated by the latter's

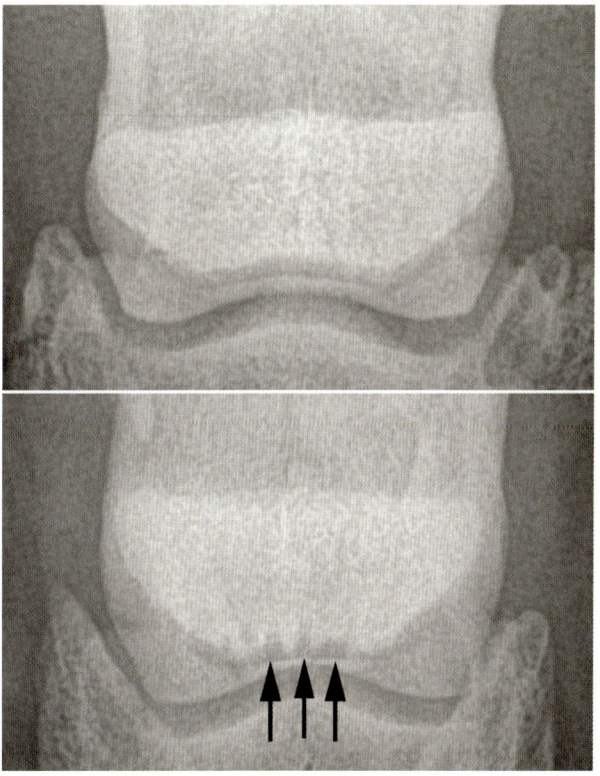

12.1 The dark spots (indicated by black arrows) on the bottom edge of the navicular bone in the lower X-ray show the "lollipop" lesions that were once thought to define navicular disease and explain chronic pain in the back of the foot. Compare this to the normal image above.

inability to lock down a diagnosis. Hence came the term "navicular syndrome," a catchall phrase that basically meant the horse was exhibiting signs of pain in the back of the foot that were thought to have something to do with the navicular bone, but no one could really say for sure.

These days, veterinarians use a slew of other terms such as *palmar heel pain, caudal heel syndrome, palmar foot pain*, or *podotrochlear syndrome* when investigating lameness that appears to be emanating from the back of the foot, and there is no clear winner in the "which term is best" debate. What has become clear is that what used to get labeled as navicular disease or navicular syndrome can actually be a number of different problems, most of which have nothing to do with the navicular bone at all. This knowledge has come to us primarily through the use of magnetic resonance imaging (MRI), which allows us to visualize soft tissue disease and damage in ways that were previously impossible, and to see bone abnormalities that do not show up on traditional X-rays.

As a result of MRI investigations into pain isolated to the foot by nerve blocks, we now know that problems such as strain or rupture of the DDFT, inflammation of the navicular bursa, lesions or inflammation of the impar ligament or collateral ligaments, edema (fluid) in the navicular bone, tiny bone chips, inflammation or arthritis of the coffin joint, wearing of the cartilage on the palmar (bottom) surface of the navicular bone, and a number of other issues can all manifest as pain in the heel region and cause a horse to show similar signs of lameness.

Signs of Palmar Foot Pain

Because there are so many different problems that can cause pain in the back of the foot, the signs can vary quite a bit. They may include one or more of the following:

• Insidious, slowly progressive lameness in the forelimbs, usually in both legs but sometimes on just one side.

• Sudden onset of lameness in the forelimbs, usually unilateral but sometimes bilateral.

• Short, choppy, or shuffling gaits.

• Lameness that worsens on hard ground.

• Pain when asked to move in a tight circle.

• Stumbling.

• Toe-first landing.

• Sensitivity to hoof testers on the central third of the frog.

• Relief from pain when a nerve block is applied to the palmar digital nerve (fig. 12.2).

• Frequent shifting of body weight when resting.

• Resting the affected foot on the toe ("pointing"), in an attempt to relieve pressure on the heels.

• Reduction in lameness with rest, but lameness returns with work.

While all of these signs can occur due to pain in the heel region, some of them may be more

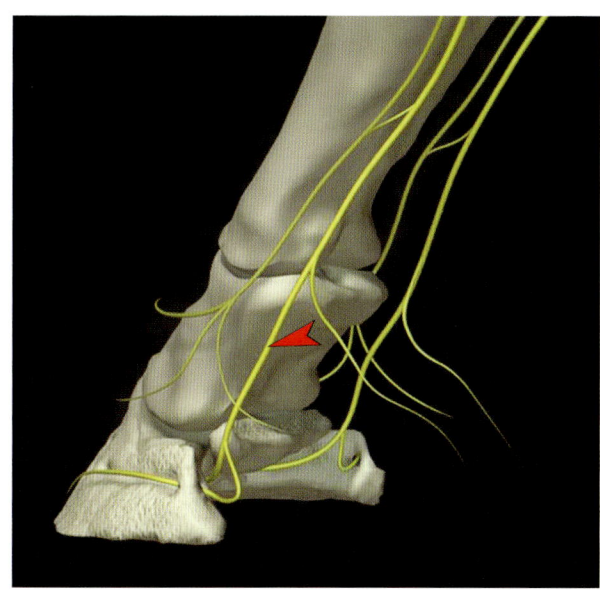

12.2 A palmar digital nerve block is meant to numb the foot below a certain point (red arrow) to allow the practitioner to determine whether the horse's pain is coming from somewhere in the foot or somewhere else. If the nerve block is performed and the lameness goes away, the problem is likely in the foot.

indicative of specific problems. Horses that show pain when asked to perform a tight circle, for example, are more likely to have damage to the DDFT than other issues. And, a sudden, unilateral onset of lameness is more likely to be an acute injury than a chronic degenerative condition.

Finding the Problem

When a horse presents with signs of palmar foot pain, a veterinarian will conduct a clinical examination looking for any unevenness in gait, as well as abnormalities in the hoof or lower limb. He or she will likely use hoof testers, and if the horse consistently shows a positive pain response when the testers are applied to the central third of the frog, your vet may then want to perform a nerve block to try to gain more information about the source of the pain.

However, we now know that the traditional palmar digital nerve block numbs sensation in a much wider region than was previously

thought—sometimes pain originating as high up as the fetlock can be blocked in this way. Thus, while this procedure can often give you an idea about whether or not pain is coming from the foot, it is not 100% reliable, and it has no ability to differentiate between various causes of palmar foot pain. There are newer, more specific types of nerve blocks that can be performed, but while these can narrow the possibilities to some extent, performing such nerve blocks takes particular knowledge and experience, and not all veterinarians have the ability to perform them correctly. False positives and false negatives can occur, not only as a result of errors in technique, but because horses can have variations in the placement of their nerves. Another drawback is that they may have to be done as a series on several separate occasions to get more detailed information, making them more expensive.

Another traditional diagnostic tool, radiography, also has limitations when it comes to palmar foot pain. For one thing, X-rays are extremely insensitive in showing bony changes, requiring a 40% change in density before anything is visible. They also can't show soft tissue problems, which are now thought to account for the majority of cases of pain in the heel region. And, as mentioned earlier, X-rays that show changes in the navicular bone do not necessarily provide an answer regarding the source of a horse's pain. Studies have repeatedly shown that the absence, presence, or degree of changes in the navicular bone have no reliable association with any specific diagnosis, so saying that a horse has navicular disease based on something seen on an X-ray is an iffy proposition. Like nerve blocks, X-rays do still have their place in investigating palmar foot pain, as they can show things like fractures of the coffin bone or navicular bone, and mineralization of the DDFT. But, horse owners need to be aware that X-rays are unlikely to provide definitive answers when it comes to palmar foot pain.

As far as other diagnostic modalities, ultrasound can be useful for imaging certain parts of the collateral ligaments, but overall, it is very limited for evaluating the equine foot, as the ultrasound waves used to create the image are not able to get through the hoof capsule. Endoscopy, where a tube with a camera at the end is inserted into a small

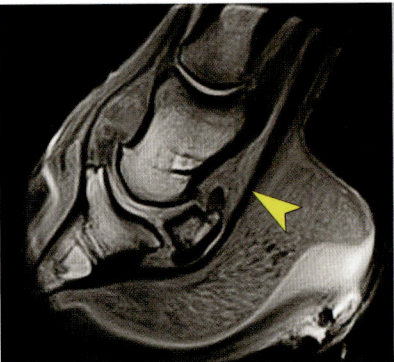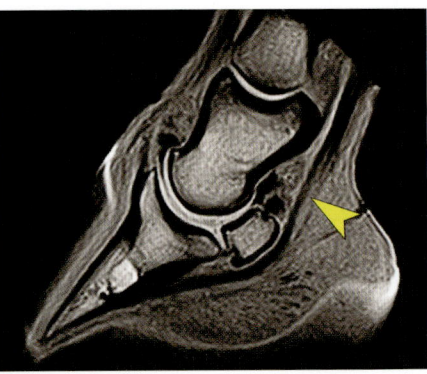

12.3 This pair of MRI images shows a normal foot (left), and one that has a tear in the deep digital flexor tendon (right). The tendon should show as completely black, as it does on the left, but on the right, it shows as disrupted and much lighter, indicating an area of damage. This injury would not show up on an X-ray and could not be fully seen with ultrasound. Without an MRI, this soft tissue injury might very well have been labeled "navicular syndrome."

incision, is occasionally suggested to get a look at the navicular bursa, but as there are so many other possible structures that can be involved in palmar heel pain, it may not be worth the risk of an invasive procedure unless there is some specific reason for suspecting the navicular bursa.

The gold standard when it comes to finding the true source of a horse's heel pain is MRI, as there is currently no other way to get a good look at the interior structures of a living hoof (fig. 12.3). The use of MRI for investigating foot pain has been a quiet revolution, as it has led to changes in the treatment of horses that would previously have been incorrectly diagnosed with navicular disease, as well as those that do indeed have it. For example, it has been found that horses with one of the more common MRI findings, tendonitis of the DDFT near the navicular bone, often improve when anti-inflammatory medications are injected into the digital flexor tendon sheath. Had these horses simply been thrown

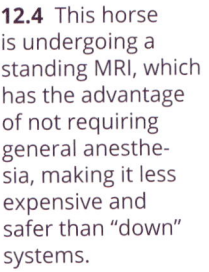

12.4 This horse is undergoing a standing MRI, which has the advantage of not requiring general anesthesia, making it less expensive and safer than "down" systems.

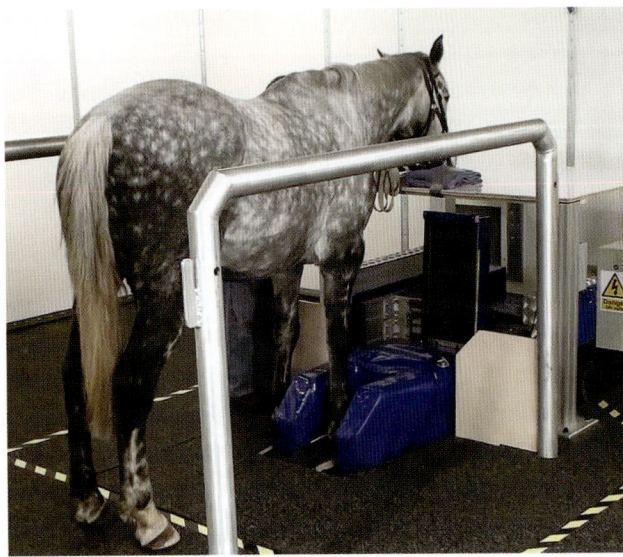

into the "navicular syndrome" heap, that treatment would never have been suggested for them. Figuring out the specific problem also helps determine whether a horse should be rested from work or not. Rest is not traditionally recommended for horses with navicular disease, but may benefit horses with soft tissue inflammation or injury.

The major drawbacks to MRI have generally been cost, availability, and the need for general anesthesia. However, more equine hospitals are equipping themselves with MRI machines all the time, increasing the chances that there is one within driving distance of your location. Many clinics are investing in standing MRI machines (fig. 12.4), which are less

Delving Deeper:
MRI and Actual Navicular Bone Disease

Of all the possibilities MRI can reveal, one of the most reliable indicators of actual navicular disease is the finding of excessive edema (fluid) in the bone (fig. 12.5). Unlike radiographic changes, which for the most part do not match up with clinical signs, fluid in the bone seen with MRI correlates directly with clinical signs, with greater amounts of fluid corresponding with more severe lameness. Edema within the bone can be caused by inflammation and/or trauma, both of which can result from the stresses the navicular bone regularly encounters.

But, MRI can go one step better, finding subtle changes even before edema in the bone occurs. One of the most commonly observed early changes is deterioration of the cartilage on the palmar surface of the navicular bone. Cartilage

gets worn away over time by repeated stresses, and this erosion triggers the bone to start accumulating fluid. If the damage to the cartilage is caught while the lesions are still shallow, therapeutic intervention may prevent further deterioration and increase the horse's chances of returning to use.

However, if the problem has been going on for some time, the lesions may be deeper and accompanied not only by edema, but also by *osteonecrosis*, which is bone damage due to reduced blood flow, and *fibroplasia*, where normal bone and marrow is replaced with fibrous tissue that leaves the bone weak. When these findings are seen, the prognosis for a return to performance is not good. Still, there is reason to hope, as researchers continue to look for novel ways to help horses with navicular disease.

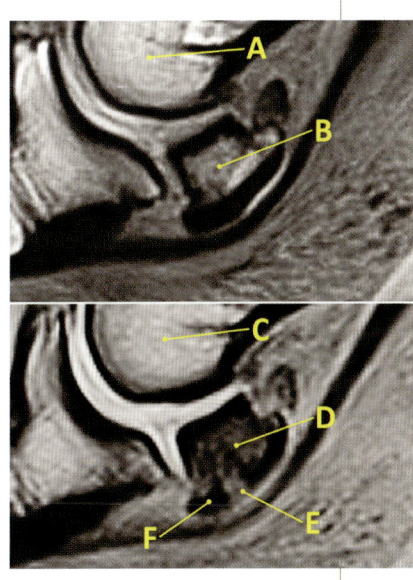

12.5 If you look at the normal navicular bone above (B), it is very similar in shading to the other bones in the foot, such as P2 (A). The abnormal navicular bone below (D) has an accumulation of fluid that makes it appear darker than the other bones (C). In addition, the light area (E) interrupting the normal dark bone of the flexor cortex (F) is a pathological erosion, meaning a lesion caused by some form of disease or injury.

pricey, do not require the horse to go under general anesthesia, and have the same 90% success rate for finding the source of lameness as larger systems that require the horse to be lying down and therefore anesthetized.

As for the expense, MRI can be quite cost effective if not used as a last resort, and it can actually save the horse owner money in the long run by providing a correct diagnosis quickly. It is very easy to spend enormous amounts of money on multiple nerve blocks, repeat exams by veterinarians, X-rays, ultrasounds, unsuccessful treatments, and inappropriate corrective shoeing, yet still be no closer to knowing what is really going on with or helping your horse. Therefore, it may sometimes make more sense to seek out an MRI early on in the process if more traditional methods are failing to provide a definitive answer. A correct diagnosis allows your veterinarian to better predict the long-term outlook for your horse and plan the most effective treatment. Many veterinarians now view MRI as the only way to ensure that they are spending their clients' money appropriately on treatment.

Finding the Cause of the Problem

Since it is now understood that palmar foot pain can be the result of many different problems, often with multiple issues going on at the same time, there is no one answer in terms of what causes these issues to occur. That said, we do know that certain factors appear to make a horse more likely to develop palmar foot problems.

One important element is hoof shape, as a majority of horses who end up sore in the back of the foot have some kind of hoof capsule distortion. As we have seen, imbalanced feet create unnatural stresses on both the exterior and the interior structures of the hoof, resulting in potentially damaging strain. Long toes and underrun heels are two common distortions known to put stress on the structures in the back of the foot, but many other imbalances can trigger heel pain as well. The upside of this is that if the problem is recognized before serious damage occurs, resolving the imbalance may return the horse to soundness.

Another possible factor is poor development of the critical support and cushioning structures of the hoof, mainly the frog, the digital cushion, and the lateral cartilages. If these structures are weak, the foot cannot function properly, and the result is often soreness in the back of the foot (fig. 12.6). Horses raised and kept in confined areas, as well as horses with long-term peripheral loading of the feet, are likely to have poorly developed or atrophied support/cushioning structures, leaving their feet much more vulnerable to mechanical strain, bruising, and degenerative changes.

Other factors associated with an increased risk of palmar heel pain are participation in activities that

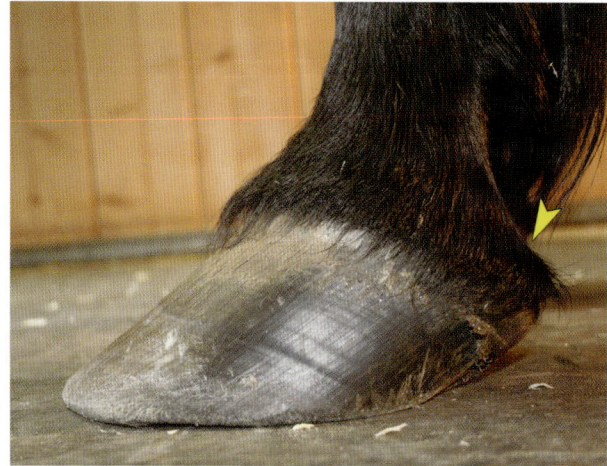

12.6 This foot is at risk for developing palmar heel pain due to its long toes and underrun heels, as well as the lack of development of the digital cushion, which gives the area above the heels an "empty" look (yellow arrow).

Delving Deeper:
Heel-First, Flat, and Toe-First Landing

Observations carried out with slow-motion video have found that sound horses, both domestic and wild, usually land flat (with the entire foot touching the ground at the same time) when walking normally on flat ground, but they start to land slightly heel first as speed increases (fig. 12.7). Unsound horses will frequently land toe first, especially if they are suffering from pain in the heel region. Unfortunately, toe-first landing is so common that many people don't recognize it as a form of lameness, but that is exactly what it is. But before you can understand why toe-first landing is a *bad* thing, you first have to understand why heel-first landing is a *good* thing.

When landing slightly heel first, the back of a healthy, functional foot expands and compresses as it contacts the ground. This correctly aligns all the bones in the lower limb as they experience the greatest loading forces, and it also dissipates energy. Energy generated by impact with the ground is also reduced by having to travel upward through the rubbery frog (which will be in contact with the ground on a correctly functioning foot) and then through the digital cushion. By the time any ground-reaction forces reach the bones, tendons, and ligaments in the back of the foot, they have been greatly dampened (fig. 12.8). A heel-first landing also helps move blood through the extensive network of capillaries within the hoof, creating a very effective "liquid cushion" in the back of the foot that further dissipates energy.

However, when the hoof lands toe first, all of that marvelous protective function goes out the window. Instead of a smooth, rolling forward motion that aligns the bony column and sends energy upward through all the shock-absorbing structures of the foot, the hoof slams down from front to back, misaligning the bones and sending concussive forces down through the coffin joint, the navicular bone, and the soft tissues around the navicular bone. If toe-first landing goes on for any length of time, the soft tissues in and around the coffin joint are likely to become inflamed and damaged. When the horse lands toe first due to pain in the back of the foot, the toe-first landing is only going to make that problem worse, and possibly add new sources of pain.

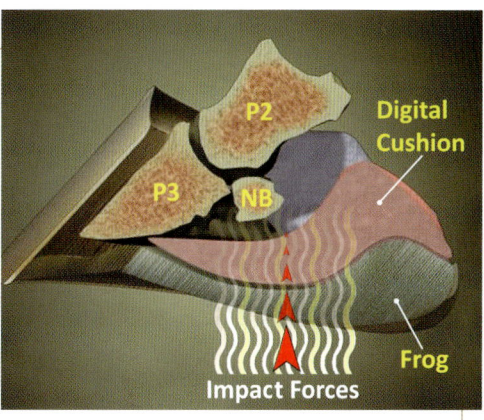

12.8 Ground-impact forces are dampened by having to pass through the frog and then the digital cushion, thus protecting the bones and soft tissues deeper inside the foot.

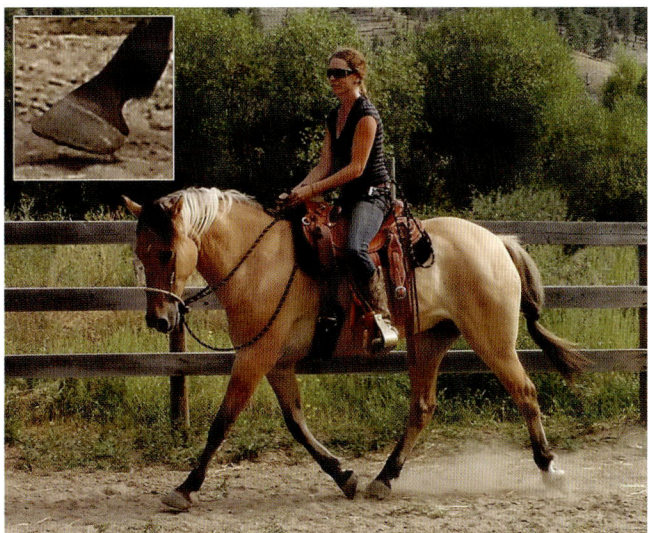

12.7 Heel-first landing, as seen here in the left front, is observed among most sound horses when they are moving faster than a normal walk.

require fast turns, hard or sliding stops, frequent circles, jumping, or working on hard ground (fig. 12.10). Horses with small feet relative to their body size and horses with upright pasterns are also at higher risk, as are horses put into intense athletic training at an early age. Some experts also think that the incorrect biomechanics of toe-first landing can cause heel pain, but the majority believes that toe-first landing is the result of pain in the back of the foot, not the cause of it. It may be that both are correct, with heel pain causing the horse to favor the back of the foot and thus land toe first, and the toe-first landing then exacerbating the original problem or causing other issues in the same region of the foot. It is not at all uncommon for a thorough investigation of palmar foot pain to turn up more than one area of concern, creating a complex web of causation that is sometimes beyond our capacity to unravel.

Learning to spot how your horse's feet are landing is a useful skill but is not always easy, especially

Master Farrier Gene Ovnicek on
Toe-First Landing

"**A**lignment of the distal interphalangeal joint [coffin joint] at the moment of ground contact is critical, and is facilitated by landing slightly heel first (fig. 12.9). It is not difficult for sound horses with well-balanced feet to land heel first. Considering this, horses that are not sound or have poorly balanced feet with hoof distortions can be easy to detect if you know how to spot a toe-first landing."

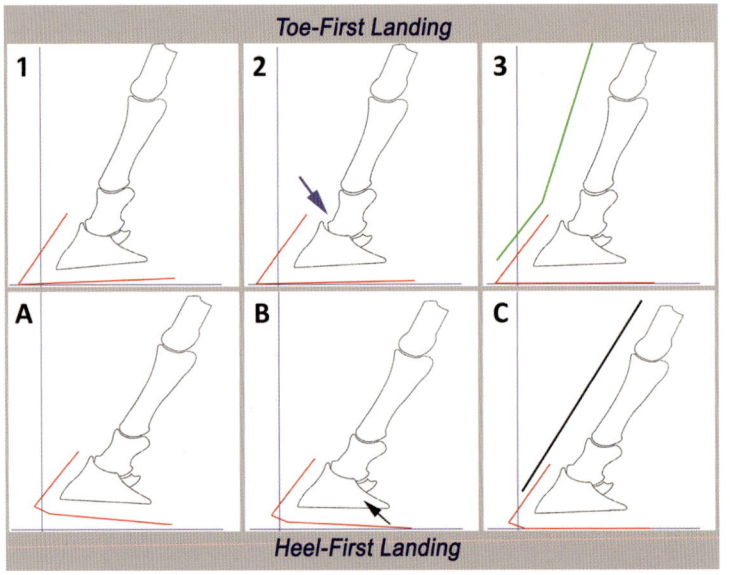

12.9 These illustrations, from Gene Ovnicek, show what happens when the foot lands toe first versus heel first. In toe-first landing: 1) the toe touches down; 2) the coffin joint "breaks" backward, sending impact forces straight into the joint, the navicular bone, and the soft tissues; 3) and when the foot is flat during peak loading, the alignment of P3, P2, and P1 is broken backward (green line). In heel-first landing: A) the heel touches down; B) shock is absorbed through the frog and digital cushion and is greatly diminished by the time it reaches the bones and soft tissues; C) and during peak loading, the alignment of the bones is correct (black line).

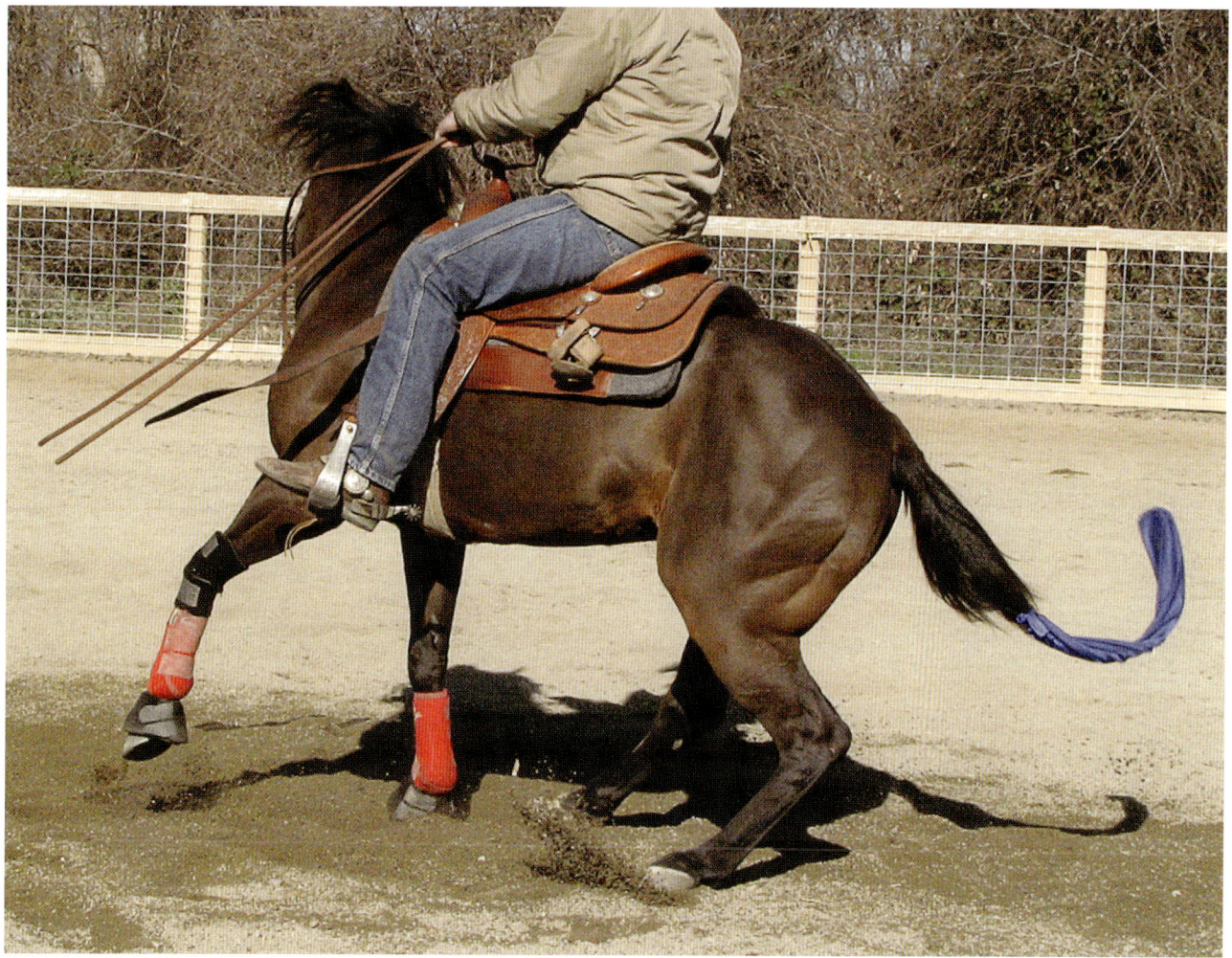

12.10 Reining horses are at high risk of developing heel pain issues due to the fast spins, repetitive circling, and sliding stops required of them. They are often put into intensive training at a young age as well, which may further increase their risk.

on soft ground. Some people find it helps to watch the hairline from the side as the horse walks past, noting whether the hairline rocks forward as the foot lands (heel-first landing) or backward (toe-first landing). You can also try focusing above the coronary band, as you may be able to notice the pastern moving backward prior to loading on some horses that land toe first. And, when you see a puff of dust in front of the toe with each footfall, this also indicates toe-first landing. If you are having difficulty,

it is extremely helpful to video the horse walking and trotting on a flat surface, then watch the video in slow motion. Keep in mind that it is normal for even perfectly sound horses to land toe first when walking uphill.

Treatment Options

Determining which structures are affected and how badly they are damaged is an absolute necessity if you want to give your horse the best possible chance to recover from palmar foot pain. Without this information, any treatment plan is at best an educated guess, and at worst, a totally inappropriate course of action that may actually cause further harm. Depending on what the problem is, treatment options may include:

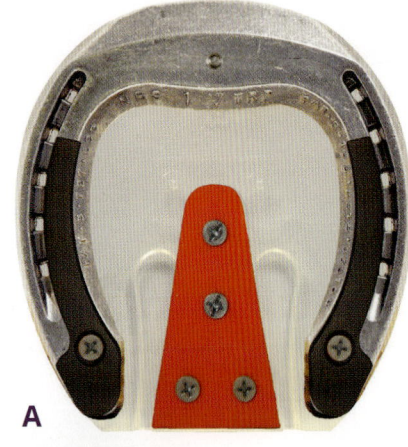

12.11 A & B A therapeutic shoeing system like the EDSS (Equine Digit Support System) set up can be adjusted with the addition or subtraction of various pads, rails, and inserts. Here you see it from the bottom (A) and from the side (B), showing the impression material used underneath it.

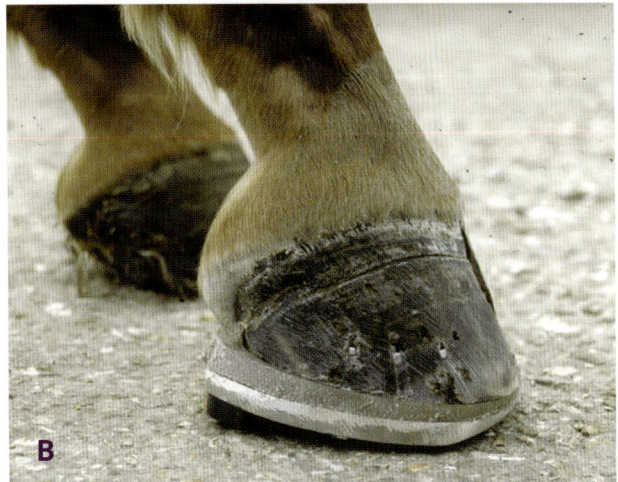

• Trim modifications.

• Therapeutic shoeing aiming to support and/or relieve pressure on the back of the foot, and to facilitate breakover (figs. 12.11 A & B). It is important to keep in mind that therapeutic devices such as wedges may place already overburdened heels under additional pressure.

• Adding impression materials, anti-concussive pads, or other shock reducing devices to shoes.

• *Non-steroidal anti-inflammatory drugs (NSAIDs)* such as phenylbutazone (bute) and firocoxib.

• *Joint injections,* most commonly corticosteroids injected into the coffin joint. Such injections may relieve pain in the coffin joint caused by synovitis or arthritis, as well as pain coming from the navicular bone and navicular bursa. Horses suffering from pain associated with the DDFT or impar ligament may also get relief from joint injections.

• *Tiludronic acid* is a relatively new drug being used to treat pain associated with breakdown of the navicular bone and osteoarthritis in the nearby tissues. Administered intravenously (IV), the drug works by inhibiting the painful process of bone resorption and remodeling. The effects last for up to four months, so if the stresses causing the bone damage can be alleviated, the drug increases the chances of the bone healing.

• *Extracorporeal shock-wave therapy (ESWT)*, an emerging form of treatment in which high-intensity pressure waves are directed at the damaged area to relieve pain and stimulate healing (fig. 12.12). The exact mode of action by which ESWT promotes healing is not yet known, but it does seem to help some horses with palmar foot pain issues and may be an option worth exploring.

• *Isoxuprine,* a drug that causes vasodilation in the extremities of humans. Some have theorized that navicular-related problems are due to poor blood supply in the navicular region, so it was thought that isoxuprine might help with that. However, more recent studies suggest that isoxuprine does not actually cause vasodilation in horses, and that blood-supply issues are not the cause of navicular disease. Still, some horses seem to improve on this drug, though no one can really say why. The track record for isoxuprine is spotty, at best.

• Rest from work.

• Confinement.

• Padded hoof boots on properly trimmed bare feet.

• Controlled exercise.

• Digital *neurectomy* (see p. 218).

The goal of any treatment plan should be to restore healthy function of the foot, which means restoring balance, trying to get the foot to land heel first at anything above a normal walk, optimizing breakover, getting the heels back to the widest part of the frog, creating a healthy hoof-pastern axis, and eliminating peripheral loading by getting the back of the frog on the ground. These principles apply to both shod and barefoot horses, and ignoring any of them is likely to influence the success of any other forms of treatment.

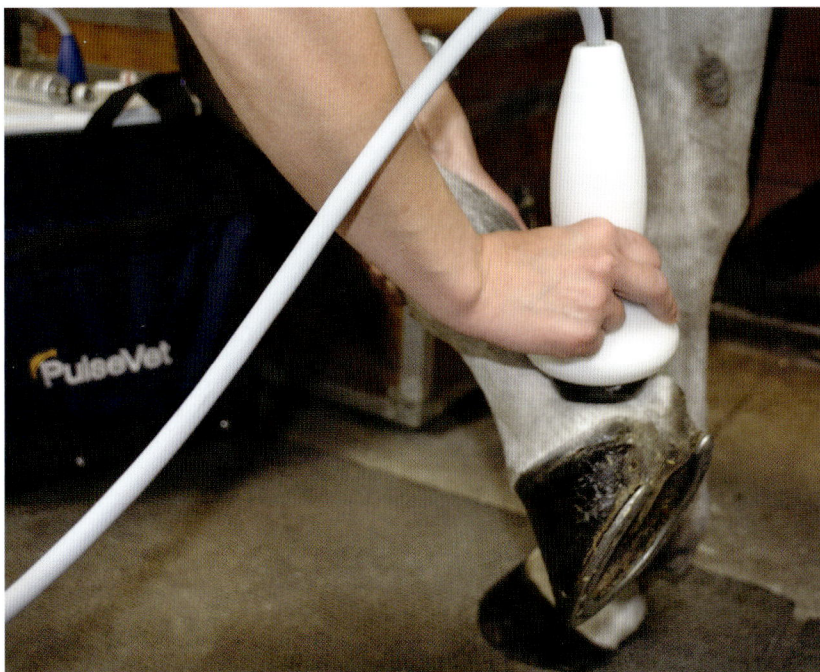

12.12 Extracorporeal shock-wave therapy (ESWT) is proving helpful to some horses with foot pain issues

It should be noted that therapeutic shoeing, which is the most common form of treatment for palmar foot pain, does not have a stellar track record, especially in the long term. In many cases, the various types of shoes, wedges, and pads provide only temporary relief, if they provide any relief at all. A significant percentage of horses treated with therapeutic shoeing will experience a downhill slide at some point, at which time retirement or euthanasia may be presented as the only options.

There are a number of reasons why the performance of therapeutic shoeing is so frequently disappointing. These include misdiagnosis of the actual problem, the use of shoeing techniques inappropriate for that particular horse (for example, bar shoes and/or wedges on collapsed or underrun heels), neglecting to address underlying hoof-capsule distortions, and failure to restore healthy hoof function (fig. 12.13). Dr. Robert Bowker states that many kinds of therapeutic shoeing merely shift the focal point of pressure, relieving the currently sore area but eventually causing the new focal point to become sore.

Because therapeutic shoeing is such an iffy proposal when it comes to palmar foot pain, some people have been seeking alternatives. There is a growing body of anecdotal evidence supporting the idea that taking a horse barefoot utilizing physiologically correct trim principles, as well as padded hoof boots to encourage heel-first landing, is sometimes able to restore function where corrective shoes could

not. Dr. Bowker not only believes wholeheartedly in this method, but has taken X-rays showing that bony changes can sometimes be reversed to at least some degree when the barefoot protocol is followed.

While that certainly appears promising and is worth exploring in many cases, there is no one form of treatment that is going to work for all horses, and the owner should still to try to determine the exact source of the horse's pain before heading down any path, barefoot or otherwise. Another point to consider is the fact that changes to a bare foot have to be made slowly, while shoeing techniques can often change the biomechanics of the foot immediately and dramatically, which may provide quick relief to some horses. Some of these changes can also be accomplished through the use of hoof boots, but there is no doubt that shoes have the upper hand when it comes to making fast changes to breakover, heel angles, the hoof-pastern axis, and the size of the ground-surface area.

When all else fails, horse owners sometimes resort to a surgical procedure called *neurectomy*, commonly referred to as "nerving," which involves severing both of the palmar digital nerves in the low pastern area. Only horses that show a positive response to a posterior digital nerve block are candidates for this surgery, and only about 70% of those will get relief from the procedure. Many vets will require an MRI prior to neurectomy to ensure that the supporting soft-tissue structures are strong enough to support the weight after all feeling has been removed. In some cases, neurectomy has caused catastrophic breakdowns due to the horse not being able to feel that his tendons or ligaments are failing under the load. If the operation is successful, the horse will no longer feel pain in the back

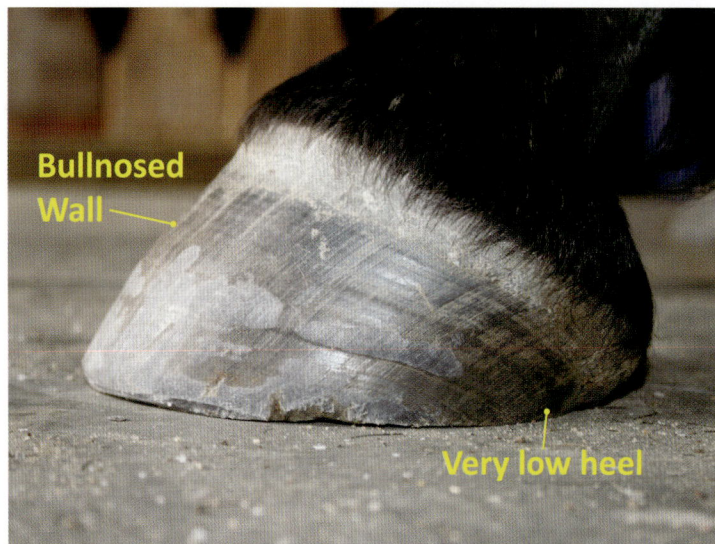

Bullnosed Wall

Very low heel

12.13 Although it is commonly done in cases of heel pain, adding a wedge to a foot like this, with a very low heel and a bullnosed (bulging outward) dorsal wall suggesting a negative palmar angle, is not a good idea. It will only put more pressure on the already compromised heels, which are bearing too much load as it is.

of the foot, but the surgery does nothing to cure the problem that is responsible for the pain.

Horse owners also need to be aware that a neurectomy is highly unlikely to be a permanent solution due to the fact that the nerves regrow over time, and when they do, the horse will once again feel the pain his condition is causing. How long a horse will get relief from a neurectomy varies from a few months to a few years, with the average being somewhere around one year. If the horse did get a reasonable period of respite but the pain eventually comes back, the procedure can be repeated once or twice, though the surgeon will have to cut a little bit higher on the nerve each time. This is why the surgeries cannot be repeated indefinitely, as cutting too high takes away feeling in the entire foot, and the horse does not function well like that.

Another consideration is that each time the surgery is performed, there is the possibility that it will cause the formation of neuromas, which are growths of abnormal nerve tissue that sometimes form on the stumps of severed nerves. Neuromas, which are the most common serious complication of palmar digital neurectomy, are themselves extremely painful, sometimes worse than the original pain the neurectomy was supposed to relieve. As there are various techniques that can be used to perform a neurectomy, your surgeon may feel that one is preferable to the others in terms of minimizing the chance of neuromas or other

unwanted complications, so this is definitely something to discuss.

A horse that has had a neurectomy can still be ridden, though some people feel there is an increased risk of the horse tripping or stumbling due to the lack of feeling in the heel region. Others assert that if a horse does stumble, it is not the neurectomy that makes this happen, but rather the problems associated with the condition that prompted the neurectomy in the first place. Either way, care should be taken when riding a horse that has had this procedure until you know how the horse performs postoperatively.

Lastly, extra attention should be paid to the bottom of the foot that has been neurectomized, as the horse will not be able to feel puncture wounds, bruises, or other injuries to the back of the foot. Daily cleaning and inspection is the best way to spot such issues, some of which can easily increase in severity if not tended to in a timely manner.

Other surgical approaches may be appropriate in some cases, and new techniques and medications to help horses with various types of palmar foot pain are currently being evaluated. In the right hands, horses diagnosed with such problems today have a much better chance at recovery than they would have in the past, and as diagnostics and treatment continue to improve, we hope we will see even more horses with palmar foot pain return to comfort and use.

13

Sidebone, Ringbone, and Pedal Osteitis

Sidebone

In a healthy foot, the lateral cartilages (LCs) remain as flexible fibrocartilage throughout the horse's lifetime. If you palpate the inside and outside of a healthy foot in the region of the quarters, just above the coronary band, you can feel these firm yet elastic structures. But sometimes, the LCs will fill in with calcium and turn into bone (ossify) as a result of cumulative stresses. This common condition

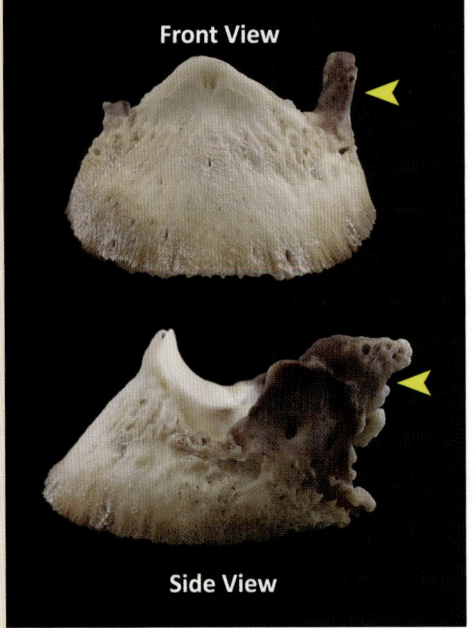

13.1 If this were a normal bone specimen, there would be no lateral cartilages on it, as soft tissues like cartilage simply dissolve away during the process of decomposition after death. The bony "wing" (yellow arrows) on one side of this abnormal specimen is cartilage that has ossified (turned to bone)—commonly called *sidebone.*

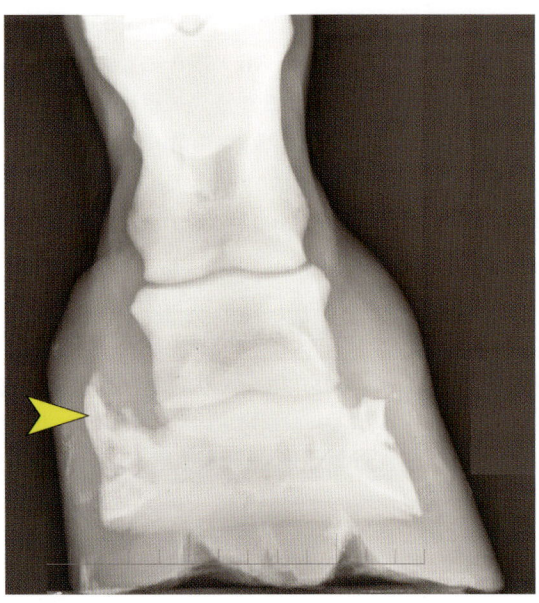

13.2 Looking at the sidebone this horse has developed on one side, it is obvious that the mediolateral imbalance of this hoof has been going on for a long time.

is called *sidebone* (fig. 13.1). Sidebone can occur on both sides of the hoof or just on one side, and it is most typically seen in the front feet. If you palpate ossified cartilages, they will feel hard and may be enlarged. The bony formation will also show up clearly on X-rays (fig. 13.2).

Because sidebone occurs so frequently, some believe that the ossification of the LCs is a normal part of aging. However, it doesn't happen to all horses, and most experts consider it a disease process. Risk factors for sidebone appear to include:

- Being a draft breed.

- Working on hard surfaces.

- Contracted heels.

- Hoof imbalances.

- Feet that are small for the horse's size.

- Short, upright pastern conformation.

- Conformational abnormalities that make the limbs crooked.

How a horse is raised may also make the horse more or less prone to developing sidebone. Raising a youngster in a small enclosure, allowing his feet to become long or unbalanced, and shoeing before the foot has fully matured can all inhibit the development of robust LCs, leaving these important structures more vulnerable to stress. Barefoot advocates believe that unshod horses maintained with physiologically correct trimming have a greatly reduced risk for developing sidebone, but evidence for this is anecdotal.

If a horse does develop sidebone, that alone does not usually cause lameness, though it may result in some stiffness and shortening of the stride. Still, even if the condition is asymptomatic, it is worth looking into, particularly if you are seeing it in a younger horse. Formation of sidebone is a physiological response to some sort of stress, and

the forces that cause the ossification of the LCs are likely creating increased stresses on other parts of the foot. Left unchecked, those stresses may indeed lead to lameness, so if you are starting to suspect the development of sidebone, talk to your veterinarian and hoof-care provider to see what might need to change in order to prevent further problems.

Another reason why you want to keep an eye out for developing sidebone is that it may be possible to reverse the process to some extent if it is caught early enough. Radiographic evidence has shown that the horse's body can actually resorb the calcifications in the LCs if they haven't gone too far, and if the problem causing the ossification is rectified. It only takes a moment to palpate your horse's LCs, and making a point of doing this every couple of months might help you nip sidebone in the bud.

Ringbone

While sidebone doesn't usually have too great of an impact on a horse's life, *ringbone* is a different story. Ringbone is the common name for a form of osteoarthritis that most often affects the pastern joint, but can also affect the coffin joint or sometimes both. When it is in the pastern joint, it is referred to as "high ringbone," and when it is in the coffin joint, it is called "low ringbone" (fig. 13.3). The

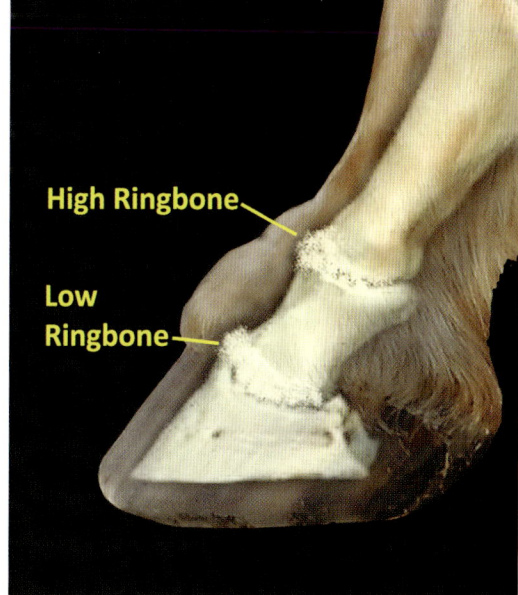

13.3 Low ringbone affects the coffin joint, while high ringbone affects the pastern joint. In some instances, horses will have both.

High Ringbone

Low Ringbone

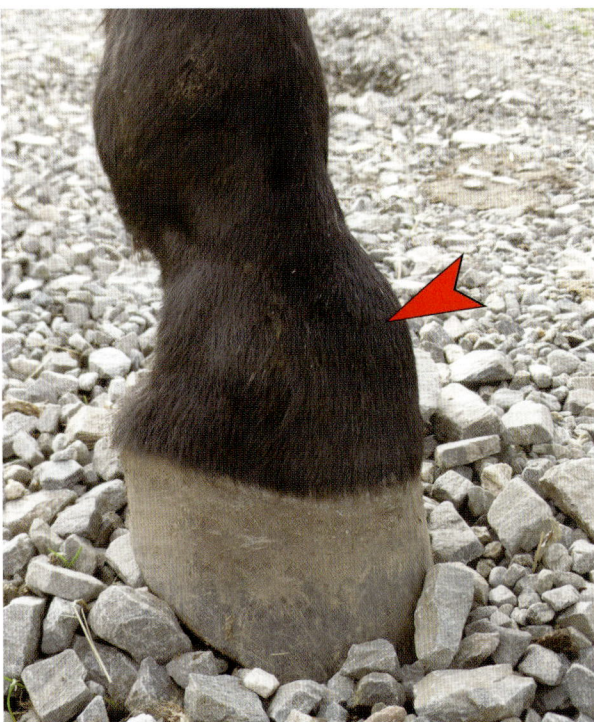

13.4 By the time you can actually see a change caused by ringbone, the disease process is well advanced. This horse's case is severe.

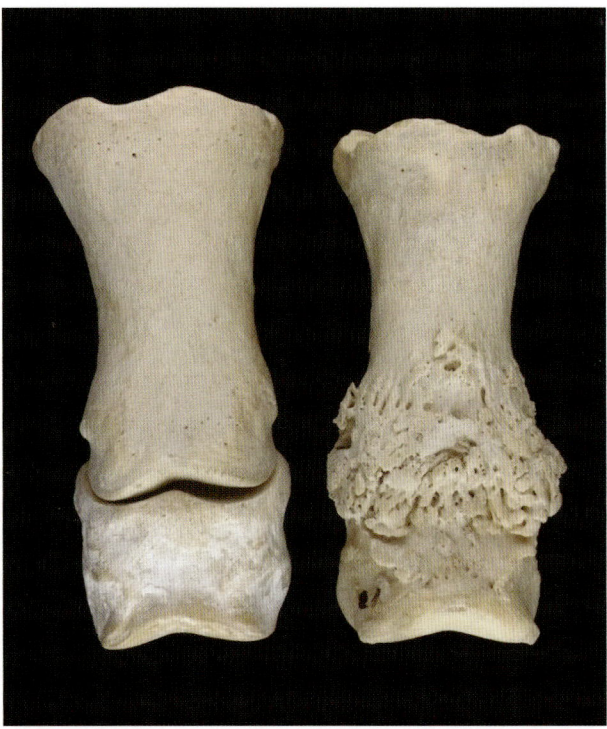

13.5 The normal P1 and P2 bones on the left are free of any osteophytes, but the ones on the right have been completely immobilized by high ringbone, which has fused the joint into one lumpy mass of bone. This degree of ringbone would have been easily visible in the limb when the horse was alive.

front limbs are usually where we see ringbone, but it can occur in any leg. The condition gets its name from the bony ring or enlargement that can form as the joint lays down spurs and lumps of irregular, abnormal bone tissue *(osteophytes)* in response to damage caused by inflammation. In advanced cases of ringbone, this bony enlargement can often be seen and felt (fig. 13.4). In addition to the growth of new bone, ringbone can also involve narrowing of the joint space, and increased density *(sclerosis)* or erosion *(lysis)* of the bone just below the joint cartilage.

In most cases, ringbone is caused by abnormal stress on the joint. As with many other lower limb and hoof issues, the root of the problem can be a conformational issue, imbalance in the foot, poor shoeing or trimming, going too long between shoeings, working on excessively hard or deep surfaces, injury, or activity-related. Horses used in sports that require a lot of turning, twisting, concussion, lateral movements, circling, quick stops, or fast changes in direction are at increased risk of developing ringbone. Ultimately, anything that causes uneven loading on the pastern or coffin joint can get this degenerative process started.

The development of ringbone begins when the increased forces affecting the joint cause microscopic damage to the joint capsule, the cartilage on the joint surface, or the ligaments associated with the joint. This damage triggers inflammation, which over time, causes even more damage. The protective fluid inside the joint breaks down, and gets thinner, and eventually, the joint starts laying down disorganized bone tissue in an attempt to stabilize itself. Over time, the entire joint may fuse, effectively immobilized by the proliferation of bone (fig. 13.5). While the fusing of a joint sounds awful, it can sometimes actually make the horse feel better, as the rough surfaces of the joint are no longer rubbing painfully against one another.

As with any type of osteoarthritis, a horse with ringbone is going to experience pain, but the degree of lameness that pain causes will vary tremendously, depending on what tissues are affected, how far the disease has progressed, and how much the horse is working or moving. Lameness may be so mild as to be barely noticeable or so severe that the horse cannot be used at all. Work is likely to increase lameness in many cases, but cooping the horse up so that he hardly moves can actually increase stiffness and soreness as well.

In addition to the different locations of high and low ringbone, there are two specific types of ringbone, *articular* and *periarticular*, and they tend to differ in the amount of pain and lameness they cause. Articular ringbone directly affects the tissues of the joint space, whereas periarticular ringbone consists of bony changes around the outside of the joint. Articular ringbone is generally more painful, as the lesions can be felt every time the joint flexes. With periarticular ringbone, joint mobility can become

limited, but it's not as painful, as the lesions are more above and below the joint. It is possible for a horse to develop both articular and periarticular ringbone (fig. 13.6). Whichever type of ringbone the horse has, it is a progressive, degenerative condition that is likely to worsen over time.

As ringbone can vary so much depending on the type and severity of the condition, the diagnostic tools needed to get a correct diagnosis will vary as well. In the earliest stages, MRI would be more likely to find the problem than radiography. Nuclear scintigraphy (bone scanning) is also good at picking up subtle changes in cartilage and bone that would

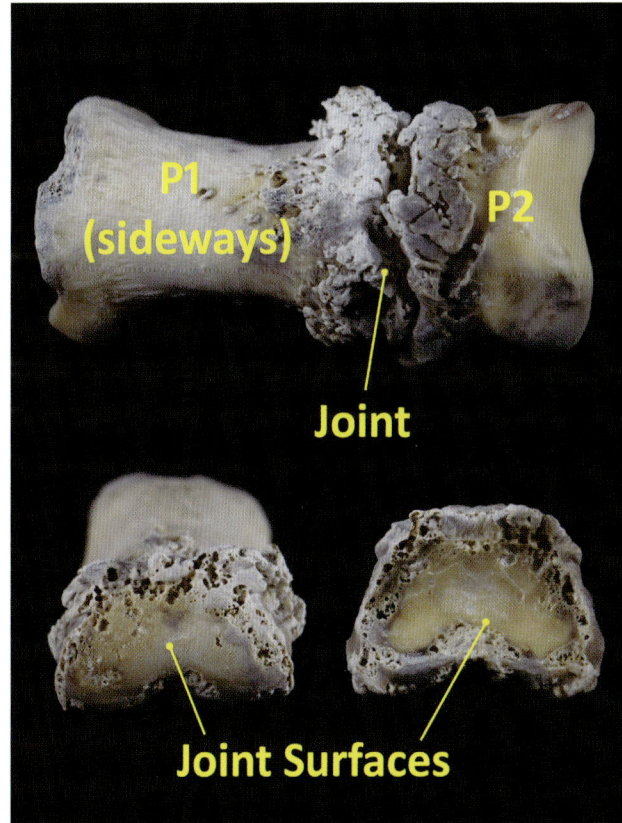

13.6 This horse had both articular (affecting the joint space and joint surfaces) and periarticular (outside the joint) ringbone, the result of long-term imbalance and overall poor hoof care.

be missed on an X-ray, so it can be very useful in the diagnosis of early ringbone. Once the disease has progressed further, changes will be visible on X-rays.

If you are able to catch ringbone early, it may be possible to halt or at least slow the progression of the disease with good hoof care that focuses on balance, easing breakover, and minimizing torque.

"You can accomplish this," says Gene Ovnicek, "by reducing the ground surface area around the center of rotation (generally the widest point of the foot). This requires reducing leverage not only in the front of the foot (long toe), but also on the sides. More importantly, you must also ensure that the heel is not too high and it does not extend too far to the back. High heels are often a major factor in coffin joint arthritis."

Joint injections are also often used to reduce inflammation and revitalize joint fluid, and some owners find that their horse's symptoms are reduced by the use of oral supplements aimed at improving joint health. In addition, there are new treatments such as extracorporeal shock-wave therapy (ESWT) that seem to help quite a bit in some cases, and you may even see the use of stem-cell therapies to treat ringbone in the not-too-distant future.

In cases where the disease is already advanced, fusing the joint surgically does a good job of eliminating the horse's pain, but there are some consequences. While the joints involved in ringbone are not designed to flex a tremendous amount, they do provide the limb with some shock absorption, and this function will be lost if the joint or joints are fused. The horse will move more stiffly, but there have been cases where horses with fused joints have continued to work and even compete successfully.

In the best case scenario, an owner will recognize the factors that predispose a horse to ringbone and do everything possible to try to prevent the disease from developing. If, for example, you have a horse with a conformational flaw that creates uneven stress on the pastern or coffin joint, places strain on the soft tissues, or increases concussion in the limb, you may want to take this into consideration when choosing the type and amount of work you do with the horse, and you will definitely want to ensure that such a horse has regular and excellent hoof care. Short or upright pasterns, long, sloping pasterns, and toes that turn in or out are just a few of the conformational issues that increase the chances of a horse developing ringbone (fig. 13.7).

Even if your horse's conformation is fine, it may pay to keep in mind the other factors that can trigger

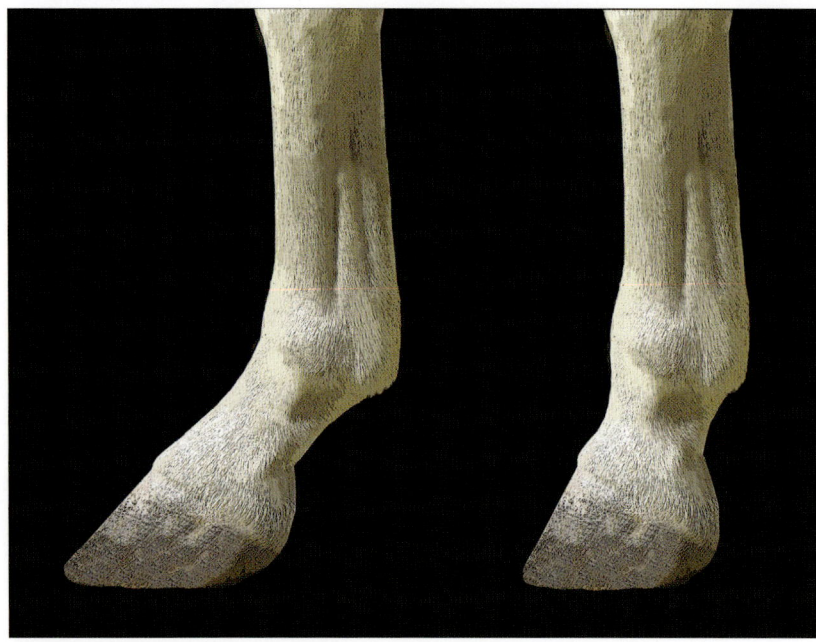

13.7 Both long, sloping pasterns and short, upright pasterns put a horse at greater risk for ringbone: the former because of excessive strain, and the latter because of increased concussion.

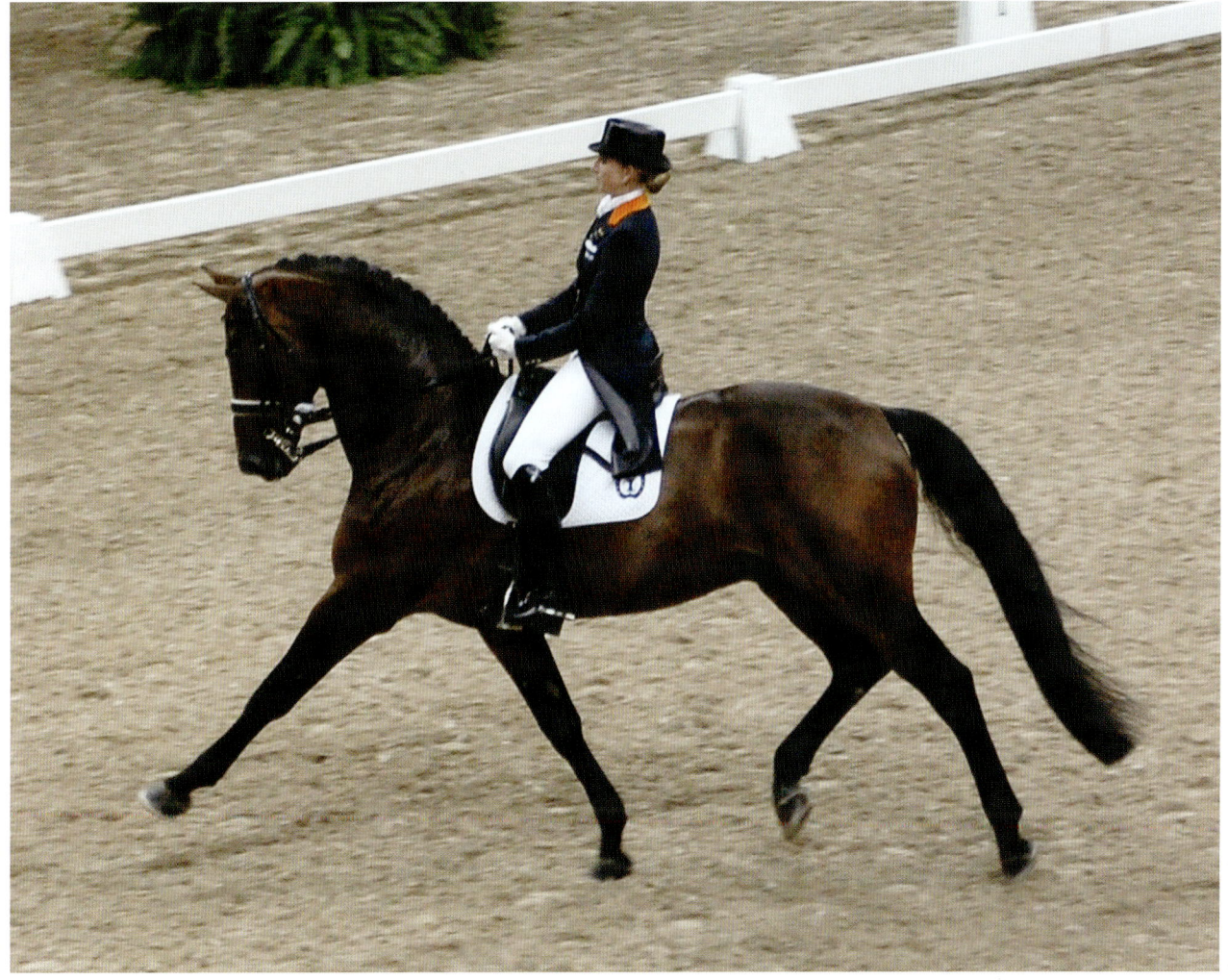

13.8 The lateral movements, collection, extension, and repetitive circling of dressage can place a surprising amount of strain on the joints and soft tissues of the horse's legs and feet.

ringbone. Whenever possible, avoid working your horse on hard footing, which increases concussion and torque, and also stay away from deep footing, which can place unhealthy strain on soft tissues and joints. Consider the fact that rigid metal shoes limit the ability of the heels to flex independently of one another, which may increase torque as well. Think about the movements you ask your horse to make and recognize what they might be doing to his joints.

And it isn't just barrel racers, jumpers, or polo players that need to increase their awareness. Though it might come as a surprise to many, the "quiet" sport of dressage actually places a significant amount of strain on a horse's pastern and coffin joints due to the high percentage of lateral movements required of the horse and the repetitive nature of the training (fig. 13.8). Dressage riders and anyone else involved in a "ringbone-risk" sport might be able to reduce that risk by incorporating more rest days and variety into their programs. Trail riding, for example, is a great way to keep a horse moving while allowing both his mind and body to recharge from intensive training. The use of flexible shoes or taking the horse barefoot may also reduce risk factors.

Mindfulness truly can go a long way in preventing or minimizing the impact of ringbone in many cases. Although there is no doubt that it can be a devastating problem, many horses with ringbone can continue to lead happy, useful lives with appropriate treatment and good management.

Pedal Osteitis

In addition to arthritic conditions like ringbone, there are other ailments that can lead to significant pathological changes in the bones of the equine distal (everything below the knee) limb. The coffin bone, in particular, often alters its shape, becomes more porous, or disintegrates in areas due to disease or mechanical processes. Generally, such changes result from abnormal pressure, compromised blood flow, inflammation, or all three.

One common finding is a demineralization (bone loss or resorption) of the solar margin of the coffin bone referred to as *pedal osteitis*. Pedal osteitis is an inflammatory condition of the coffin bone that shows up on X-rays as changes to the solar margin of the bone. While sometimes spoken of as a condition in and of itself, pedal osteitis is more correctly a result of other conditions such as laminitis, very thin soles, excessive concussion, or chronic high heels. Pretty much anything that puts chronic or repeated pressure on the tip of the coffin bone can lead to this problem.

An X-ray of a coffin bone with pedal osteitis will show bone loss in part or all of the lower rim of the bone, as well as increases in the size of the vascular channels that go through the affected areas of the bone (fig. 13.9). Instead of being smooth, the edge of the bone may have a ragged appearance due to the resorption of bone along the margin. This leaves the coffin bone in a weaker state, making it more susceptible to fractures and bone chips.

We see pedal osteitis more frequently in the front feet than in the hind, and often if one foot is

Holes (Loss of Density)

Bone Loss

Loss of Density (fading)

Normal Solar Margin

13.9 In pedal osteitis, the bone will have areas and little holes where the bone has demineralized (lost density), and the solar margin may change shape, have pieces missing, or become ragged due to bone loss. In the X-ray on the left, the coffin bone has normal density and its solar margin is rounded and fairly smooth. In the X-ray on the right, there is a loss of density that shows most noticeably in the faded, ragged solar margin and the small holes pocking the bone itself.

affected, the adjacent one will be too. When a horse has this condition, the degree of lameness is quite variable. It can range from mild to severe, and may be intermittent to constant. Most commonly, the horse will walk with a stilted gait that is frequently worse on a circle.

There are two kinds of pedal osteitis: *septic* and *non-septic*. Septic pedal osteitis means that there is an infection associated with the condition. The infection could be a result of chronic abscessing, a foreign object getting lodged in the foot, a penetrating injury opening the gates for bacteria to get in, necrotic tissue from laminitis, severe white line disease, or any other cause of internal infection. The infection burrows into the coffin bone, causing the cascading effect of inflammation and demineralization.

Non-septic pedal osteitis, which is far more common, is caused by mechanical forces, with no infection involved. Non-septic pedal osteitis can be caused by many things including bruising, excessive concussion (for example, lots of jumping or too much work on hard surfaces), toe-first landing, conformational faults, laminitis, and poor farriery—particularly leaving the heels too high.

Treatment depends on what kind of pedal osteitis is affecting the horse, though in either case the goal is to reduce inflammation. If it is non-septic, reducing concussion with pads and packing material under a shoe, or hoof boots with pads, is the first line of treatment options. Keeping the horse on a soft surface and giving time off to rest are also important. If sepsis is involved, antibiotic treatment may be attempted, but it can be difficult for the medication to effectively fight the infection in the foot. Frequently, surgery is necessary to remove the infected tract or portion of bone in order to adequately defeat the infection and prevent further inflammation and demineralization of the coffin bone.

Section Four:
Creating Healthy Hooves

As the previous chapters have shown, there is an astonishing variety of things that can go wrong with the equine foot. Avoiding those problems—or rehabilitating a foot that has issues—may seem like a daunting task, but you, as the horse owner, can have a tremendous amount of influence over the health of your horse's feet. One of the most important things you can do is ensure that you have a solid grasp of the factors that promote good hoof health. This section will examine the cornerstones of creating a healthy hoof and help orient you in the right direction if management changes are necessary.

How Hooves Get Healthy and Stay That Way

Nature vs. Nurture

When you look at certain breeds of horses such as Morgans and Arabians, you see that most individuals in these breeds have strong, solid feet (fig. 14.1). Conversely, when you look at Thoroughbreds and Quarter Horses, you see large numbers of individuals with problem feet. This would seem to indicate that genetics is an extremely important factor in the creation of good hooves. However, current research and a wealth of anecdotal evidence suggest that in most cases, what happens to a horse's hooves *after* he is born has far more influence than any genetic contribution. In fact, it may be mostly the management and training practices commonly used with horses of a given breed that lead to the differences seen among breeds. Still, there is undoubtedly genetic variability in hoof size, conformation, and quality, and it only makes sense to give horses the best start possible by breeding for good feet.

Conscientious breeders take hoof quality into serious consideration when making breeding decisions. They will do their best to avoid breeding horses solely on the basis of bloodlines or

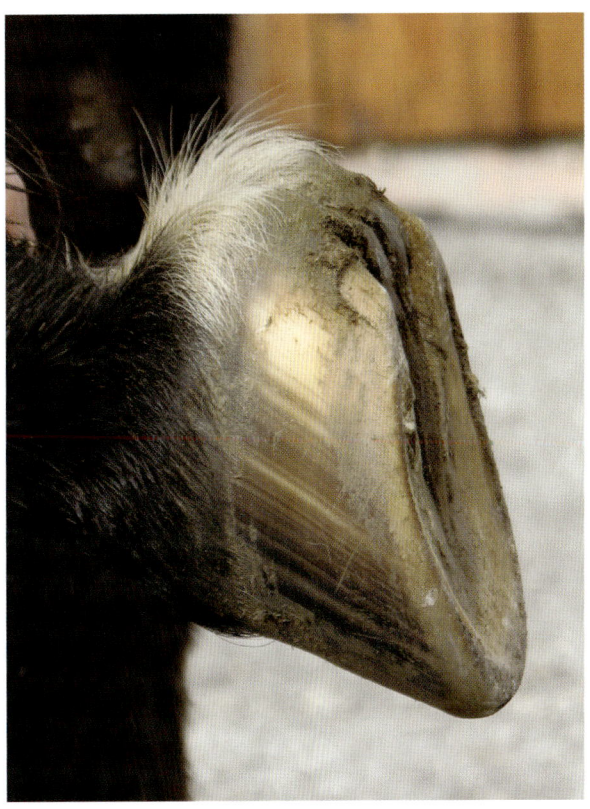

14.1 This Arabian, like many of his breed, has strong, solid, healthy feet. Is this the result of genetics or how most Arabians are raised and used?

show records if the horse has hoof problems that are thought to be heritable. These include club feet and long, sloping-pastern conformation that causes a tendency toward underrun heels and long toes. Thoughtful breeders will also avoid harmful trends like breeding halter horses to have huge, muscular bodies with tiny feet. They understand that if horses from their breeding program are constantly plagued with foot problems, it is going to reflect on the breeder in the long run.

Most hoof problems, however, are made, not born, so you have to look at other factors. Take Thoroughbreds, for example, a breed widely believed to have weak feet. They are certainly being bred without much consideration of heritable hoof quality, but at the same time, these horses are often confined in small spaces, loaded with grain, shod at an early age, and put into hard training extremely young, all of which can seriously compromise even a very healthy hoof.

Furthermore, the first consideration of the trimming and shoeing methods used on racing

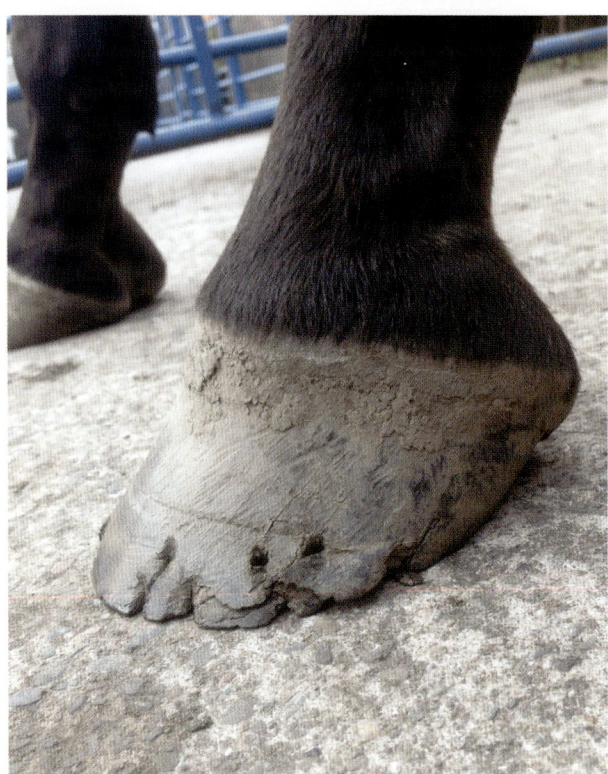

14.2 Many Thoroughbreds have feet that look like these, with crumbling, "shelly" walls, thin soles, long toes, and underrun heels. However, hoof-rehab specialists will tell you that most can have much better feet with proper care.

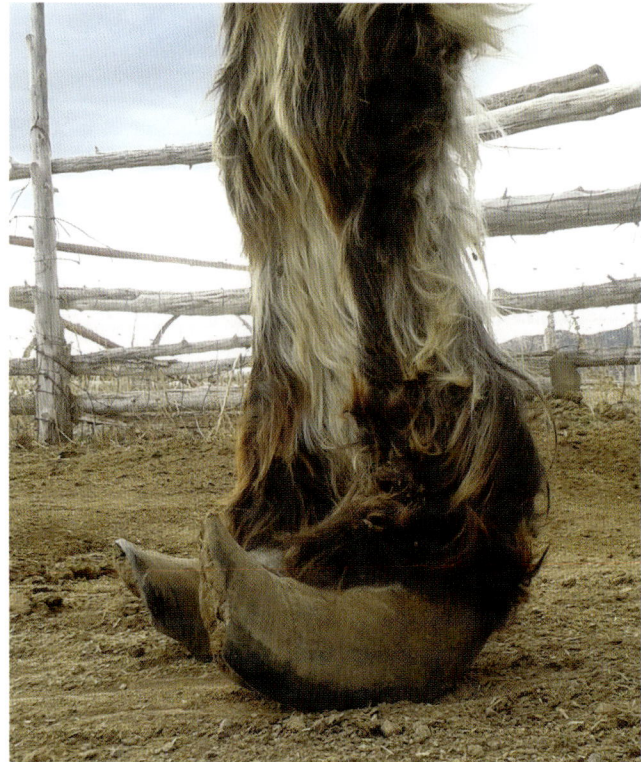

14.3 Many people think that wild Mustangs have great feet because of their "survival-of-the-fittest" genes. However, their feet often deteriorate quite quickly once they are in captivity. This neglected, laminitic mare is an extreme example, but an inappropriate diet and insufficient movement cause problems for many Mustangs that come off the range with strong, healthy feet.

Thoroughbreds is to maximize speed, not hoof health. As a result, there is a virtual epidemic of long toes and low heels on these horses. Some say that is simply the natural hoof conformation of a Thoroughbred, but others point out that leaving the toe long is thought by many trainers to make the horse just a tad faster, although it can increase their chances of injury. The fact that you can take many "typical" Thoroughbreds and completely rid them of shelly walls and long-toe/low-heel syndrome with good, physiologically correct hoof care would seem to argue for the "nurture camp" (fig. 14.2).

This, of course, is true for other breeds as well: make the appropriate changes to trimming/shoeing, diet, and lifestyle, and a majority of horses with so-called "bad feet" can end up with healthy, fully functional feet. While some hooves may simply be too damaged to recover, most feet are capable of bouncing back to a remarkable degree, given the right conditions.

The reverse is unfortunately also true, meaning that you can take a fabulous foot and turn it into a diseased, crumbling mess in almost no time at all. This is a common problem with wild Mustangs taken into captivity. They usually come off the range with strong, healthy feet (fig. 14.3), but many of them quickly start to develop flares, cracks, thrush, laminitis, and all the other problems that plague so many of our domestic horses. Since we know that their naturally selected DNA didn't suddenly change, we have to look at what *has* changed, with the usual suspects being diet, hoof care, and the amount of movement they get on a daily basis.

The Importance of Movement

A healthy hoof, whether wild or domestic, has certain characteristics that allow it to function properly over a lifetime of use. These include thick, tough walls and soles; strong, well-developed lateral cartilages; dense, fibrous digital cushions; robust frogs that make contact with the ground at the back; short toes; and heels that are wide and relatively low but not underrun. Whether or not a horse's feet develops and maintains these characteristics will depend to a very large extent on how much movement the horse is afforded and on what kind of terrain that movement takes place, starting on Day One of that horse's life. Even if you don't raise young horses, knowing how a healthy hoof develops in a youngster can help you understand how movement can improve hoof health in mature horses, whether they have obvious foot problems or not.

Horses in a free-roaming environment spend 16–20 hours per day foraging, which means they are moving almost continually (fig. 14.4). Though most of this movement is accomplished at a walk, it nonetheless has profound benefits for their hoof development and ongoing hoof health. As we mentioned in the anatomy section, when a horse is born, the internal and external structures of the hoof are relatively soft and unformed—perfect to support the weight of a newborn foal, but *only* the weight of a newborn foal. In a natural or free-roaming environment, the foal is up and moving within hours, often surprisingly long distances, so his feet immediately start adapting to this work load. Every step a young horse takes helps transform his feet by stimulating the soft, fatty digital cushions to become thick and fibrous, helping the tube-shaped

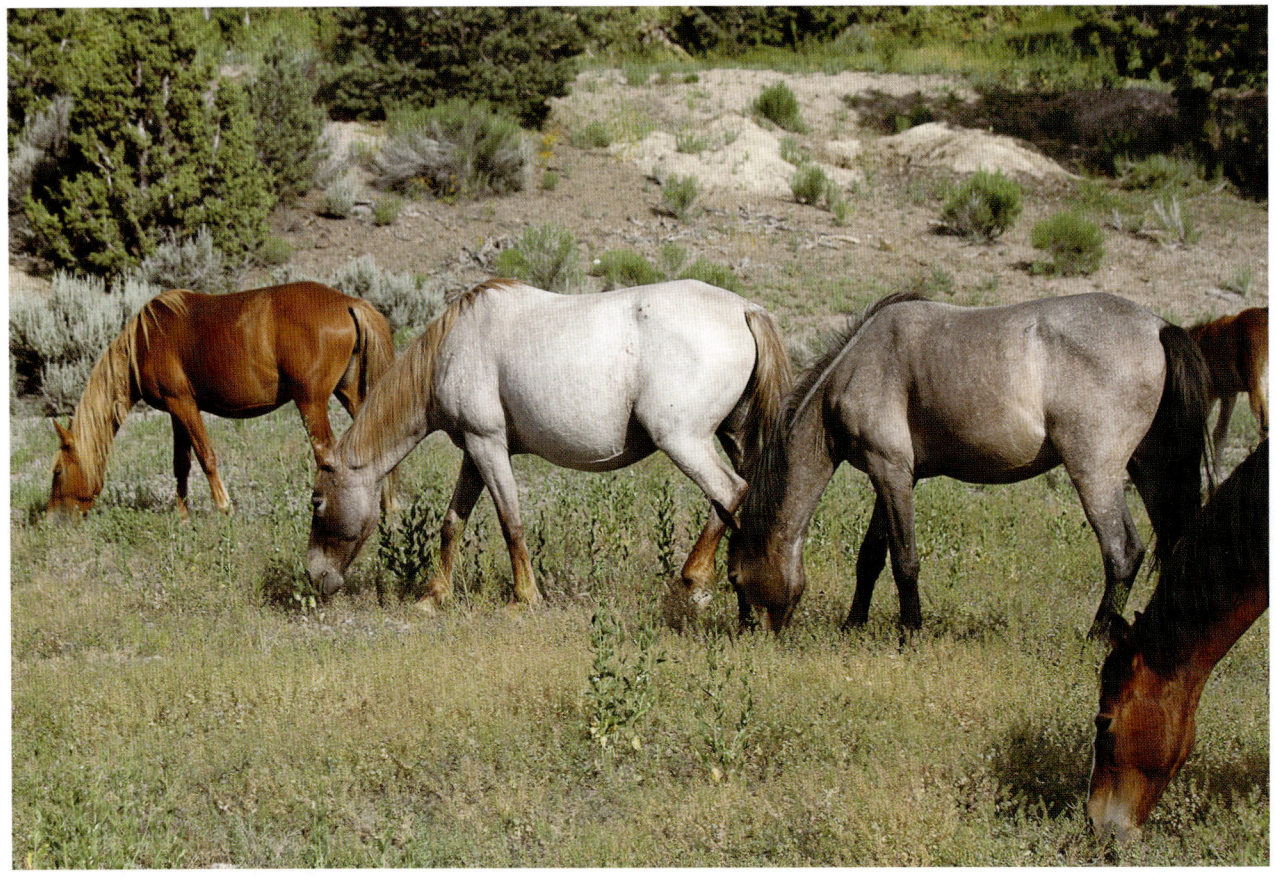

14.4 Horses in a natural environment spend the vast majority of their time grazing, which usually involves nibbling a bit, then walking, then nibbling, then walking. They are thus moving almost continually throughout the day, which helps them develop strong, healthy feet.

baby hoof to spread into a stronger conical shape, strengthening the lateral cartilages, and toughening the other structures of the hoof.

As the horse grows and becomes heavier, his feet are designed to adapt to be able to support the increased stress put on them by a heavier body. As long as the horse is allowed plenty of movement on varied terrain, including a fair amount of firm terrain, the feet will continue to develop in size and strength well into the fifth year of life. This may be the single most important factor in the development of healthy hooves in a growing horse.

It follows, therefore, that management practices that restrict a young horse's movement will retard hoof development, especially if the horse is kept on soft footing (fig. 14.5). Numerous studies have shown that exercise is imperative for normal musculoskeletal development and maintenance, and this includes the bones and soft tissues of the feet. If the tissues are not stressed adequately through exercise, they will be weaker than they should be. As little as three weeks of stall confinement has been shown to have measurable negative effects on the skeletal development of a young horse, and it has similar effects on adult horses, who experience a loss of bone density when they don't move enough.

Ironically, because movement is so critical to healthy hooves, we often see bad feet in some of our most valuable horses because the more expensive horses tend to have more confinement early in their lives. Sadly, a horse deprived of appropriate movement as he is growing is going to be more likely to suffer from lameness issues down the line, regardless of breed or pedigree.

Some people try to compensate for a lack of turnout by longeing a young horse, especially if they are trying to condition the youngster for show. Unfortunately, this is far more likely to do harm than good. Activities like longeing, which involve repetitive movements and lots of circling, can easily overload developing tissues and lead to injury. In order for tissues (bone, muscle, tendon, ligament, or hoof) to develop strength, they need to be stressed by exercise and then have time to heal and strengthen in response to that stress. It has been shown that bone can have an adaptive modeling response to specific stress with as little as 30 cycles of a given stress—this means that as few as 30 strides of galloping exercise will stimulate a young horse bone to adapt specifically to galloping.

However, if the young horse was galloped 300 strides every day, this would overload the musculoskeletal system and allow insufficient time for tissue recovery, which is likely to result in injury. Young horses can also develop degenerative problems like arthritis when they are worked too hard, too young. While most of us think arthritis is only found in older horses, it is not at all uncommon to X-ray an actively working three-year-old and find arthritis already impairing the joints in the feet and lower limbs.

Rather than longeing, the type of exercise that is needed is typical of young horses at play—short bursts of galloping, romping around, running up and down hills, and so on (fig. 14.6). Because it is difficult to mimic the varied influences of play exercise with a training program, it is healthiest

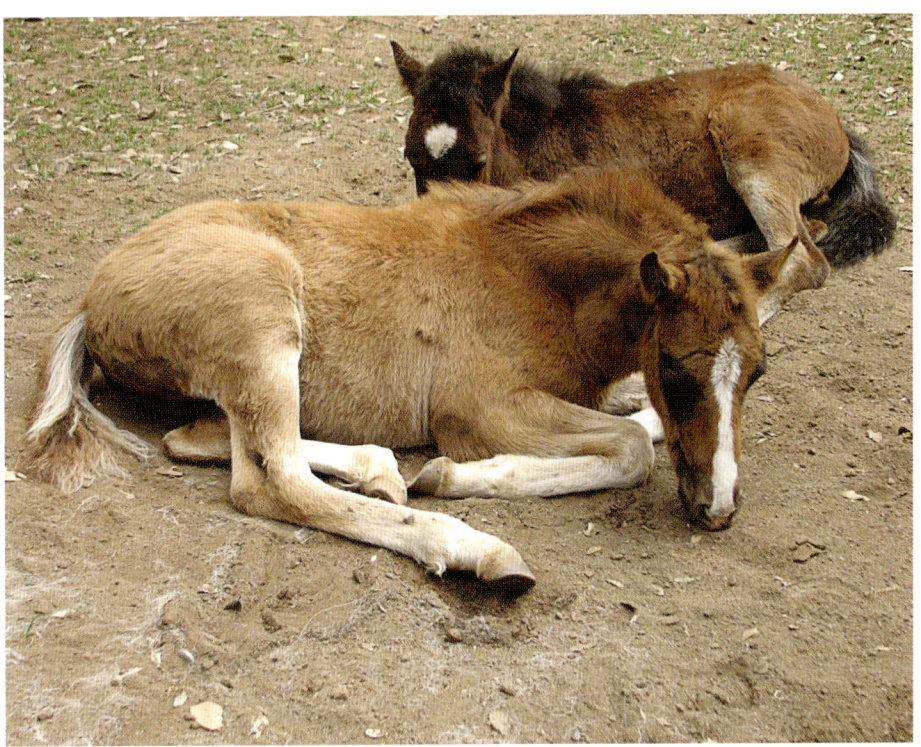

14.5 The soft dirt and grass of the paddock these foals live in makes for a nice comfy bed, but it is not the best footing to help young feet develop optimally.

for young horses to be turned out in a large space with other youngsters on varied terrain so that they can engage in natural movement. The more space they can be turned out in, the better. Ponying a foal from his dam or another calm horse is another good way to exercise a baby, though it is important to start off slowly and gradually increase the duration of such sessions. Even hand-walking a foal (or better yet, jogging with baby!) can improve hoof health for a foal that lives in a more confined space, and it is a great way to start training, build your relationship, and get a youngster used to the world (fig. 14.7).

When working with an adult horse, you don't have to worry about dealing with developing joints, but excessive longeing is still problematic, as the continual circling puts torque on the joints

and may contribute to the development of arthritic conditions like ringbone.

The principles about the benefits of movement for young horses definitely apply to mature horses as well. Many problems, particularly those that can result from poor development of the structures in the back of the foot, will often improve significantly if you can get the horse moving more and moving correctly, meaning slightly heel first at gaits faster

14.6 When they have enough space, foals like this Dartmoor pony will exercise themselves in natural movements that are ideal for the development of their feet.

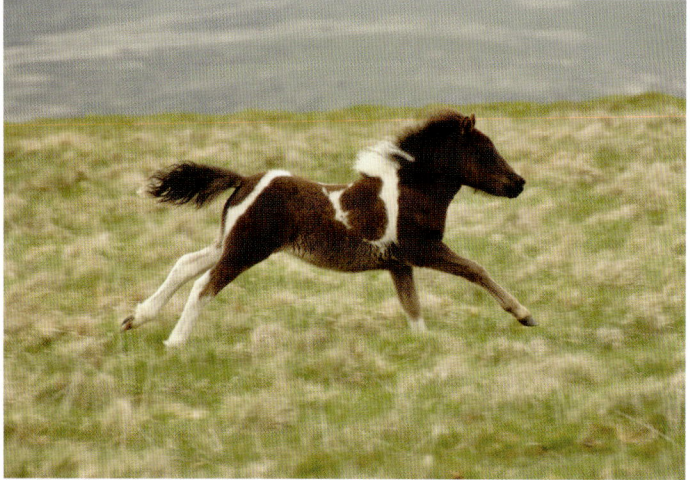

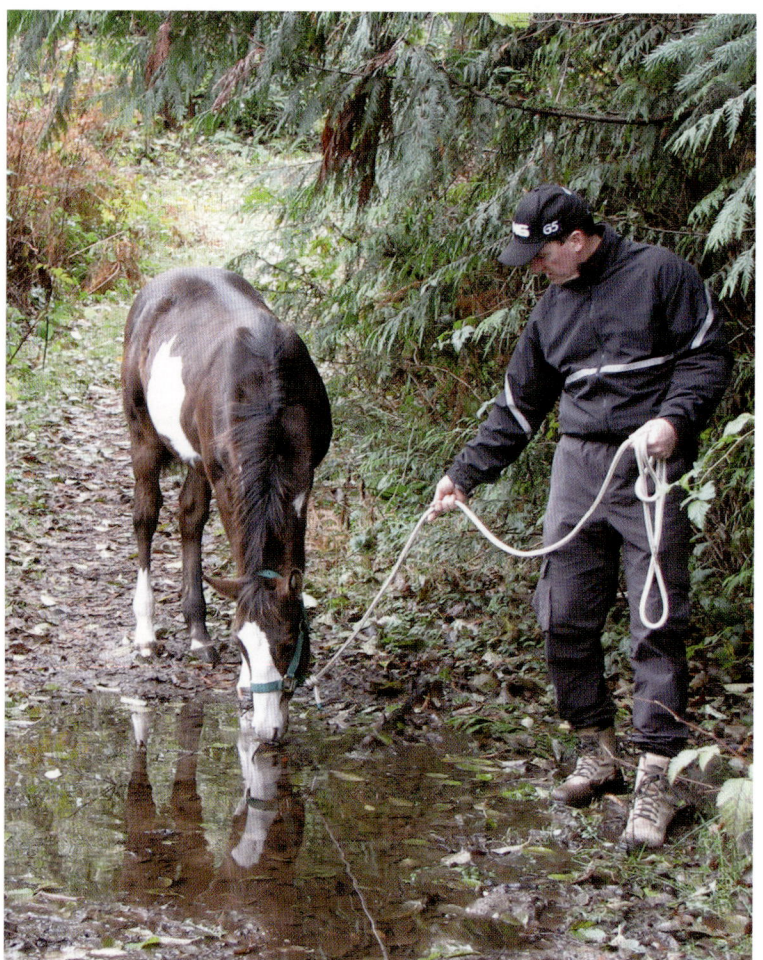

14.7 Hand-walking a young horse out in the world is not only good for hoof health, but a great way to bond with and start training a foal.

than a normal walk. These changes alone can make a huge difference in overall hoof function and blood flow within the foot, which in turn help the internal and external structures of the hoof to improve. When horses start moving the way they are meant to and their hoof care is optimized, it is quite possible to see soft, fatty digital cushions become more fibrous and supportive; thin walls and soles become stronger and thicker; flat soles lift and develop concavity, and shriveled, diseased frogs become full and springy.

The horse's living arrangements can play a big part in improving a horse's feet through movement. The more space he has to move in, the more improvement you are likely to see, and if you can avoid keeping him in a stall altogether, that is definitely a plus (fig. 14.8). While stalls may be convenient for us, there is no getting around the fact that standing around for hours on end, especially with continual exposure to manure and wet bedding, does not promote good hoof health and is therefore likely to hamper your efforts to improve your horse's feet.

The ground your horse moves on also makes a difference when it comes to improving hoof health. Most horses enjoy footing that will conform to the bottom of their feet, but if the footing is too soft, it doesn't provide enough of the stimulation that comes from the pressure and release feet get on firmer footing. An ideal turnout area will therefore have varied footing—some firm, some softer, and will be arranged in such a way that the horse uses both.

Many people report seeing noticeable improvements in hoof health after creating areas of pea gravel or crushed rock, with pieces small enough to easily sift through a manure fork and not get

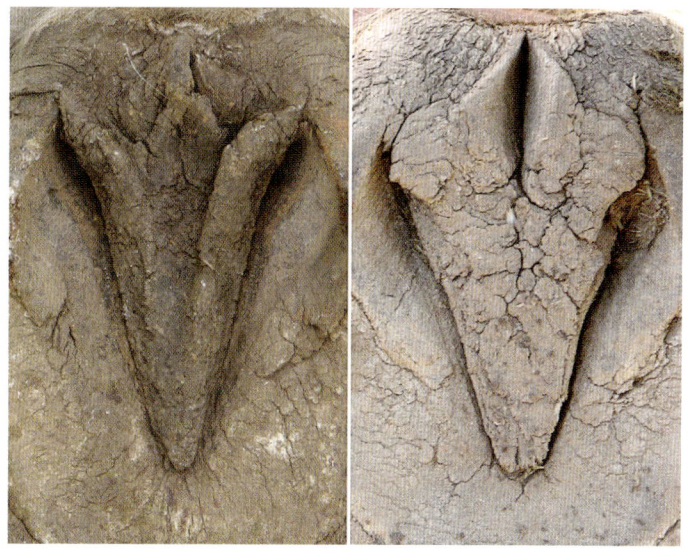

14.8 This is the same frog, only four months apart. On the left, it is shriveled and essentially non-functional, but it is coming back nicely on the right. The main change that accomplished this was moving the horse from a facility where she lived most of her life in a stall, to an acreage that afforded her 24/7 turnout in a large, firm paddock with other horses to encourage movement.

jammed up in the horse's feet. This kind of footing is both conformable and supportive, and seems to be helpful in various types of hoof rehabilitation.

If the horse's current environment can't provide 24/7 turnout that stimulates movement on varied ground, it is worth thinking about moving him to a place that does if you are serious about hoof health—it really is that important. If that is not an option, you can make even a relatively small paddock more pro-movement by creating mazes or tracks of interior fencing that force the horse to travel longer distances to get to food and water. Installing a number of feeding stations in different areas of the paddock will also increase the amount of movement your horse gets. Jaime Jackson's book *Paddock Paradise* (Star Ridge Publishing, 2007)

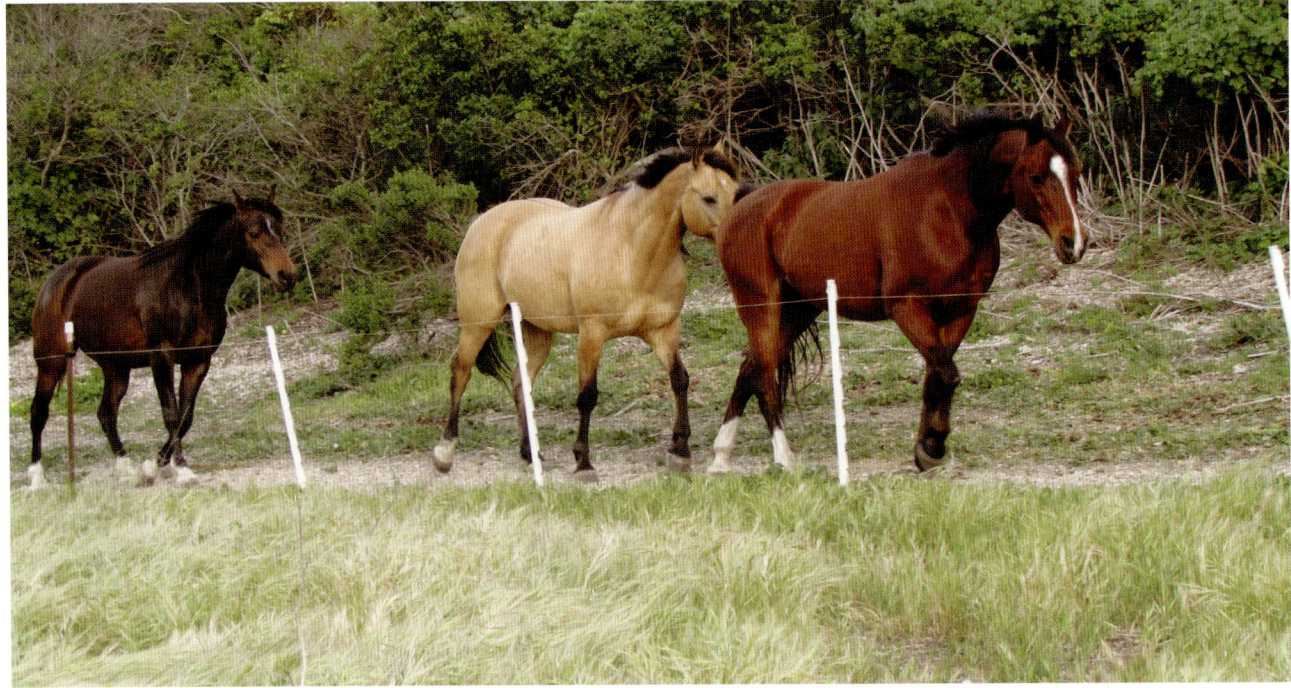

14.9 These horses are walking on a track that is part of a "Paddock Paradise" set up by Jaime Jackson at the headquarters of the Association for the Advancement of Natural Horse Care Practices.

contains many such ideas, centering around the principle that by creating a space that approximates the lifestyle of free-roaming horses living naturally in the wild, you can provide a more stimulating environment that gets your horses moving and promotes good mental and physical health (fig. 14.9).

More intense exercise, such as riding or short periods of longeing on a line or free longeing in a round pen, is certainly also beneficial when trying to improve the quality of an adult horse's feet, though as with youngsters, you don't want to overdo it when the horse is unfit or not used to a particular activity. Also recognize that if you are rehabilitating a horse that has painful feet, the horse may be too sore to do much moving around at first, though this can be mitigated in many cases by the use of

anti-concussive materials under his shoes, or with padded hoof boots for a barefoot horse. You never want to force a horse to move if doing so might cause further damage, but if your vet or hoof-care professional gives you the go-ahead for exercise, realize that it could be a critical aspect in improving your horse's hoof health.

Feeding the Foot

Another extremely important component of hoof health for horses of any age is diet. In fact, diet is so often at the root of a horse's hoof problems that it should be one of the very first avenues of inquiry with any horse that has non-injury related issues with his feet. In addition to laminitis, issues such as being tenderfooted, having flat soles, shelly walls, or white line disease, flaring, and many other common hoof problems can all be related to what the horse is eating. Solving these issues almost always goes more easily when the dietary concerns are addressed (fig. 14.10).

Usually, making the horse's diet more foot friendly ends up being a matter of "less is more." Ask any vet or equine nutritionist and he or she will tell you that far more problems—hoof and otherwise—are caused by overfeeding horses than by underfeeding them. It may make us feel good to put our horses out on lush pasture, feed them rich hay, top them up with grain, stuff them with carrots and apples, and pile on the supplements designed to improve hoof quality, but all these things have the potential to be extremely detrimental to our horses' hooves and overall health.

Providing a diet that promotes hoof health should be an absolute must for all horse owners, but if you have a horse with a known metabolic disorder, or hoof issues that even *hint* of laminitis (remember the subtle signs!), controlling the horse's diet can make the difference between soundness and a life of problems, pain, and debilitation. Countless horses endure prolonged suffering simply because their owners have not been made aware that what they are feeding is a major factor in their horse's foot problems, or they have been made aware but are not taking this issue seriously enough.

When it comes to feeding and hoof health, what we really need to be looking at, in most instances, is how to keep things *out* of the horse's diet that weaken the hoof—specifically, too many simple sugars and starches, what we might call "quick"

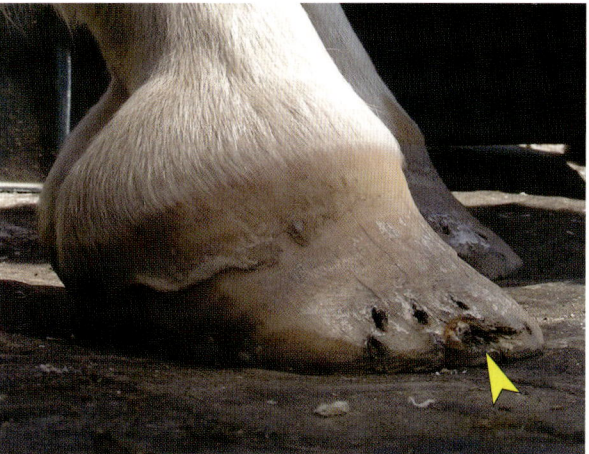

14.10 Many hoof problems, including crumbling walls, white line disease, and flaring, can, at least in part, be related to diet. Thus, if all else is in order, changing the diet may be the missing piece of the puzzle. The hoof in this photo, with its flared, crumbling, and white-line-infected toe, could be chronically weakened from a diet too high in simple sugars and starches.

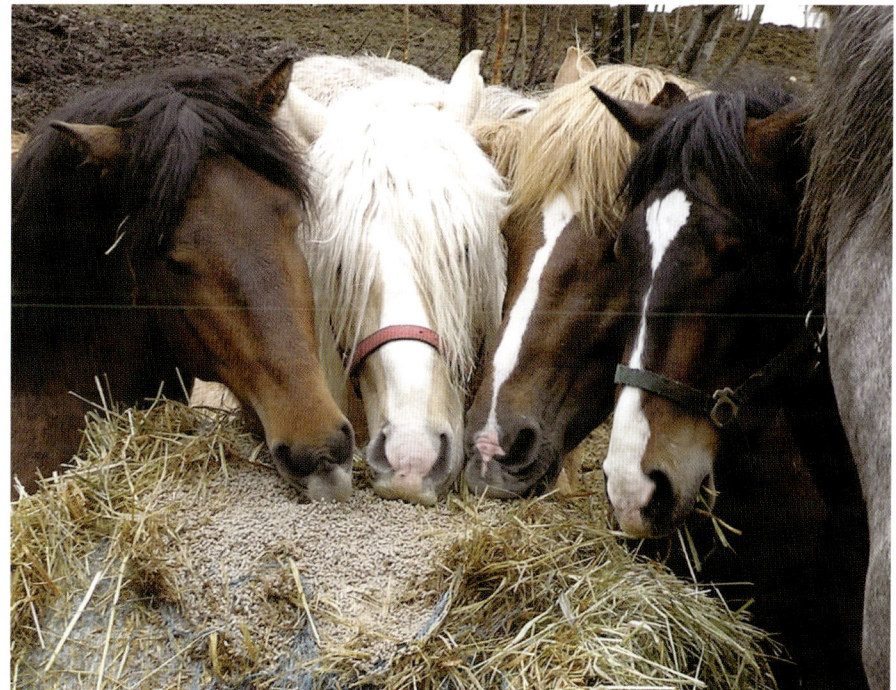

14.11 Many people consider grain-based feeds a staple for their horse's diet, but horses are not designed to handle large amounts of grain. In many cases, long-standing hoof problems will finally resolve once the horse is taken off grain and other sources of quick carbs.

carbohydrates (fig. 14.11). There is a mounting body of evidence that sugars and starches that convert quickly into glucose in the body result in damage to the laminae, which as we've seen can have all sorts of consequences, some of them devastating.

Obvious sources of quick carbs are grains and anything sugary or coated with molasses. Less obvious and often overlooked sources are hays high in ESCs (ethanol soluble carbohydrates) or starch, and pasture with elevated levels of sugar due to seasonal changes or stresses such as overgrazing, frost, or drought. Non-native or "improved" grasses—varieties of grass designed to put weight on cattle—can also be problematic, as can those beloved carrots and apples for some horses (fig. 14.12). In addition, some horses react to high protein diets the same way they would to a high carb diet, so care should be taken when feeding high protein feeds or hay containing alfalfa.

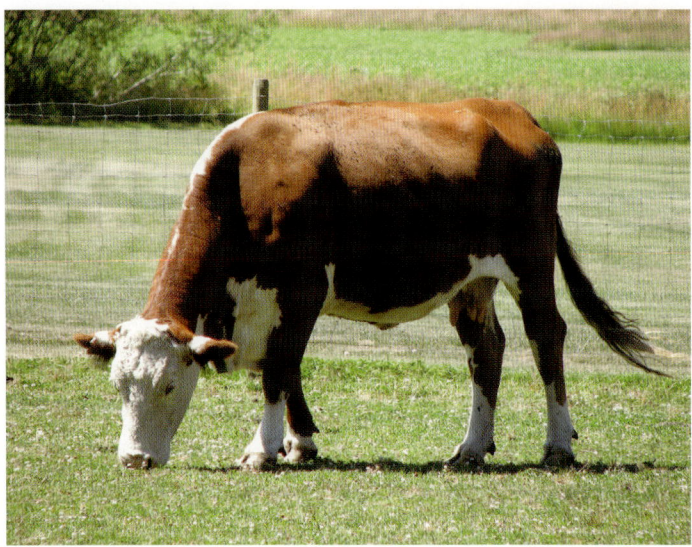

14.12 Improved grasses designed for the cattle industry can sometimes be much too high in carbohydrates to be healthy for horses.

Any horse that is known to be prone to laminitis or exhibits any of the subtle signs that can indicate subclinical laminitis, as well as horses that gain weight easily or have been identified as having metabolic problems, should be put on a strict, low-carb diet free of all grain and grain products, sugary substances, apples and carrots (both of which contain a surprising amount of sugar), and anything else that might load them with simple sugars or starch, including fresh grass, which is always a risk for carb-sensitive horses. The ideal diet for such horses consists mainly of low-carb, moderate protein hay that has been analyzed, as there is truly no way to know the nutrient profile of any hay that has not been tested.

A diet lower in simple sugars and starches may actually be beneficial to all horses, as we now understand that the equine digestive system is not set up to handle sugary or starchy feeds in significant amounts. Diets too high in these substances are known to be a major factor in the formation of gastric and hind gut ulcers in horses, an extremely common health problem that often goes unrecognized. All of this doesn't mean that you should necessarily cut out all grain, grass, and sweet treats from every horse's diet, but it does mean that you should be careful and observant when using such feeds, and make sure that your horse is not showing any symptoms of laminitis, ulcers, weak/thin walls, or obesity—another very common problem in the horse world today.

And, if you think those extra pounds are really no big deal, think again. The feet of a horse that is overweight are subject to both metabolic and mechanical stresses, making them much more prone to problems. One study by researchers at Virginia

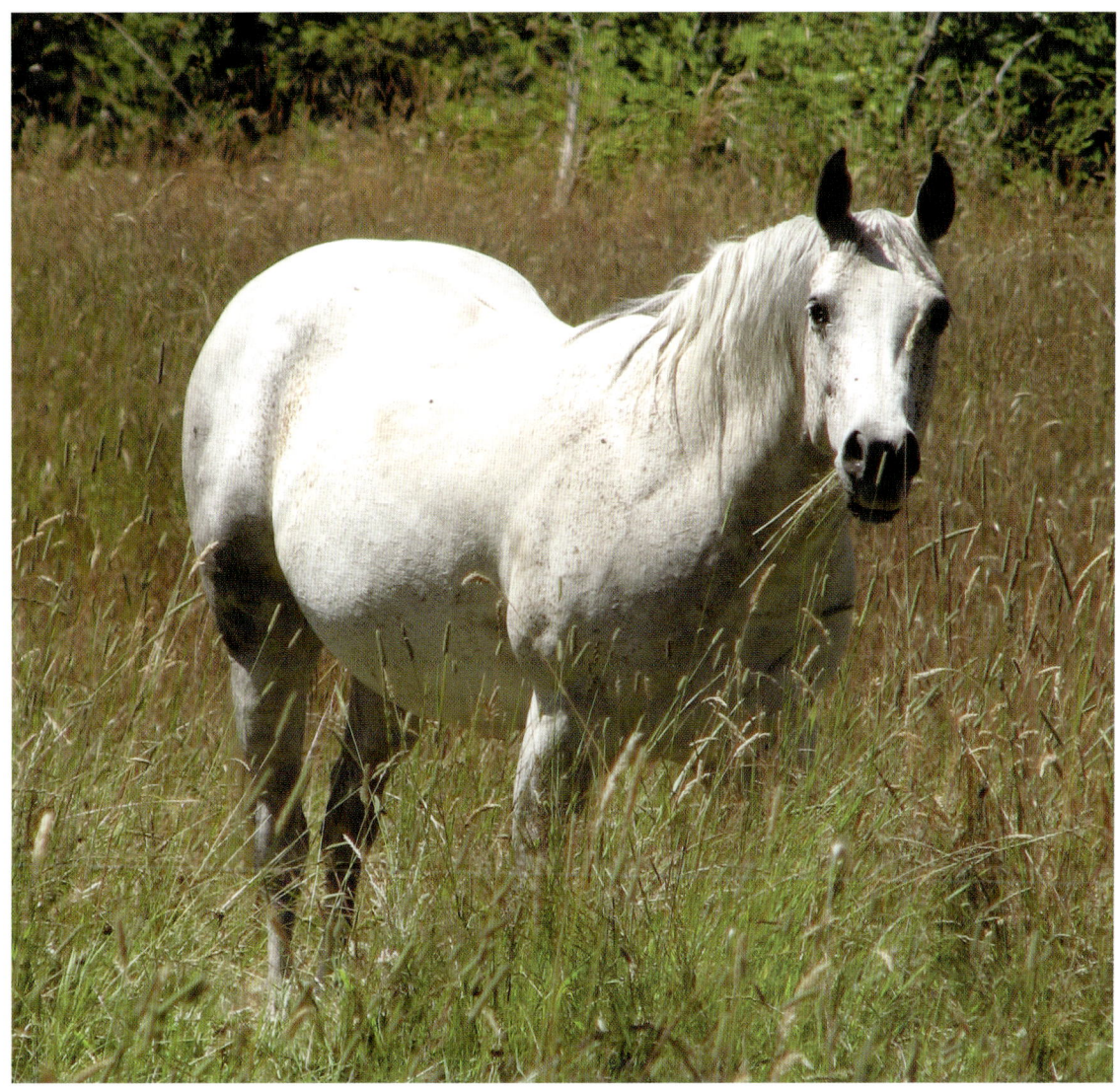

14.13 This obese horse's feet and body are experiencing both metabolic and mechanical stresses.

Tech found that overweight horses are vulnerable to chronic inflammation, oxidative stress, insulin/glucose imbalances, heat stress, reduced performance levels, and increased bone, tendon, and joint injuries (fig. 14.13). They concluded that obesity is a major health concern in horses that has been widely underreported.

Unfortunately, many of us have horses that are overweight and we don't even know it, due to widespread misconceptions as to what constitutes a healthy weight. Equine nutritionists generally say that you should be able to see a hint of ribs on a horse until he is two or so, and after that, you want to be able to easily feel, but not see the ribs. It is also useful to get familiar with the *Henneke scale,* a rating system for equine body condition that uses specific markers to determine where a horse falls on a scale of 1 to 9, with 1 being emaciated and 9 being extremely obese. The ideal body condition for most horses is around 5 on the Henneke scale (fig. 14.14). Ultimately, it is the owners' responsibility to educate themselves on what is a healthy weight for their horses and to monitor their horses' body condition.

A good diet for most horses—average to easy keepers—will be forage based and will consist mainly of hay that is moderate in simple sugars and protein, with a balanced vitamin/mineral supplement as needed, access to salt, and little if any grain.

Hard keepers or hard-working horses may need more calories in their diet than grass hay can provide, but many equine nutritionists are now recommending the addition of calories in the form of fats, such as vegetable oils or rice bran, instead of loading the horse up on starches and sugars. Fats are easily digested and utilized by the horse, whereas sugars and starches can not only damage the feet, but also wreak havoc with the digestive system.

Whenever possible, opt for hay that has had a nutritional analysis done so that you know what you are feeding. If you are aiming for "low-carb hay," look for hay that has an ESC (simple sugars) plus starch total of no more than 10%. While even this

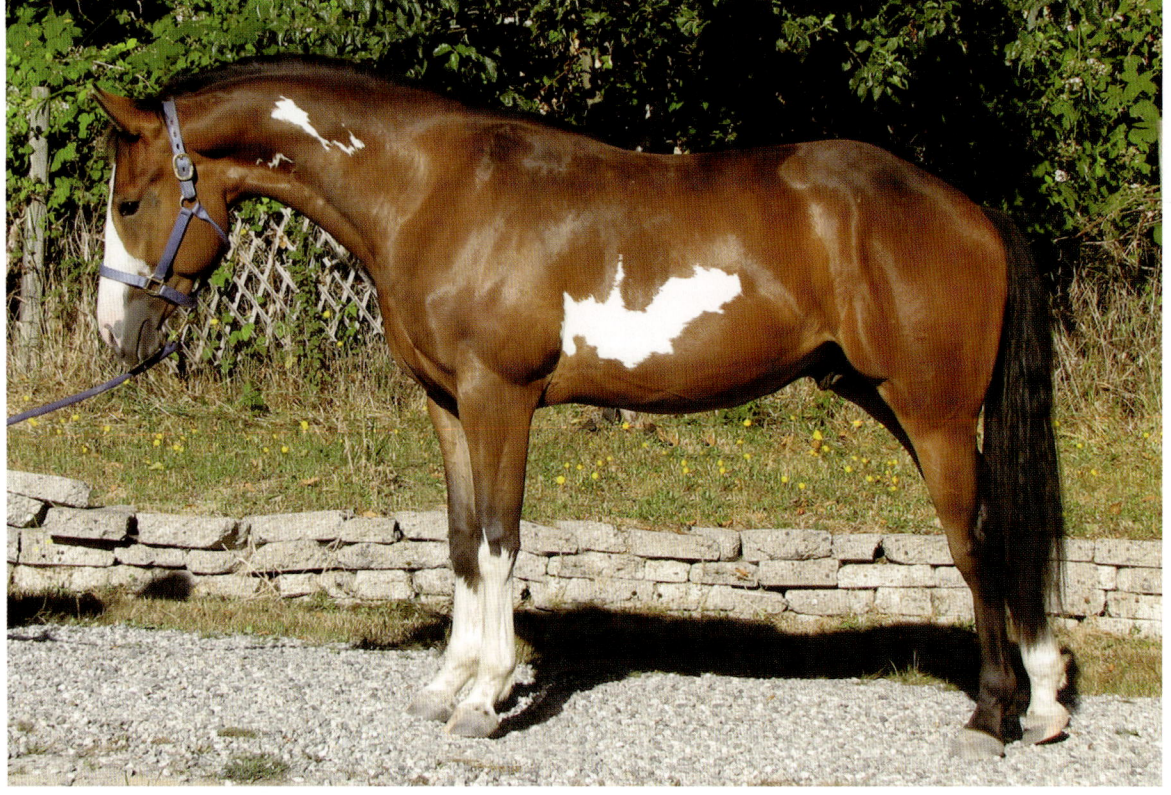

14.14 This horse would rate right around 5 on the Henneke scale for equine body condition (1–9), which is just where you want a horse to be.

Delving Deeper:
ESC vs. WSC

When looking at a complete hay or pasture analysis, there are two figures that refer to sugar content. One is *ESC* (ethanol soluble carbohydrates), and the other is *WSC* (water soluble carbohydrates). ESC is *simple sugars,* while WSC contains both simple sugars and a more complex type of sugar called *fructan.* There has been some debate regarding which number to pay attention to if your horse is prone to metabolically-related laminitis. Most people have found that using the ESC number, as recommended by equine nutritionist Eleanor Kellon, VMD, is the best way to gauge whether or not a hay is appropriately "low sugar" for such horses, yet some don't trust that figure.

The confusion stems from the fact that researchers have used a chicory-derived fructan called *inulin* to induce laminitis in horses for experiments, so some people have extrapolated that fructan in general is a danger for carb-sensitive horses. It would follow that a hay (or grass) high in fructans would increase the risk of laminitis. However, a couple of facts need to be clarified.

First, in order to induce laminitis in their experiments, the researchers gave the horses a massive dose of pure inulin via stomach tube. This produces a type of laminitis that results from overloading the hindgut bacteria with sugars, not the type that has to do with glycemic spikes and insulin, which are the main things we are trying to control when devising a low-carb diet for a metabolically challenged horse.

Second, as Dr. Kellon has explained, the type of fructan found in grass is primarily *levan,* not inulin, and no study has ever shown that consuming levan can cause laminitis. Even

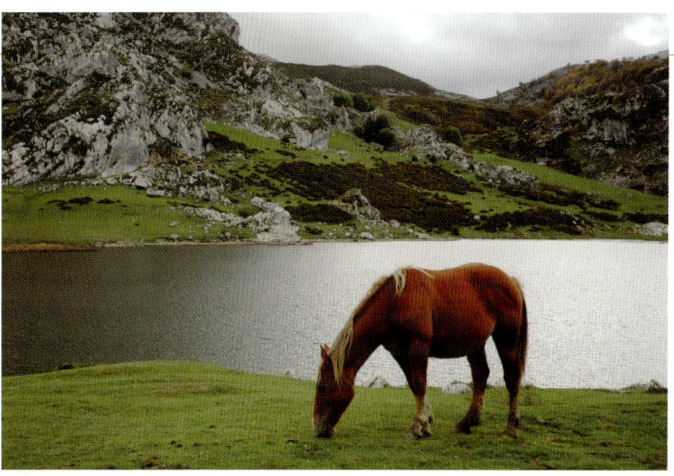

14.15 While fructans may not be the source of the problem, "grass founder" is a major health issue in domestic horses, so much so that any horse considered at risk for laminitis should be allowed to graze only with extreme caution—or not at all.

if levan could cause laminitis, a grass or hay would have to be 37% fructan to equal the experimental doses of inulin used, and the horse would have to somehow extract this substance into a pure form while avoiding the ingestion fiber or other components that would slow the absorption of the fructan. In real life, that simply doesn't happen.

However, this doesn't mean that horses can't get laminitis from eating grass—they can and often do (fig. 14.15). It *does* mean that it isn't the fructans causing the problem. What *is* causing the problem are the simple sugars that cause rapid rises in blood glucose levels, which in insulin-resistant horses also cause abnormally high insulin levels. While we don't yet fully understand how high insulin causes laminitis, we now know that it does, so this is why it is so important to control the simple sugars in the diet of metabolically at-risk horses.

That said, there are people who have found that a WCS plus starch number of over 10% will apparently cause problems for their horses, even if the ESC plus starch number is under 10%. Although unusual, this is certainly something to keep in mind if you are feeding "safe" hay and still having problems.

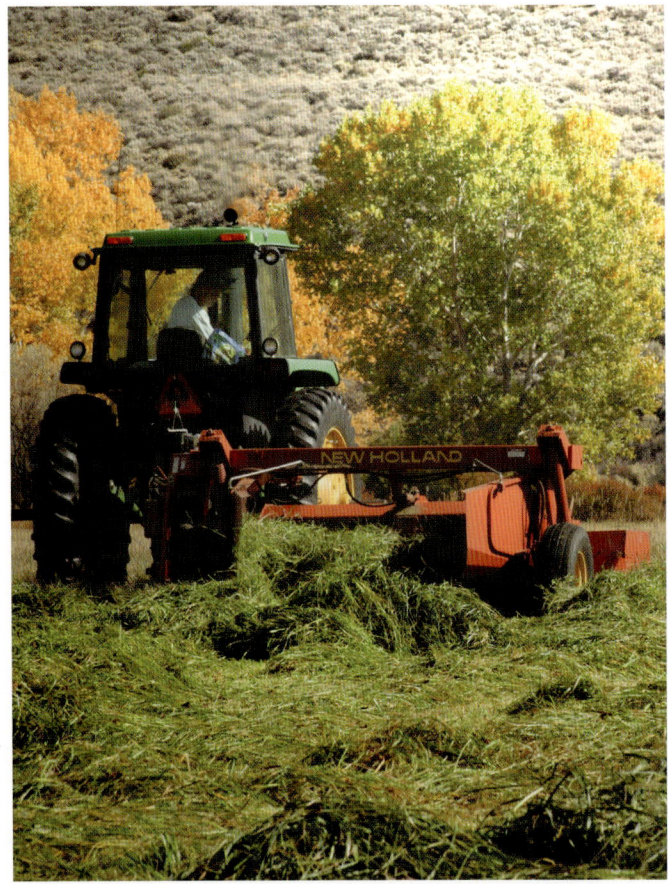

14.16 Sugars accumulate in grass during daylight hours, then drop after the sun goes down. Hay cut in the evening will thus be significantly higher in sugar than hay cut in the morning.

number may be too high for some very carb-sensitive horses, it is a safe and nutritionally adequate number for most. Protein should be around 8% for average horses, up to 12% if they are working hard. Weanlings and nursing mares have slightly higher protein requirements. And, as we mentioned, keep in mind that overfeeding protein can have a similar effect to feeding too much sugar in some horses, as protein is turned to glucose in the body (a process called *glucogenesis*). This is why

some horses show signs of laminitis on high protein diets, even though the sugars in their feed sources are low.

If you decide you want to know more about what you are feeding but tested hay is not available in your area, you may want to consider getting your hay analyzed yourself. The most widely used laboratory for the horse industry is Equi-Analytical Labs, in Ithaca, New York. Their website (equi-analytical.com) has all the information you need about testing and how to get a good sample, which is not as simple as grabbing a handful from a few flakes and sending it in.

Equi-Analytical also has a very useful online library of past analyses that can give you an idea of the nutritional values of different types of hay. Keep in mind, though, that the library provides only general information, and to know what is in your specific hay, you have to test it. Hay from the same field will vary from year to year, cutting to cutting, and even from the same cutting done at different times on the same day.

Sugars in hay are particularly variable, as the amount of sugar hay contains depends on a number of factors, including:

• *Sunlight during growth:* Growing grass produces sugar in the presence of sunlight, with more sun equaling more sugar. Hay that is cut from grass that has been growing during a stretch of cloudy days or in the shade will therefore be lower in sugar.

• *Time of day it was cut:* Grasses start to produce sugar when the sun comes up, then they utilize that sugar for growth after the sun goes down. This means that grass contains the highest amount of sugar just before the sun goes down, and the lowest amount just before the sun comes up. If you were to cut a very uniform grass in one field on a sunny day, some in the afternoon and some very early in the morning, the morning cutting would contain less sugar (fig. 14.16).

- *Stage of growth:* When grass is young and short, sugars tend to be low, then they increase until they peak at the flowering stage. After that, sugar levels generally fall off as maturity increases. A hay cut from a field that is very mature will therefore tend to be lower in sugar than hay from the same field had the cutting been done just before or during flowering.

- *Stress:* Any form of stress will generally cause sugar levels in grass to rise. Grass can be stressed due to lack of nutrients (not enough fertilization), overgrazing, drought, or freezing temperatures (fig. 14.17).

- *Drying time:* Once grass is cut, it will lose some sugar during the process of drying. Grass that dries very quickly will "lock in" a higher amount of sugar than hay that dries slowly. For example, cutting hay on a hot, sunny day will produce a higher sugar hay than the same grass if it were cut on a cool, cloudy day.

- *Rain after cutting:* Sugars in freshly cut grass (or dry hay) can be "leached out" to a certain extent by water, and getting wet will also extend the drying time. Hay that has been rained on will thus have a lower sugar content than it would have had it not been rained on. Other nutrient values such as protein and minerals are virtually unchanged by

rain, despite the fact that it may lose color. So, while rained-on hay often doesn't look "pretty," it can be an excellent choice for horses with metabolic issues or carb-related laminitis, as long as it was allowed to dry properly and is not moldy.

Having an accurate nutritional profile not only allows you to choose hays that are most appropriate for different horses based on factors like sugar and protein, it also lets you see which minerals are too

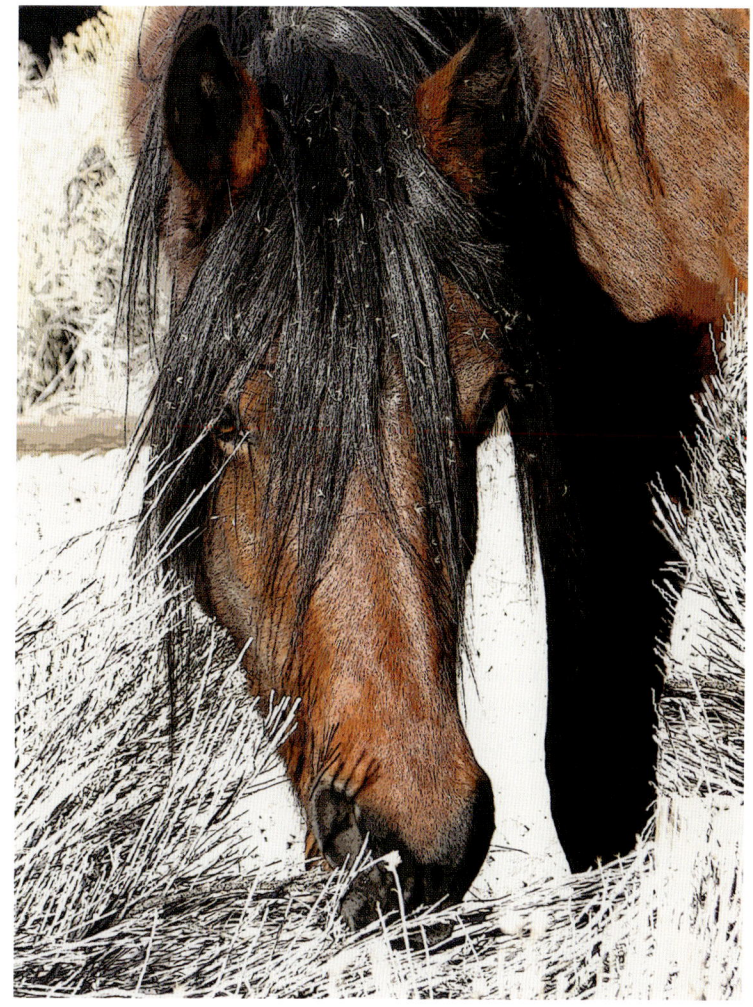

14.17 Grass may look like it has "nothing in it" late in the season, but frost can actually shoot sugar levels up to extremely high levels, adding a surprising amount of carbohydrates to the horse's diet. This is why the incidence of laminitis is higher than average in the fall.

low or too high, thus giving you the chance to supplement safely in accordance with what your horse actually needs. Too often, horse owners throw a random vitamin/mineral supplement into their horse's diet without having the slightest idea about what the mineral numbers are like in their hay. This can lead to excess supplementation, which can be dangerous in some cases, and it can also lead to mineral imbalances that can leave the horses worse off than if they were given no supplements at all. For example, many hays have high iron and low copper content, and as iron interferes with the body's ability to utilize some other minerals, including copper, a supplement that adds additional iron to the mix (as most do) is going to make the copper deficiency already present even worse.

Having an appropriate diet, including correctly balanced minerals, can make an enormous difference in hoof health, and in your horse's overall health as well. The more that we, as horse owners, can start requesting and insisting upon hay analyses from local hay growers and feed stores, the more common hay testing for horses will become.

Hoof Supplements

There are a dizzying number of supplements on the market that are touted to improve hoof quality and eradicate all sorts of hoof ailments, from chipping walls to laminitis. Hoof supplements are alluring because they offer a silver bullet for what are often frustrating problems, and we all know that believing in a quick fix is a lot easier than taking a hard look at what we are doing and possibly having to make some real changes. Unfortunately, most hoof supplements generally do little, if anything, to actually

benefit the hoof, though they might make the horse owner feel better for being "proactive."

Whatever ailment they are aimed at, hoof supplements purport to provide something that your horse needs, usually something assumed to be insufficient or missing from his diet. But, while it is certainly true that mineral deficiencies and diets too low in protein can affect hoof quality and growth, the amount of relevant substances present in most hoof supplements are usually inadequate to make up for any real dietary imbalance. If you are serious about correcting possible imbalances, you will need to get a thorough laboratory analysis of everything the horse is eating, figure out what the deficiencies actually are, and work with a qualified equine nutritionist to balance the deficiencies without upsetting other mineral ratios—a common problem with random supplementation (fig. 14.18).

Add to this the fact that the equine-supplement industry is completely unregulated, and tests have shown that many products do not contain the amounts of supposedly "active" ingredients they claim, and you can see why many experts consider hoof supplements to be a waste of money. The one possible exception *might* be biotin, which some studies have shown to have a positive effect on hoof growth and horn quality. Other studies have reached the opposite conclusion, but anecdotal evidence suggests that some horses may indeed benefit from biotin supplementation. It is certainly not going to hurt your horse in any way to try it, but don't hope to see any results for at least six to eight months, as it takes that long for new growth to be far enough down the hoof to make a noticeable difference.

One other caveat: in order to be certain that biotin or any other supplement is indeed making

	As Sampled			Dry Matter	
	%	g/lb.		%	g/lb.
Calcium	.33	1.49		.35	1.59
Phosphorus	.20	.89		.21	.95
Magnesium	.35	1.57		.37	1.68
Potassium	.85	3.84		.90	4.08
Sodium	.046	.206		.048	.219
	ppm	mg/lb.		ppm	mg/lb.
Iron	95	43		101	46
Zinc	25	11		26	12
Copper	8	4		9	4
Manganese	67	30		71	32
Molybdenum	.5	.2		.5	.2

14.18 These numbers are the mineral percentages in a basic hay analysis. To correctly supplement your horse's diet, you would need to know all of these figures and more from your hay, exactly how many pounds of hay your horse is consuming daily, all other sources of minerals, what your horse's daily requirements are, and what the ratios of all the minerals should be. Take all that into consideration and it becomes clear why the average hoof supplement is highly unlikely to provide what your horse actually needs—if he actually needs anything at all.

a difference in a horse's feet, all other possible influences would have to remain 100% constant, including the weather, feeding, trimming, exercise, overall health, lameness, or any of the other myriad factors that can affect hoof health. Any one or a combination of these factors could affect the hoof, for better or for worse, and therein lies one of the difficulties for horse owners in assessing the value of hoof supplements.

More from Dr. Bowker: Physiologically Correct Hoof Care

It is easy to get confused these days when it comes to what constitutes good hoof care. Different farriers and barefoot practitioners advocate an array of methods that generally sound logical enough when you listen to each individual, yet their techniques often stand in complete contradiction to one another. Fortunately, a few intrepid souls are trying to come up with definitive answers through hard science—and their findings are starting to find their way into mainstream hoof care.

We've previously mentioned Professor Emeritus Robert Bowker, VMD, PhD, former director of the Equine Foot Laboratory at the College of Veterinary Medicine at Michigan State University. Dr. Bowker's groundbreaking research on the physiology and biomechanics of the equine foot has led him to define what he calls the "physiological trim," a set of trimming guidelines that is being utilized with great success by hoof-care professionals in a variety of camps, on both barefoot and shod horses. While Dr. Bowker's approach may seem strange to some, much of what he advocates is not really new at all. What *is* new is that his work has helped to illuminate why and how these trimming parameters may be helpful in the prevention and treatment of hoof-related lameness.

What Is it?

The goal of the physiological trim is to allow the foot to dissipate energy with maximum efficiency, while at the same time providing maximum support (fig. 14.19). To achieve this, Dr. Bowker outlines these basic principles:

• The back of the frog should be in contact with the ground. This usually means that very little if any frog tissue is removed during a trim.

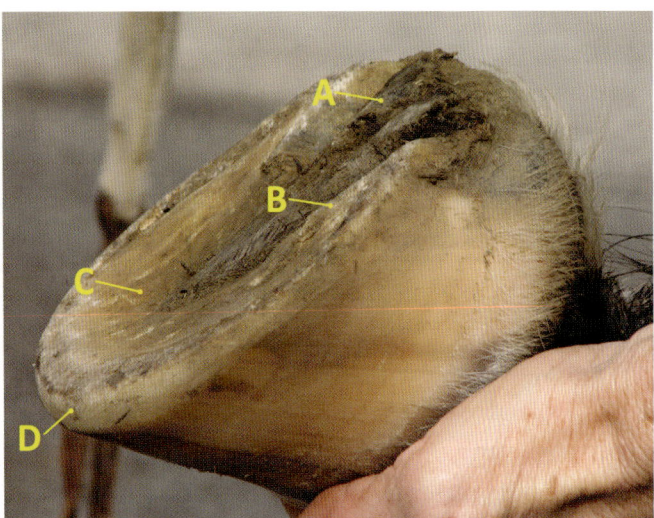

14.19 This foot is maintained following Dr. Bowker's physiological trim principles. The back of the frog makes ground contact (A); the bars share in weight bearing (B); the sole is not lowered (carved out) (C); and the toe is short and bevelled to facilitate breakover (D).

• The bars should be weight bearing on a conformable surface, just a millimeter or two shorter than the level of the hoof wall, on average. Most horses will require little if any trimming of the bars if hoof care is performed at appropriate intervals.

• The live sole should not be "lowered" or removed. The sole, particularly the outer part nearest the wall, should share in weight bearing, along with the frog and bars, when the horse is standing or moving on anything other than a hard, flat surface.

• The toe should be short, with approximately ⅓ of the hoof in front of the true apex of the frog, and ⅔ behind the apex. This also generally equates to approximately 50% of the hoof mass in front of the widest part of the foot and 50% behind it.

• The toe should be bevelled to facilitate breakover, and the point of breakover should be close to the tip of the coffin bone.

• The coffin bone should be slightly higher (2–5 degrees) in the back, which allows the coffin bone to be ground parallel when the hoof lands slightly heel first, as it is meant to do in most gaits. That is the moment of greatest impact.

• Horses should be kept barefoot whenever possible; if shoes are necessary for certain events or activities, remove them afterward.

• All changes aimed at achieving this or any trim should be made gradually.

In addition, Dr. Bowker recommends that horses be kept on a surface that has enough give to conform to the solar surface of the foot (engaging all structures in weight bearing), but enough firmness to provide the beneficial pressure/stimulation we've mentioned previously. Many hoof-care professionals are finding that the combination of the physiological trim with plenty of movement over the right kind of footing is the best way to create a foot with optimal biomechanical function, a foot that protects the bones and soft tissues from injury while enduring tremendous thrust and load-bearing forces.

Though Dr. Bowker's studies have led him to conclude that the most optimal hoof form and function is achieved when horses are left barefoot, farriers who apply his principles to shod horses report excellent results.

One of the main reasons why the physiological trim makes such a difference is that when it is put into practice, the foot, whether shod or barefoot, will not be peripherally loaded. States Dr. Bowker, "I don't know where the idea got started that the walls are meant to be the primary weight-bearing structure, but all I can say is that the data we have gathered seems to indicate otherwise."

While that is stating it gently, Dr. Bowker and many other experts are, in fact, adamant that the equine hoof is not designed to "hang" from the laminae, and is prone to an alarming host of problems when it is forced to do so. The excessive strain on the laminae affects the strength of their connection, circulation within the foot is altered and compromised, support structures may be damaged and prone to atrophy, the sole becomes thinner, the wall becomes thinner and weaker, and the coffin bone may be driven downward within the hoof capsule—to name just a few.

Unfortunately, it is extremely common to find peripheral loading in shod horses, and it can happen in barefoot horses, as well, though it is

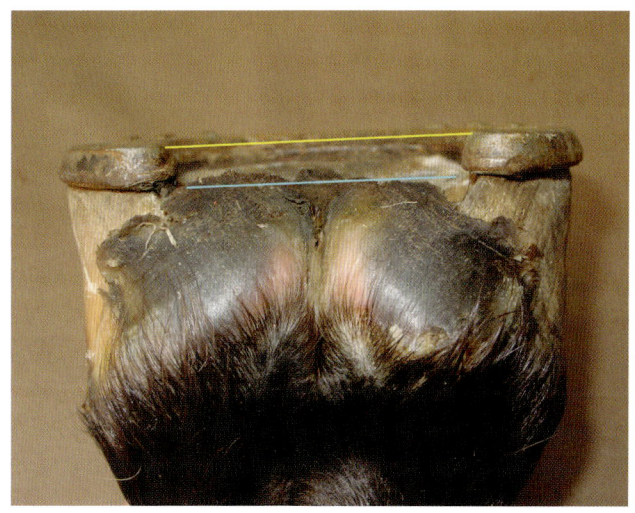

14.20 This horse lives in an area where the ground is soft and moist most of the time. On such footing, this foot would not be peripherally loaded, even though the frog does not reach down to the bottom of the shoe. Notice the gap between the level of the frog (blue line) and the level of the ground surface of the shoe (yellow line). If this horse lived elsewhere or worked on firmer footing, the hoof might be peripherally loaded to some degree.

less common, as their walls will tend to chip off if they get long enough to take on the majority of the weight bearing. But barefoot or shod, the degree to which peripheral loading affects the foot will vary depending on the conformability of the footing the horse is on (fig. 14.20).

When the footing is soft enough to fill in the bottom of the foot and support the other structures, as it is in many arenas, any excess height from an overlong wall and/or a shoe will be somewhat mitigated by the way the foot sinks into the ground. However, if the footing is firmer, the frog, sole, and bars can be lifted right off the ground, rendering them unable to perform their functions of support and energy dissipation.

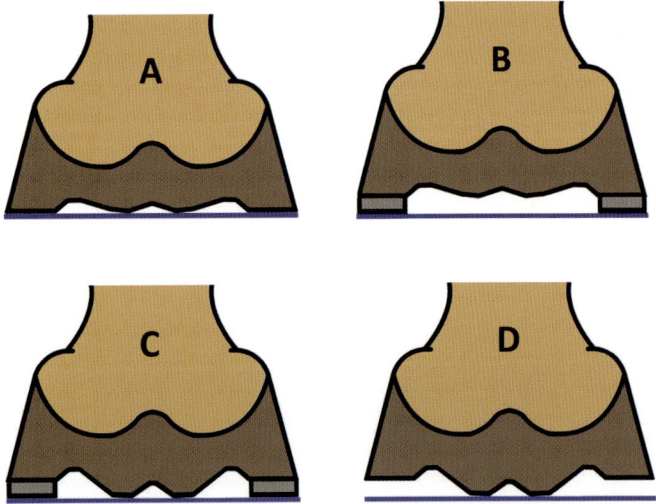

14.21 A–D A barefoot hoof doesn't need a lot of frog height to make contact with the ground (A). But, if you took that same hoof and added a shoe, the height of the shoe would lift the frog out of ground contact, creating peripheral loading unless the horse is always on soft footing (B). In order for the frog to make ground contact on a shod foot, it has to grow to accommodate the height of the shoe (C), but if you take the shoe off a foot with a frog like that, the frog would be too high and would require trimming (D).

Physiologically Correct Trimming for Shod Horses

One of the biggest benefits of horses going barefoot is that it is fairly easy to get the average bare hoof set up so that the back of the frog is in contact with the ground. Shod horses, on the other hand, are often deprived of this benefit, possibly because their owners and hoof-care providers don't realize what a huge hoof health booster it is, and perhaps because the providers are not exactly sure what one would do to get the frog on the ground in a shod horse, even if they wanted to. Fortunately, more and more farriers are discovering the drastic difference that

engaging the back of the foot can make, and they are making it happen successfully.

To do this, it is necessary to first understand that getting the frog on the ground is not an isolated element you can extract from Dr. Bowker's principles while leaving everything else unchanged. *All* of the principles of physiologically correct trimming must be in place or the frog is unlikely to be healthy enough to grow down to the ground on a shod foot. Problems like contracted heels and dorsopalmar (front to back) imbalance will work against the creation of a robust frog, so any such problems need to be addressed.

In addition, it is critically important for the farrier to stop trimming away healthy frog material. If it seems necessary, a very minimal removal of flaps and edges to keep the collateral grooves open is okay, but otherwise, the frog must be left alone to grow and develop. One reason you need to maximize frog growth is that the frog must actually be longer than the walls in order to make contact with the ground on a shod horse (figs. 14.21 A–D). While this may look strange before the shoe is put on, it works beautifully once the shoe is in place (fig. 14.22).

It is also absolutely essential that hoof-care providers (and owners) recognize the difference between a *prolapsed* frog and a healthy frog that has grown down to meet the ground (fig. 14.23). While the two can look rather similar, there are very important differences in form, function, and origin. A healthy frog has internal structures that are well suspended within the hoof capsule, covered with a layer of elastic frog horn on the solar surface. When the frog grows down to meet the ground on a healthy shod foot, the layer of frog horn simply grows thicker, but the position of the internal structures does not change.

When a frog is prolapsed, the internal structures have dropped out of their normal position, moving the whole frog downward. While the frog may indeed make contact with the ground, it has not arrived there by growing thick and strong, but rather by being pushed from within when it is already thin and weak. In such a state, the back of the foot is not able to function properly at all. In fact, the horse is very likely to get sore due to the pressure of the prolapsed frog touching the ground.

Too often, the cause of a prolapsed frog is a well-meaning hoof-care provider who over-trims the heels, sometimes in an attempt to get the frog in contact with the ground. Ironically, the effort to improve the health of the back of foot is the very thing making it worse, for by taking the heels down too far, the HCP is lowering the palmar/plantar angle of the coffin bone to the point where it is pressing down on, and damaging, the internal structures in the back of the foot.

When the frog has actually prolapsed, you can be fairly certain that the coffin bone has a negative palmar/plantar angle (see sidebar, p. 25), and will likely have other features reflective of that (fig. 14.24). A foot can have a too-low palmar/plantar angle without a prolapsed frog, so you want to learn how to recognize the external features that indicate the angle of the coffin bone (figs.14.25 A & B). Whether the frog is prolapsed or not, a negative or even ground-parallel palmar/plantar angle will compromise the frog, digital cushion, blood vessels, and other structures in the back of the foot.

When the foot has a good palmar/plantar angle, and the frog is not being excessively trimmed

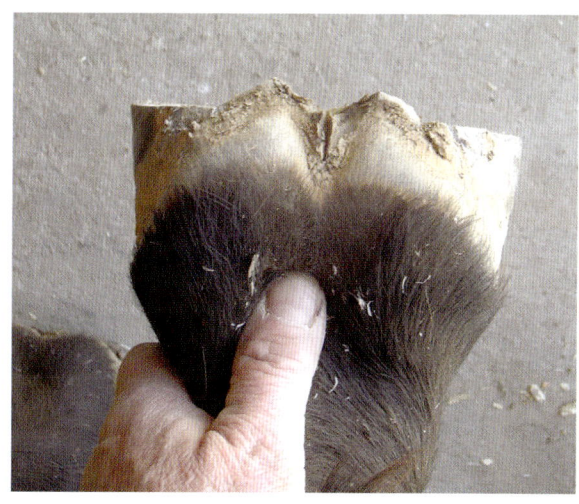

14.22 This is what a healthy frog grown to be in contact with the ground on a shod foot looks like before the shoe is put on.

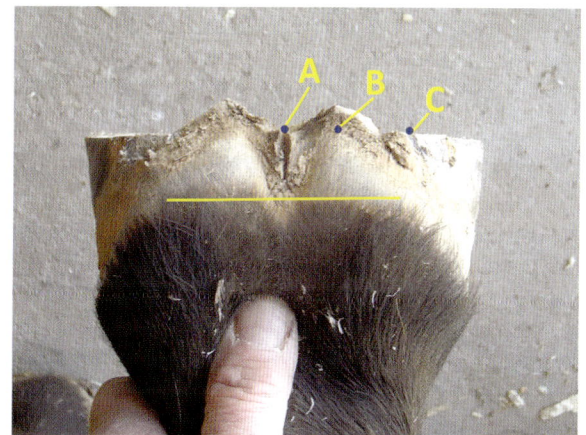

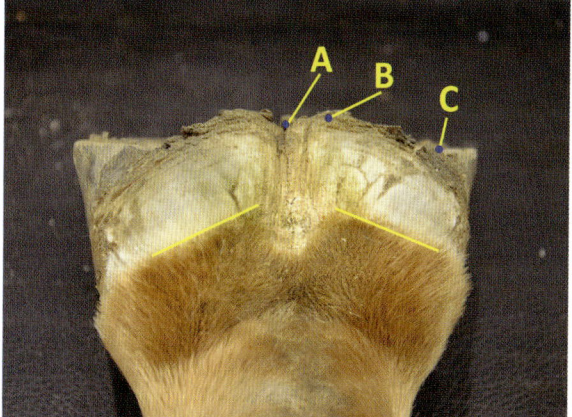

14.23 At first glance, the healthy frog (above) and the prolapsed frog (below) look fairly similar. But there are at least three significant visible differences: 1) Compare the level of the central sulcus (A) with the level of the heel (C)—they should be on the same plane. 2) Compare the bottom of the heel bulb (B) with the level of the heel—they should also be on the same plane. 3) Look at the hairline across the heel bulbs— it should be relatively straight, not sharply angled. You can imagine that the structures creating the A-B-C line on the healthy foot are like a tightly pulled sheet, while those in the unhealthy foot are like a sagging hammock.

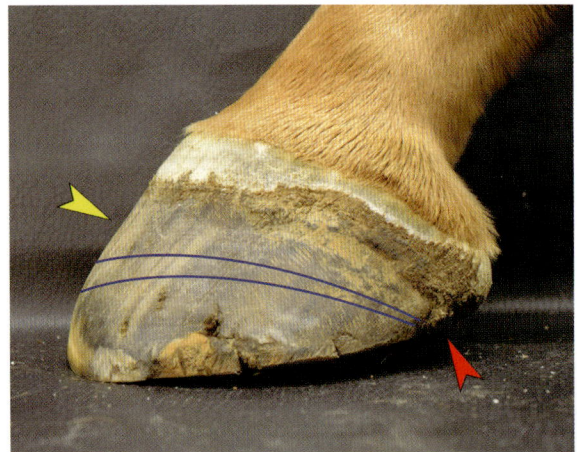

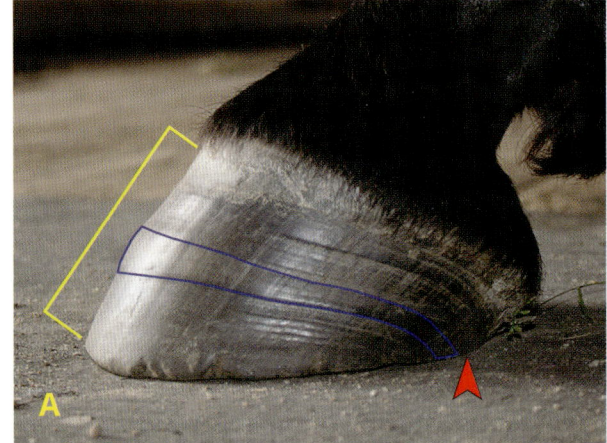

14.24 This hind foot is up off the ground due to a prolapsed frog and the shoe having been removed. Several aspects of the foot point to a probable negative plantar angle. First is the crushed heel (red arrow). Then there are the growth lines, which are significantly farther apart at the toe than the heel—they are faint thus hard to see in a photograph, so we've highlighted a couple of them with blue lines. There is also the slightly convex profile of the foot, exacerbated by the dubbed toe.

(meaning nothing more than loose shreds and minimal amounts along the edges are removed), but the frog is still not growing enough to make ground contact, it may help to pack the bottom of the foot with "clean" dirt or artificial support material and keep it that way (don't pick it out) between farrier visits. This will provide missing support and stimulus to the bottom of the foot, and very likely, when that material is removed at the next visit, the farrier will find that the frog has grown. It should be noted that applying frog pressure (sometimes called frog support) in the form of inflexible devices such as a heart bar shoe or rigid frog pad is not the same thing as having the frog on the ground and may be

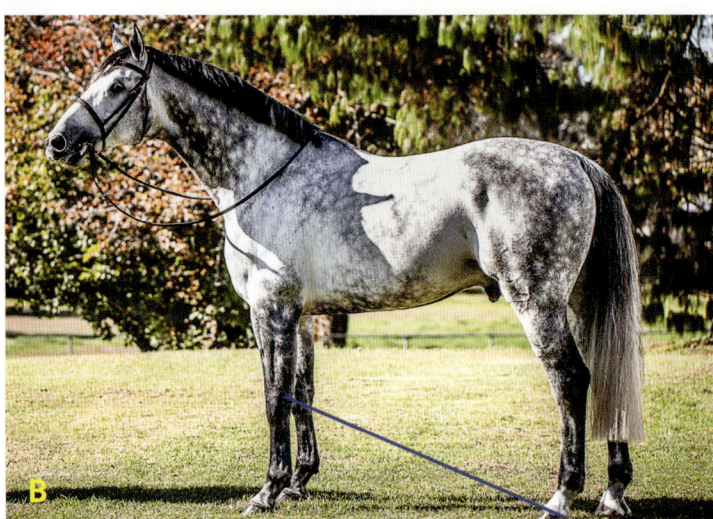

14.25 A & B While the foot in A does not have a prolapsed frog, it has other features indicative of a negative palmar (or plantar, if it is a hind foot) angle. Like the prolapsed foot in figure 14.24, it has a bulge in the dorsal wall (yellow bracket), a very low heel (red arrow), and growth rings that are wider at the toe than at the heel (example outlined in blue). One way to gauge the plantar angles of the coffin bones of the hind feet is to stand the horse square on level, firm ground, making sure the hind cannon bone is perpendicular to the ground. If you draw a line following the hairline forward, it should ideally strike the front leg at the level of the knee, as it does on the gorgeous Holsteiner stallion, Cassiago (B). When the coffin bone has a negative plantar angle, the line will strike well above the knee.

counterproductive, as the pressure is more constant and thus biomechanically somewhat different than the pressure and release most beneficial to frog and overall hoof health.

Lastly, owners and farriers who want to implement physiologically correct hoof care on shod horses need to be aware that they may have to shorten the time between resetting the horse's shoes. Since the walls cannot wear down under the shoe, they will lift the frog away from the ground as they grow, so to keep the frog where it needs to be, shoes may have to be reset in as little as three or four weeks, if the feet are growing fast. Still, owners and farriers who make the change to this style of hoof care are typically very impressed with the improvements in overall hoof health they see, and its popularity is growing.

The Role of Perfusion and Hoof Mechanism

When the frog is on the ground and working as it should, it is able to play its important role in protecting the foot. However, it is only one part of the shock-absorption system in the equine hoof. Another key factor in the efficient reduction of impact energy is *perfusion*—the delivery of arterial blood to the vast network of microvessels in the hoof. Good perfusion is crucial to diminishing the tremendous forces experienced by the foot, as passing energy through moving fluid is one the most effective ways to dampen that energy.

In the hoof, maximum perfusion is achieved through a process referred to as *hoof mechanism,* which, as mentioned earlier, is the expansion and contraction of the hoof in response to loading and

unloading during movement. While it was long believed that blood was forced *out* of the foot by positive pressure (compression) during loading, Dr. Bowker's work has shown that there is actually negative pressure inside the foot during loading, meaning that it is moving blood *into* the foot during the loading phase.

This remarkable feat is thought to be due to the outward expansion of both the heels and the lateral cartilages, as well as the downward movement of the coffin bone that occurs when the foot is loading, all of which effectively creates a vacuum that sucks blood into the foot (fig. 14.26). This blood that flows through the foot's vast network of blood vessels acts like a thick, cushy insole, so you put that on top of the "gel pad" created by the digital cushion and the frog, and the horse's feet are very well protected. When the foot is unloading, the heels and

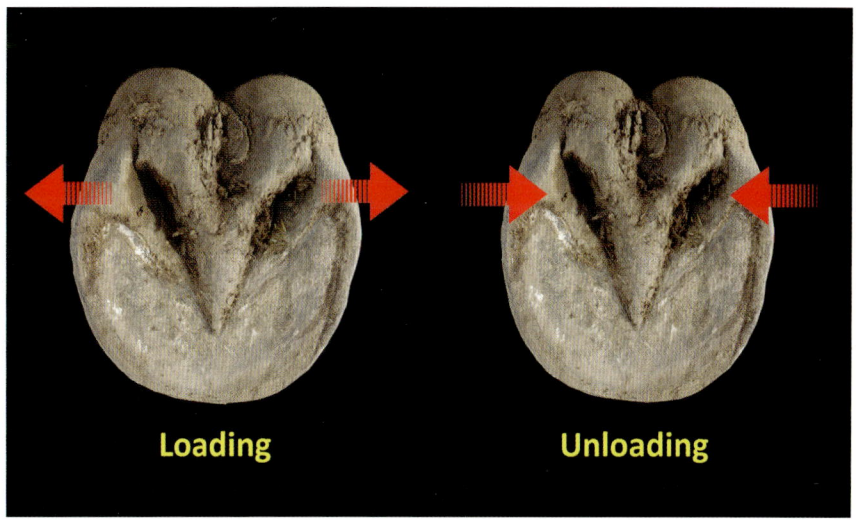

Loading   **Unloading**

14.26 The foot expands when it is loading, creating negative pressure that sucks blood into the foot. The foot then contracts as it unloads, shooting blood back up the leg. Note that the bottom of the foot actually becomes wider during the loading phase (left).

lateral cartilages snap back together, pushing the blood back out of the foot and boosting it up the leg. In this way, the feet of the horse act like four extra hearts.

Of course, all of the structures involved have to be functioning as they are designed to for maximum benefit. Dr. Bowker's studies on blood flow in the equine foot have demonstrated that the best perfusion is achieved with the frog, bars, and solar surface all sharing in weight bearing on a conformable surface. According to Dr. Bowker, correctly trimmed barefoot horses demonstrate greater perfusion than shod horses, but how much a shoe diminishes perfusion varies depending on the trim, type of shoe, and application of the shoe. Having the frog of a shod horse on the ground, as described earlier,

definitely helps increase perfusion, though even if the foot is not peripherally loaded, shoeing may decrease perfusion by reducing the ability of the foot to expand and contract.

Says Dr. Bowker, "We don't entirely understand how shoeing affects the biomechanics of the foot at this time, but we do know that perfusion is different in a shod versus a barefoot horse, even on the same surface, and we know that peripheral loading decreases perfusion."

Ultimately, a foot lacking good perfusion and a properly functioning frog is at greater risk of injury. Dr. Bowker states, "When the foot hits the ground, whatever energy is there is going to be dissipated. It's just a question of whether it's being done by the correct tissues or not. Say you're in an automobile accident and you hit the window with your face and thus stop moving forward. This means all the energy of your momentum has been absorbed (fig. 14.27). The problem in this scenario is that the face is not designed to dissipate energy.

"When the horse's foot hits the ground correctly with all the structures doing their job, there is maximal efficiency for the dissipation of energy. However, if the energy is not dissipated, high frequency energy moves into structures that are not designed to deal with it. Human biomechanical studies have shown that it is the high frequency energies that are so deleterious to bone and connective tissues. That's why we like sneakers for running, because they help dissipate that high frequency energy."

Metal horse shoes, by contrast, appear to raise impact energies to higher frequencies. Exactly what effect this may have on the bones and other interior structures of the foot has yet to be determined.

"There is still much that we don't know," says Dr.

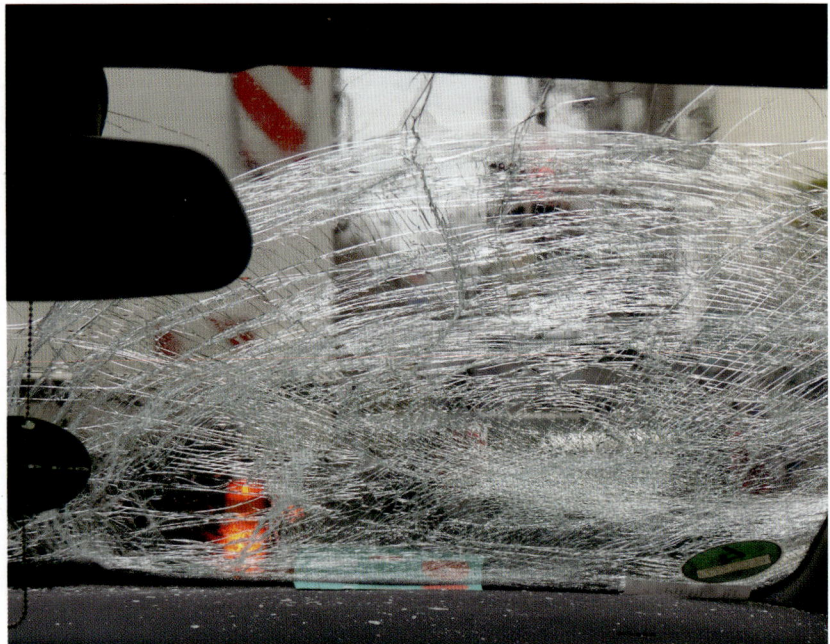

14.27 Dr. Bowker uses the metaphor of a face hitting a windshield to explain why forcing the wrong parts of the foot to dissipate energy is problematic.

Bowker, "but we do know that peripheral loading creates the most pressure per square inch of weight-bearing surface, due to smaller surface area, whereas spreading the load over the entire solar surface means less pressure per square inch. This definitely changes how the foot experiences impact energies."

Dr. Bowker is certainly not alone in his conclusions about the back part of the foot, blood perfusion, and energy dissipation. Pete Ramey has been following Dr. Bowker's work for years and could not agree with him more.

"Every aspect of the back part of the foot is designed for energy dissipation," states Ramey. "The foundation is cartilage instead of bone, there are miles of 'extra' blood vessels for hydraulic energy dissipation, and the back of the foot is designed to twist, flex, and conform to the ground. The frog is a very important, yielding structure that should be the front-line shock absorber for the whole system.

"All this combined creates an easier, safer 'ride' for the joints, ligaments, tendons, and muscles—much like the difference between rubber tires versus steel wheels on a truck. Additionally, horses with poor development in the back of the foot (bare or shod) tend to land toe first. Toe-first impact is an important contributor to coffin bone rotation, most wall cracks, white line separation, and issues with pain in the back of the foot. The key point should be prevention. By understanding the importance of the shock-absorbing qualities of the back of the foot, you start to realize how many problems horses may actually endure due to excess shock (fig. 14.28)."

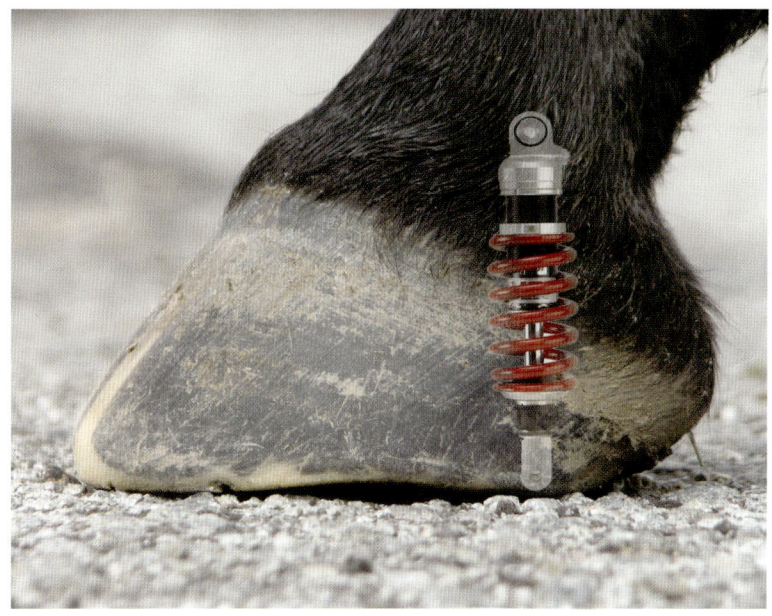

14.28 Everything about the back of the foot is designed for energy dissipation, making it the shock absorber for the horse.

Footing and Peripheral Loading

While it is difficult to argue with the logic and science behind Dr. Bowker's conclusions, some might quite reasonably point out that the frog and bars don't need to be "on the ground" if the horse is kept in softer footing, as the foot will sink into the footing enough for the back parts and the sole to make contact.

To this Dr. Bowker says, "If the frog is not quite on the ground but the horse is always on a conformable surface, it may not be a bad thing, but there is still a great deal to learn here. I'm starting to notice that when the horse's frogs are deeply recessed, there are differences in the connective tissue inside the frog. There is basically nothing inside of these feet (fig. 14.29). Even though they have a frog, it's

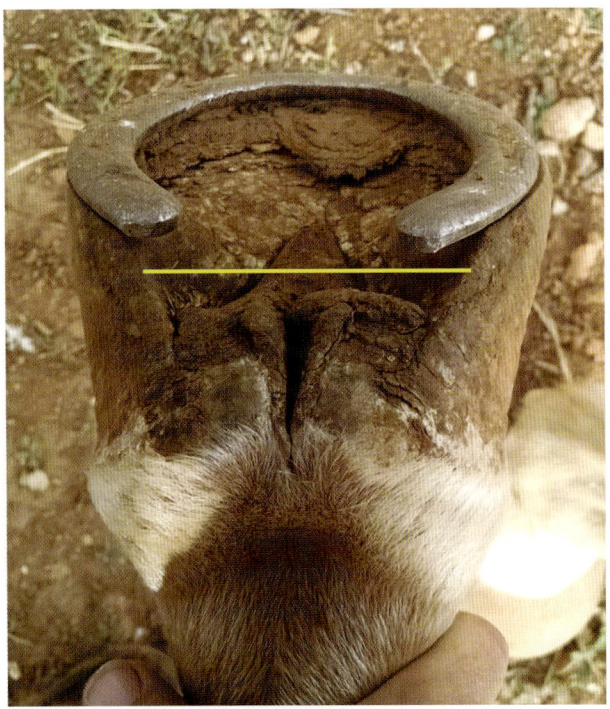

14.29 Dr. Bowker has found that a foot with a deeply recessed frog will lack the internal fibrocartilage that gives a normal frog its shock-absorbing capacity. This foot has overgrown walls and heels that make the frog look more recessed than it is, but even if the heels were at a reasonable height (yellow line), you can see that the frog is still quite a bit below that level—and some frogs are much worse than this.

"When you have peripheral loading," he explains, "the hoof wall is the main thing dissipating the energy, and bone is not being compressed. You can mitigate the problem of energy dissipation to some extent with soft footing, but you still face the problem with the bones, which need the compression that occurs when the entire solar surface is correctly engaged to become dense and strong."

This is why Dr. Bowker speaks of a "firm yet conformable" surface like pea gravel as optimal for the promotion of hoof health, rather than a soft one such as spongy grass.

When to Shoe, If to Shoe

When, if, and how long to shoe are also important considerations for hoof health. According to Dr. Bowker, you are more likely to have a horse with good feet if you delay shoeing a young horse as long as possible, and then only keep shoes on for brief periods, if they are used at all. Dr. Bowker's post-mortem studies on thousands of horses' feet led him to observe that the internal structures of horses shod for the majority of their lifetime often look more like those of immature horses. He also found that horses with this lack of development of the key support structures in the back part of the foot are at much greater risk of developing tenderness and problems in that area.

While Dr. Bowker's observations have given us a tremendous amount of insight, his assertion that it is best not to keep shoes on a horse indefinitely is hardly unique. Read any farrier textbook and you will find a statement about hooves needing a break from shoeing to "recover" from the effects that rigid metal shoes have on the hoof (fig. 14.30).

just the horn there—there is no fibrocartilage or fibrous tissue inside the frog."

Such observations add weight to the "use it or lose it" argument that Dr. Bowker makes about the frog, and to the idea that the external development of the frog reflects the robustness—or lack thereof—of the internal structures.

Dr. Bowker also points out that while soft footing helps in some ways, it is often too soft to provide the frog pressure and release necessary to develop the internal structures of the foot.

Some people are aware of this and take it to heart, often removing their horse's shoes for the winter when the horse is being ridden less. Dr. Bowker's recommendations go a bit further, suggesting that if people feel they need to shoe their horses for specific training or shows, they should remove the shoes immediately afterward, allowing the horse to go barefoot most of the time.

However, there are many who would argue that shoeing allows you to make changes or support a foot in ways that you simply cannot accomplish barefoot, and there is no doubt that this is true in some instances. For example, there are cases where it is necessary to move the point of breakover back significantly to relieve leverage on the toe, and you may be able to move it back more substantially in one go with a shoe than you could if you were just trimming the toe back on a barefoot horse. Still, with the ever-improving array of hoof boots and treatment tools like hoof casting, the world of "it can't be done without shoes" is ever shrinking.

But barefoot hoof care requires commitment to an overall lifestyle for your horse to maximize its success, and that just won't work for some owners. Others remain convinced that their horses are simply better off in shoes for a variety of reasons. If you are on the fence about whether or not to shoe your horse, or whether you need to make some kind of change in your hoof-care program, the one whose opinion ultimately matters the most is your horse. Take a look at his feet and level of soundness, and let that guide your decision. If his feet are well-formed, robust, and healthy, and the horse comfortably does everything you need him to do, your hoof-care regimen is likely just fine. If the feet are anything less than healthy, you might want

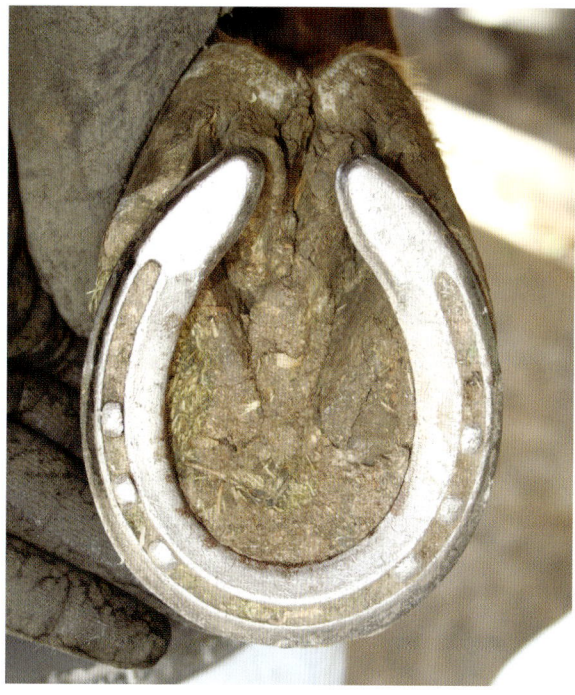

14.30 Some "time off" from being shod would likely be the best way to help this unfortunate foot de-contract and develop healthier structures—both internally and externally.

to try something different. Someone once defined insanity as doing the same thing over and over again but expecting a different result. This definitely applies to hoof care! In the end, it isn't about shod versus barefoot, it is about healthy, sound hooves and happy horses.

Shoe Size

If you do opt to shoe your horse, there are other factors—in addition to the style of trim—that an owner should be aware of. One of these is ensuring that the shoe size being used is the right size for your horse. There are a number of factors your farrier must consider when choosing the correct shoe, including hoof shape and size, how much the hoof can be expected to grow between shoeings, and

Master Farrier Gene Ovnicek on
Shoeing Horses

"**M**ost people shoe horses just because they think that's what you need to do. However, I believe that as a general principle it is healthier for the equine foot to be barefoot, and that most horses could go barefoot if their owners were willing and able to make the commitment it takes for that to succeed. In reality, that just isn't going to happen, so that leaves us shoeing a lot of horses, and we end up with a lot of problems.

"But keep in mind that it's not the shoes necessarily that create the problem, but how they're applied. Shoes that create imbalance—meaning they artificially impose balance that is different than that of a healthy, naturally worn foot—cause the foot to become distorted. And, taking the frog off the ground is a major problem as it doesn't allow the foot to function optimally. When I shoe horses, the whole idea of that frog and that

foot next to the ground is of paramount importance and is never left out of anything I do, either for routine hoof care or as a treatment modality (fig. 14.31).

"To make that happen, the heels are trimmed routinely so that the frog is on the ground as adequately as it would be if the horse were barefoot. The frog makes that adjustment in a fairly decent way, and overall hoof health for horses shod in this manner can be very good. I don't think it's *as* good as being barefooted, but it does let us offer horse owners something that will allow their horses to be sound in the best possible way with shoes.

"Ultimately what matters most is the trim under the shoe, where the shoe is placed around the coffin bone, getting the frog on the ground, and getting the horse to land heel first—all these are the factors that contribute to the creation and maintenance of a sound, shod foot."

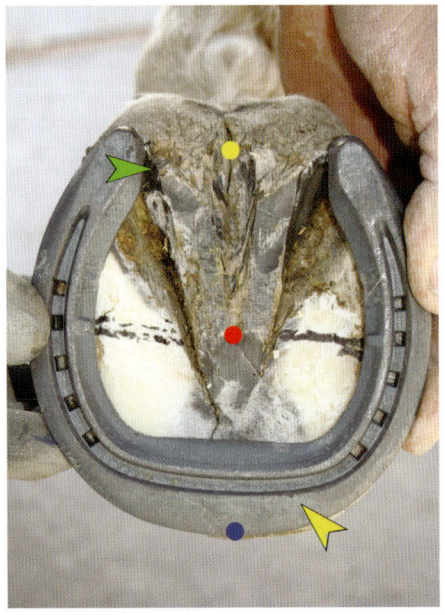

14.31 Gene Ovnicek considers Dr. Bowker's physiological trim principles to be of paramount importance for shod horses, as well as barefoot horses. Though hard to see from this solar view, the back of the frog (green arrow) of this shod foot makes contact with the ground, even with the shoe on. You can also see that this foot has good dorsopalmar balance, meaning there is about as much mass in the front of the foot (red dot to blue dot) as in the back of the foot (red dot to yellow dot). This indicates that the toe is nice and short, as a long toe is likely to stretch forward, creating more mass in the front of the foot than in the back. There is also a bevel in the shoe (yellow arrow), taking the place of the beveled edge Dr. Bowker recommends for a barefoot wall.

even the skill level of the rider, as horses ridden by well-balanced riders are less likely to interfere with their own shoes. Good farriers are aware of these considerations and take care to ensure a proper fit for every foot on every horse. Nonetheless, it is not uncommon to find horses with shoes that are not the right size for the feet they are on.

While it should be obvious to any professional that applying undersized shoes is a bad idea that can lead to contraction and other issues, it happens. When it does, you will see some or all of the hoof extending over the edge of the shoe. One practice, called "short-shoeing," involves a shoe that is not long enough for the foot (fig. 14.32). This may mean leaving the heels hanging over the back, or the front edge of the shoe may be set behind the toe.

While some farriers would have to concede that they have occasionally applied a too-small shoe simply because they didn't happen to have the right-sized shoe in their truck, there are other reasons why this might happen. Farriers may resort to short-shoeing the heels if they are attempting to keep a horse from pulling off his front shoes by stepping on them with his hind feet. Regardless of why it is done, short-shoeing can cause bruising, tearing of the laminae, and underrun and crushed heels, along with all the strain and damage to the internal and external structures that go along with these problems (fig. 14.33).

Short-shoeing the toes is sometimes done in an attempt to move the point of breakover back, especially in horses with long-toe/low-heel hoof conformation. When the toe is short-shod, farriers will also sometimes file down the lower portion of the front of the hoof wall to match the placement of the shoe, a process called "dubbing the toe." However, it

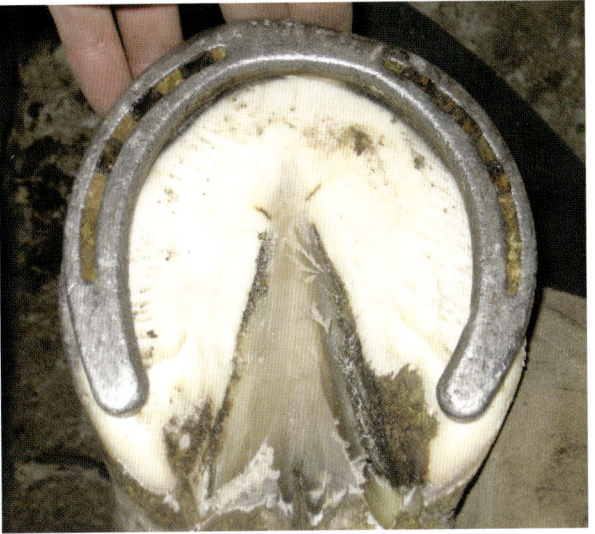

14.32 This ridiculously short shoe was removed from this foot. The farrier who removed it (not the same one who had put it on) then trimmed the foot to put on a correctly sized shoe. After deciding to take a photo, he held the shoe in place to show how wrongly fitted it was.

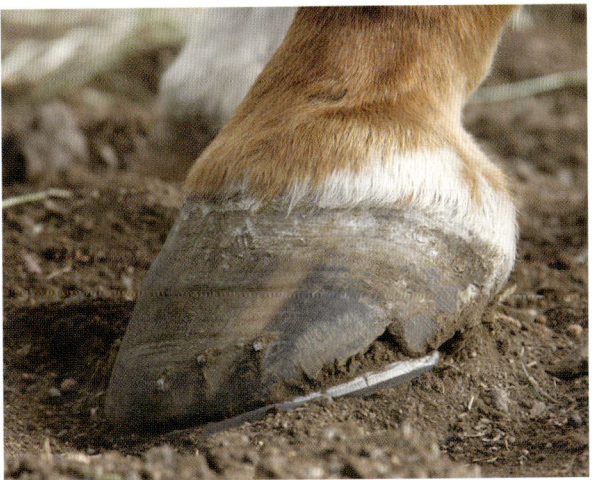

14.33 This horse's badly underrun heels and damaged quarters were likely caused, at least in part, by short-shoeing.

should be understood that both short-shoeing and dubbing the toe compromise the function of the strongest part of the hoof wall, which means that less strong parts—the quarters and the heels—have to pick up the slack. The resulting strain can lead to quarter cracks and flares, as well as bruised or crushed heels. For this reason, it is generally preferable to roll or rocker the toe of the shoe rather than short-shoe, or to use shoes specifically designed for this purpose that already have the rocker built in.

Just as undersized shoes can cause problems, shoes that are too big are also a potential source of harm. Not only does an oversized shoe make it more likely that the horse will hit himself or step on his own shoes, but it also changes the biomechanics of the foot. The size of the shoe plays a role in how the foot impacts the ground, how it loads, how much leverage it has to overcome before it lifts off the ground, how much torque is placed on the foot and the tissues of the lower limb, and more. The larger the shoe, the more it is going to alter the physics of the way the foot interacts with the ground.

A shoe can be too large in either length, width, or both. Shoes that are too long most often have the back of the shoe extending out behind the heels. This may be done in an attempt to "support" weak, underrun, or collapsed heels, or to move weight bearing farther back. What actually happens, in both

cases, is that the long shoe increases leverage and, therefore, increases pressure on the heels, making the situation worse in many ways, not better (fig. 14.34). And, you can't shift weight bearing back by extending the shoe behind the heel, as the heel itself is still the part that has to bear weight, and its position has not changed. Some of the problems that can result from long-shoeing the heels include bruising, collapsed heels, sheared heels, and damage to the internal structures in the back of the foot.

As for shoes being too wide, this is a bit of a tricky subject. It has long been thought that using a wide-webbed shoe or fitting a shoe a bit on the wide side was a good way to give the horse a strong base of support, but once again, there are consequences to altering how the foot travels in the air and how it interacts with the ground. The wider the shoe, the more the foot will be forced to tip side to side when the foot moves in any way other than perfectly straight forward. This lateral leverage, though it may be subtle, is now thought by some experts to be a factor in collateral ligament injuries and damage to the coffin joint. Think about how the hoof moves when a horse turns—rolling to one side or the other—and you will be able to see why making the shoe wider can place the bones and ligaments under unnatural strain.

How to Find (and Keep!) a Good Hoof-Care Provider

Finding a good hoof-care provider (HCP) can be a challenge. Many horse owners believe they are simply not knowledgeable enough to judge the work of a farrier or trimmer, and that is certainly true in a lot of cases (fig. 14.35). If you have ever felt that

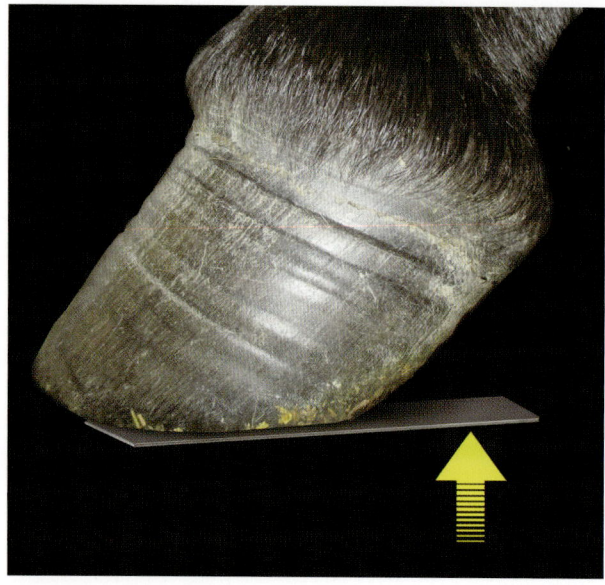

14.34 Imagine putting a metal bar under a horse's foot, then pulling up on the back of the bar to lift the heel. The leverage from your lifting would put a lot of pressure on the heel where the bar touches it. A long shoe sticking out behind the foot has a similar levering effect when the foot pushes down into the ground.

way, rest assured that if you have made it to this point in this book, you are now far more knowledgeable than most! Using this knowledge to look around at the feet of the horses in your area will be one of the best strategies you can employ if you are looking for a new HCP. When you see some feet that look strong, well-balanced, and healthy, find out who does those feet and give that person a call.

High on the list of other strategies that may be helpful in finding a new HCP is good ol' word of mouth. Ask other horse owners in your area about who they use, and if they are happy with that provider's work. Ask if their horse has ever had any hoof-related issues, and if so, what the provider did to correct the problem, and what the outcome was. If a lot of people are reporting that their horses are consistently sound and happy under a particular HCP's care, or that their horse used to have problems but is doing great with this provider, these are always good signs. You do have to keep in mind, however, that hoof problems may have nothing to do with the HCP, and that he sometimes gets blamed for things not his fault in any way. (Note: For grammar's sake, we are using the pronoun "he" when talking about HCPs, but we just want to acknowledge that there are many wonderful women HCPs out there, and they have our undying respect for doing a very tough job!)

When you do call a hoof-care provider, don't be afraid to *politely* ask questions. Understand that some longstanding professionals may take offense if it sounds as if you doubt their expertise, so how you

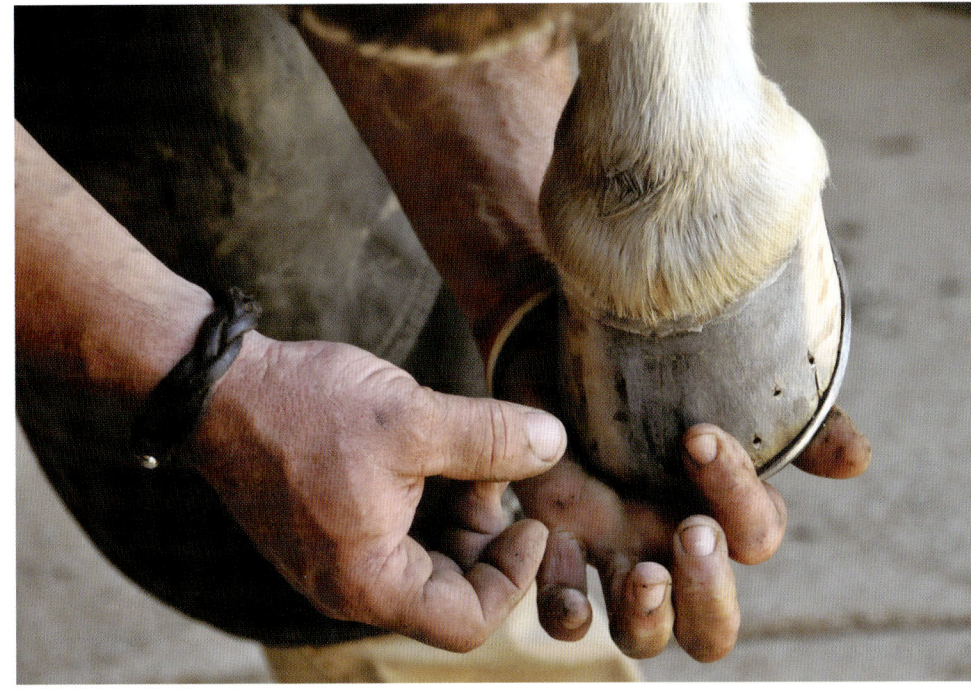

14.35 Good farriers are part artist, part scientist, which makes many horse owners feel inadequate to judge their work.

come across can make a difference. It can be helpful to lead with something like, "I've heard you are excellent, so I'd like to learn more about you—I hope you don't mind if I ask you a few questions." Then, find out if the HCP has any certifications or is a member of any organization, and what he does for continuing education. Does he attend conferences? Lectures or webinars? Read hoof-care journals or scientific papers? Find out how long he has been in the hoof-care profession, full or part time, and how he got his education. Some educational programs are just a week or two, and some are much more extensive. Ask if he might have client referrals you can contact. Inquire if he has worked with any veterinarians.

If the HCP bristles at your inquiries, this could be a sign that he would be difficult to work with should you ever have questions or concerns about your

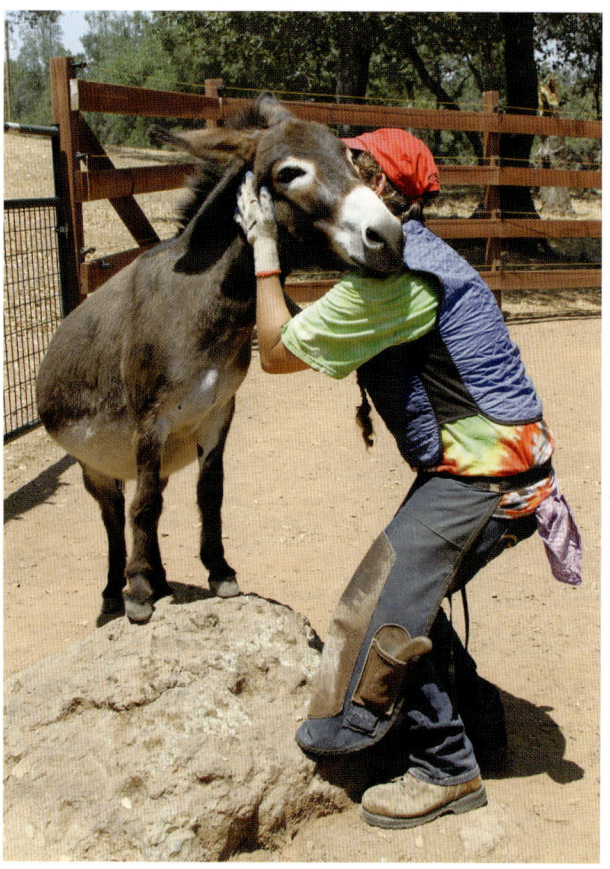

14.36 The best hoof-care providers truly love the animals in their care, and it shows!

issues or concerns. Observe how good he is at listening to you and answering your questions, as this will not only give you information about how well you will be able to work with him, but how well he, if needed, can work with a veterinarian.

Also note how he is with your horse. Some HCPs are great horsemen, but others are not. The best farriers tend to have a deep and abiding love for the animals they work with, and it will show in everything they do (fig. 14.36). An HCP doesn't necessarily have to be a horse whisperer to provide good hoof care, but if he is unreasonably harsh or impatient with your horse, that does not bode well.

That said, you, as the horse's owner, need to understand that it is your responsibility to ensure that your horse is safe and easy for the HCP to handle. It is not the job of the HCP to train your horse to behave while getting his hooves worked on, and when your horse won't keep still, pulls his feet away, kicks, flails, bites, or leans on the provider, the provider may not be willing to keep working on your horse. Trimming and shoeing horses is difficult, dangerous work, and poorly behaved horses increase the risk to an HCP exponentially. When you understand that one bad move from your horse could literally cost your HCP his career (or his life), you will get why you need to take this aspect of training very seriously.

To gauge whether or not your horse is "farrier-friendly," try holding up each one of your horse's feet for a length of time, like the HCP would have to do. If your horse is jerking around or leaning on you, you will quickly feel why farriers don't want to work on horses like that. What looks like a little yank from the horse can actually have profound repercussions on the HCP's body. If you don't know how

horse's feet in the future. And, if you run into the "I've been doing this for 20 years so I know what I'm doing" type, don't let that sway you. Just because someone has been doing something for a long time doesn't mean he's been doing it well, and there are unfortunately plenty of HCPs out there who make a living despite having less than optimal knowledge and skills.

If you like what you are hearing when you talk to a new HCP, offer to pay for a consultation so that the provider can come to your barn, take a look at your horse's feet, give an evaluation, and suggest how he would take care of the horse's feet and any to train your horse to behave well for the HCP, it is well worth the money to work with a professional trainer and get the job done (fig. 14.37). Your horse cannot get the best care if his feet won't keep still, and you may have trouble keeping a good HCP if your horse is a problem.

In addition to training your horse, there are other things you can do to make the HCP's job as easy as possible and encourage him to want to keep you as a client:

• *Put the cell phone away and pay attention to your horse!* The owner is the farrier's first line of safety, and distracted horse handling can result in farrier injuries (fig. 14.38). Hoof-care appointments are not the time to catch up on emails, phone calls, texts, or Facebook. This is a very common complaint you will hear from HCPs.

• Have a clean, covered, and well-lit area for your professional to work in. Working in deep muck, exposed to the elements, or in poor lighting does not help him do his best work. Muck, mud, and rain also damages tools, in addition to making the HCP unhappy.

• If flies are abundant, put fly spray on your horse so he doesn't yank the HCP around because the bugs are annoying him.

• Clean and dry your horse off as best you can before the HCP arrives, especially his feet and legs. The provider has to get up close and personal with

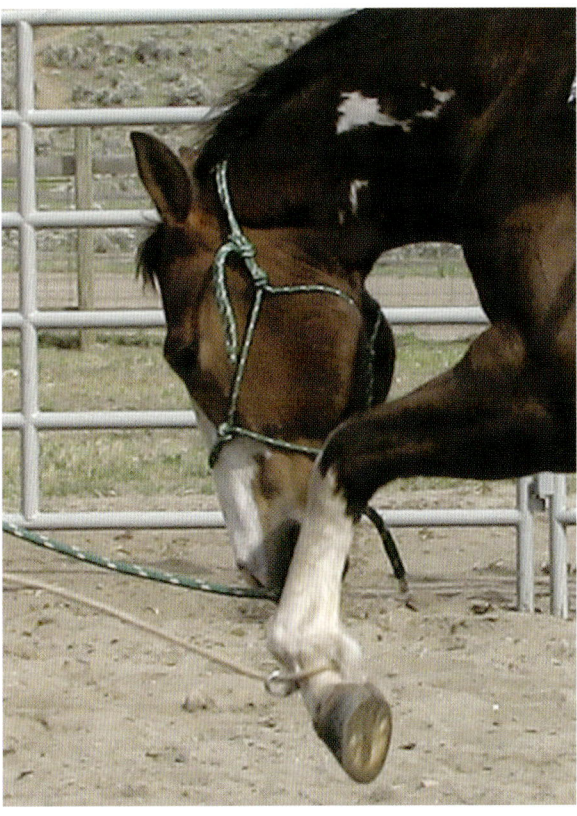

14.37 This young horse is learning to be tolerant and calm while his feet are being handled, an extremely important aspect of training.

14.38 This woman is putting her farrier at risk by talking on the phone and clearly not paying attention to her horse-handling duties. The loose dogs are a potential disaster waiting to happen, as well.

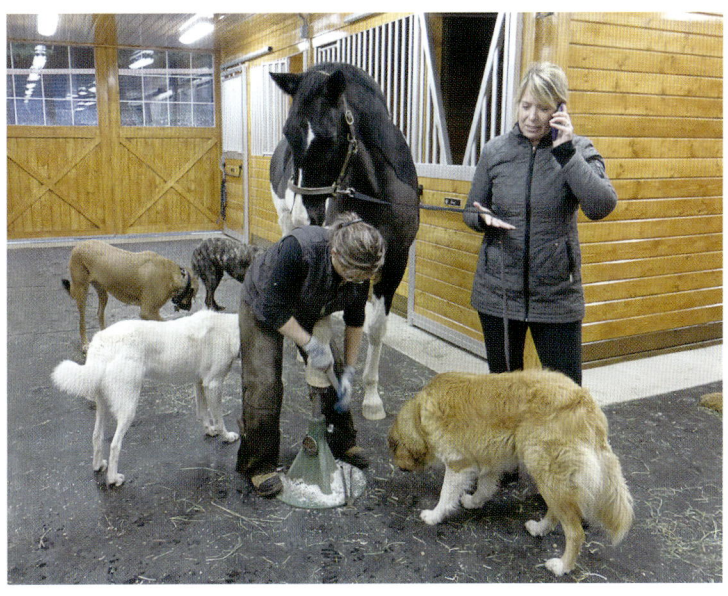

14.39 It is your job, not your hoof-care provider's, to get feet like these clean—and it is best to do this before the HCP arrives.

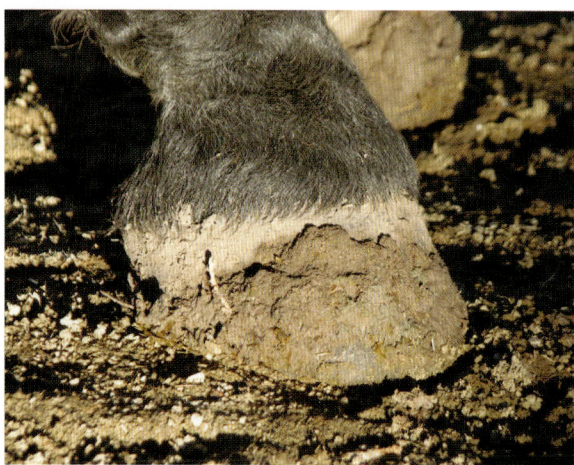

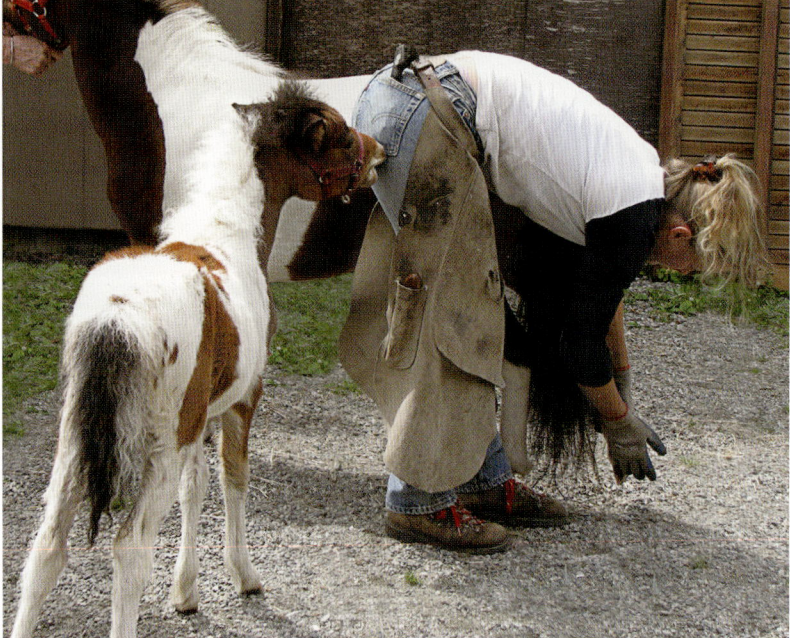

14.40 This hoof-care provider is about to get goosed, a distraction that could cause an accident. While not likely to be a disaster with wee horses like these, a situation like this could become deadly serious in an instant with a larger animal.

your horse to work on him, and he will not appreciate it when your horse is covered with grime and slime. Dirty feet also dull the HCP's tools, which doesn't thrill him either (fig. 14.39).

• Have your horse caught, clean, and ready by the time your HCP arrives. The moment he pulls up is not the time to head out into the 60-acre field to fetch your hard-to-catch horse.

• The work area should be quiet and free of children, roaming dogs, and other animals that might get underfoot or cause a distraction, either of which can create a dangerous situation (fig. 14.40).

• Pay your provider promptly. HCPs don't like hunting down payment from clients any more than do electricians or plumbers.

• Ask what trimming/shoeing schedule he recommends for your horse, and stick to it. Some horse's feet grow so fast that they need to be trimmed/shod every 4 weeks for optimal care, while others grow more slowly and do well on an 8-week cycle. Get feedback from your HCP on what is best for your particular situation. Realize that if you extend the cycle longer than what is suggested, the overgrowth may cause chipping, splitting, flaring, and other problems that might otherwise not happen. The HCP can't bring out the best in your horse's feet if he is not able to work on them at optimal time intervals.

There is an expression, "The best customers get the best service." If you want good hoof care for your horse, the provider needs to be a quality professional, and if you as the client are a considerate customer, you'll be likely have a long and beneficial relationship with your HCP.

Going Barefoot

"This whole barefoot movement is the most important thing that has ever happened in the horse industry. It has had widespread effects, even among farriers who use shoes, as it has forced them to look more closely at their work, and with more depth. We have learned so much from studying the bare foot and how it functions, and so much of this is applicable and beneficial to shod horses as well." —Master Farrier Gene Ovnicek

More and more horse owners are choosing to maintain their horses without shoes these days, for various reasons. Some are attracted by the fact that it is less expensive, others are comforted knowing they will never lose another shoe, and some feel safer with the increased surefootedness of a barefoot horse (fig. 15.1). But for most, the main reason to "go bare" is that they believe there are substantial health benefits, not just for the hooves, but for the entire horse.

Many experts agree about "going bare," and the work of scientists like Dr. Bowker certainly seems to support their assertions. Even Dr. Stephen O'Grady, a leading equine podiatrist who in the past was not seen as being particularly "barefoot friendly," has actually published an article in the *American Farrier's Journal* in which he states, "The equine foot with healthy structures is superior in its natural or barefoot state as opposed to the shod state with regards to accepting the weight of the horse, shock

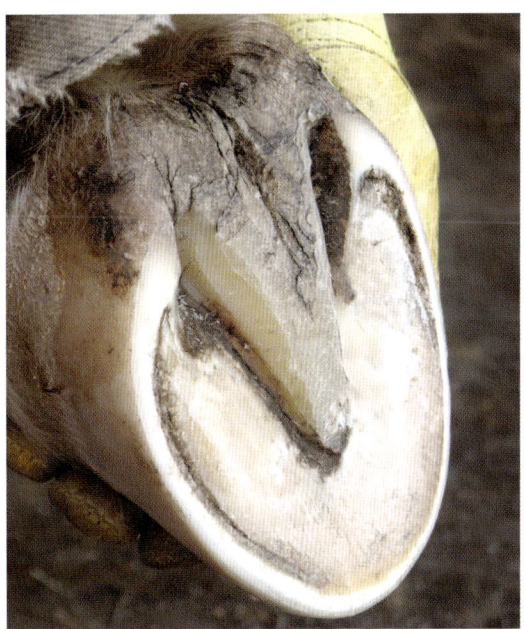

15.1 Owners of barefoot horses often report feeling safer due to the fact that bare feet have such excellent traction. If you compare the textures of the wall and frog to that of a steel shoe, then couple that with the natural flexion of a bare hoof, you will understand why the barefoot horse feels so able to grip.

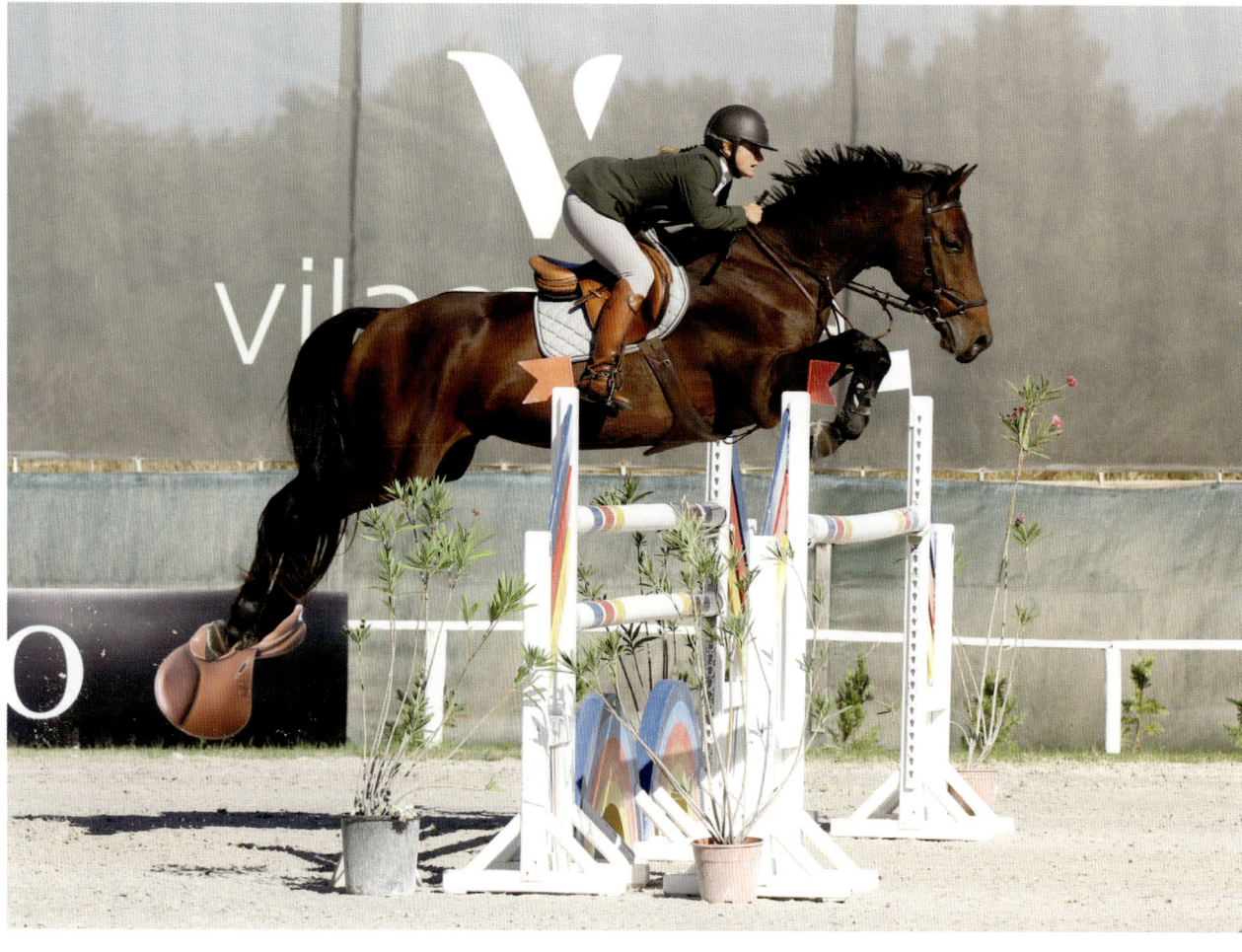

15.2 Sandra Gaspar Carreira loves the fact that her horses' feet are so much healthier now that they are barefoot, but she is also strongly motivated by the fact that they simply jump better without shoes.

absorption and dissipating the energy of impact."

However, there is still a perception among many in the horse world that barefoot only works if you don't actually *do* much with your horse. Nothing could be further from the truth, as witnessed by the continually growing number of riders in disciplines ranging from endurance to eventing, from Western performance to dressage, at levels from pleasure riders to Olympic competitors, who are discovering that not only *can* their horses do what they do

barefoot, they can do it *better*, and they are sounder than ever.

Those who doubt that barefoot horses can be serious performance horses should talk to British Olympian Emma Hindle, who has found that her dressage horses are not only sounder but move more correctly barefoot, in part, she believes, because they can feel the ground better. They might also want to chat with Grand Prix showjumper Sandra Gaspar Carreira (fig. 15.2), who has been so successful with her barefoot jumpers that many other international competitors—including several Olympians—are now bringing her their horses to get them on a barefoot program. Carreira says that for her, the bottom line is results, and as she sees more clear rounds and healthier feet now that her horses are barefoot, she is convinced that this is the best way for a horse to compete.

The Western sports are also seeing a rise in barefoot competitors, in part due to the success of people like two-time Women's Professional Rodeo Association (WRPA) World Champion barrel racer Leslie Maynard (fig. 15.3), who says, "I love competing on barefoot horses—they just feel so confident on the ground." Previously the last person to ever think barrel horses could be successful barefoot, she has found that they actually have excellent traction, even in muddy conditions, and she has been able to rehabilitate several barrel horses that were considered "lost causes," bringing them back to success in the arena using barefoot methods.

Then there is the Houston Police Mounted Patrol Unit that ended up taking their entire squadron of hard-working horses barefoot after one of their best mounts, who had been diagnosed with navicular disease and was failing to improve with therapeutic shoeing, was able to return to active duty after they decided to try barefoot trimming as a last ditch effort. The squad now reports that since they made the switch to barefoot, they have far fewer problems with lameness, fewer injuries, and that the incidence of general illness has decreased as well—a "side effect" they were not expecting (figs. 15.4 A & B).

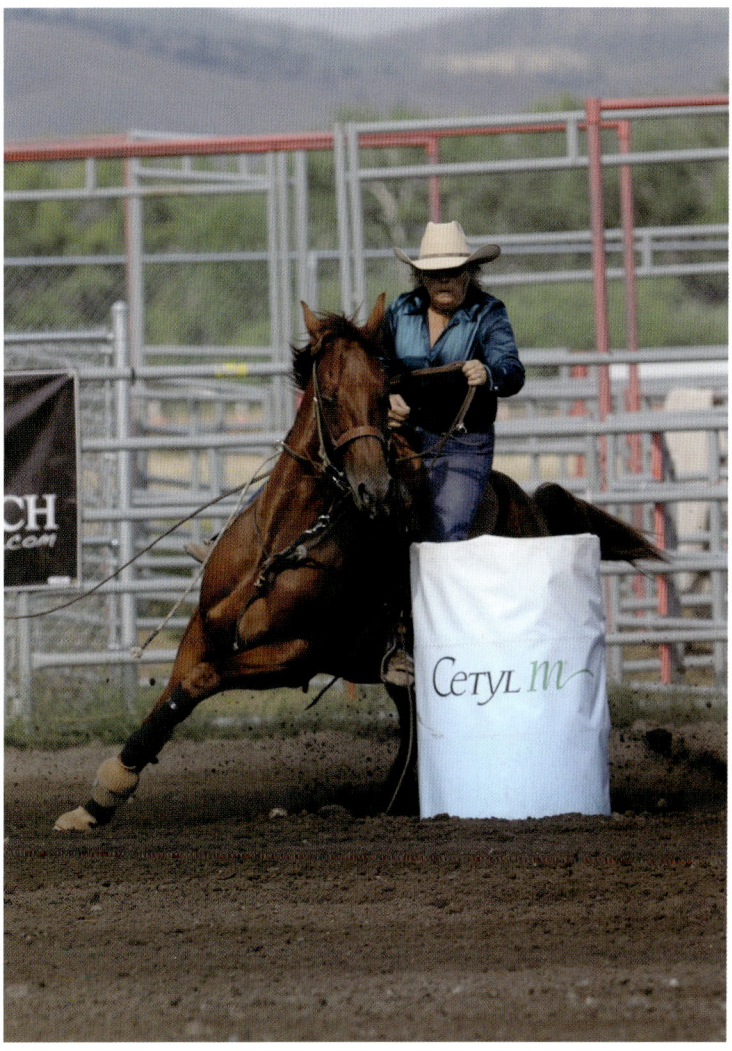

15.3 Leslie Maynard competing on her barrel racer LRM Rockstar George, who was third in the 2011 WPRA World Champion 1D Futurity Standings and who won the 2011 WPRA World Champion 2D Futurity Title.

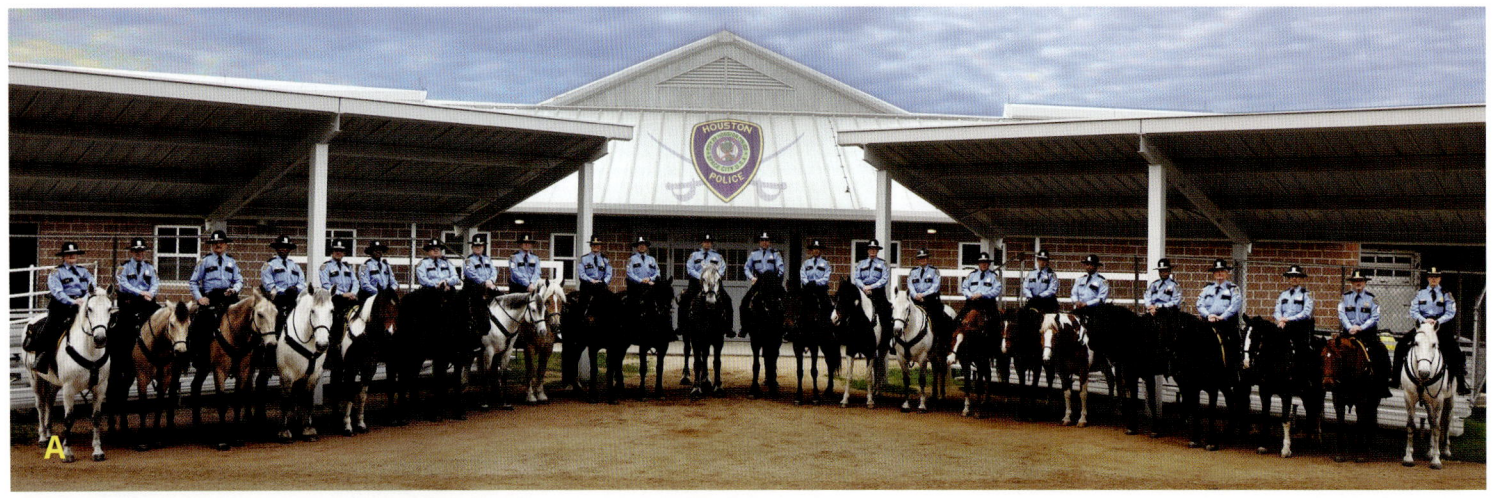

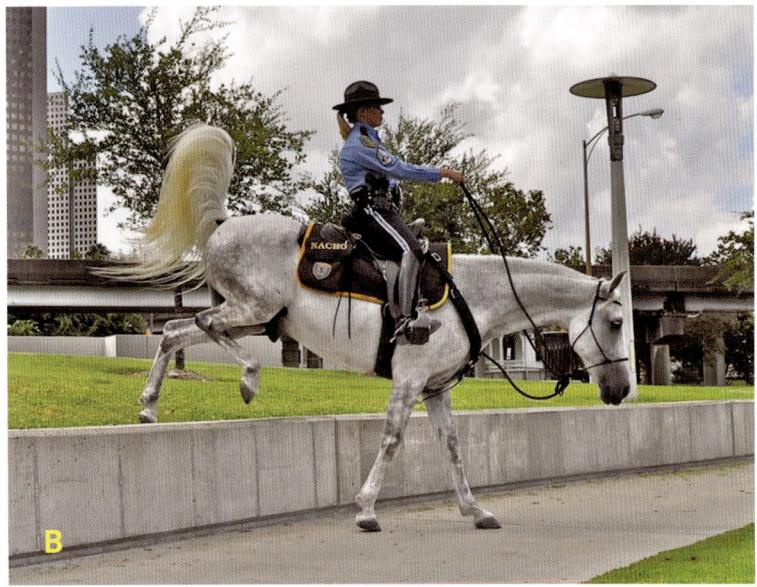

15.4 A & B After discovering the benefits of barefoot hoof care through an experiment on one horse, the Houston Mounted Police Unit decided to take the entire squad barefoot (A). The results have been extremely positive, as the horses now experience far fewer hoof problems and better overall health. Another benefit the Houston Mounted Police enjoy because their horses are now barefoot is improved traction and performance on a variety of surfaces. You would never want to do what you see in B with a horse wearing metal shoes, as the horse would almost certainly slip on the concrete. (Authors' note: Although not relevant to hooves, we would like to say that we are also impressed by this officer's good hands that allow her horse complete freedom of movement, and the fact that she is doing all of this in just a rope bridle. Beautiful horsemanship, trust, and connection.)

However, if you are considering making the switch from shod to barefoot, it is important to know that the process is often more involved than simply pulling the shoes and riding off on your merry way. While it is certainly possible for the vast majority of horses to make the change to barefoot, the transition is much more likely to be smooth and successful if you know what to expect, what you need to do, and how to make it all happen. You need to understand that it can take time and commitment, and you must consider the various factors that will have an effect on whether the transition goes well or not. As a starting point, it may help to ask yourself the following questions:

1 *How healthy are my horse's feet?*

If your horse has thin soles, a damaged coffin bone, weak digital cushions, contracted heels, or other significant concerns, going barefoot is likely to take more time, effort, and knowledge than it would for a horse whose feet are relatively healthy (fig.15.5). This is not to say that if your shod horse has hoof problems you shouldn't try going barefoot—many would

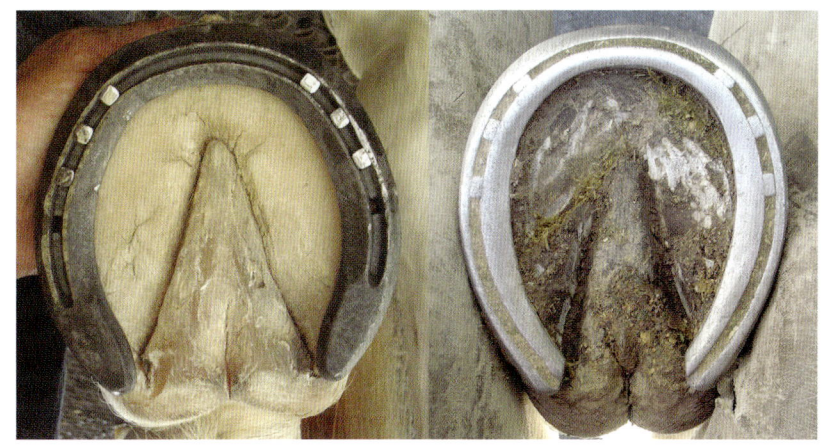

15.5 The healthy foot on left, with its broad, strong heels, and robust frog, would probably have little trouble making the transition to barefoot. The contracted foot on the right will have weak interior as well as exterior structures, so it is likely to need more time to adjust.

say that the fact that your horse has hoof problems is the very reason you *should* try barefoot. You do need to be aware, however, that a foot with preexisting challenges may require more attention and patience to make the switch, so just be ready for it.

2 *Am I willing to make use of hoof boots?*

Many horses, especially if they have been shod for a long time or have compromised feet, are going to need some support in the form of boots and possibly pads for a while after the shoes come off. Padded hoof boots have been shown to make a huge difference during the transition period, allowing the foot to remain comfortable while it develops and strengthens. How long the boots will be needed is completely individual. Some horses will need them for a brief period and only while being ridden, while others will need 24/7 protection for a very long time. Some horses will eventually become true all-terrain dynamos, while others may always need boots to ride out on rough ground, especially if they live on softer footing (fig. 15.6). The bottom line is that the worse off your horse's feet are before you pull the shoes, the longer it is likely to take before you can dispense with boots, and the more attentive you will need to be to ensure that the horse is comfortable during the transition.

But for hoof boots to work, you have to be willing and able to use them, as boots do require a bit of time and effort from the horse owner. If your

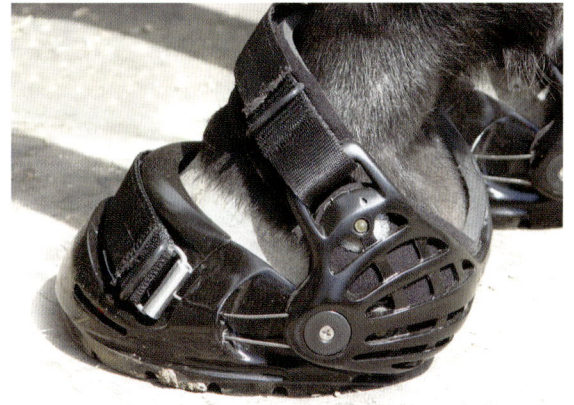

15.6 This previously foundered Morgan gelding does very well barefoot in most terrain, but as he has metabolic challenges that make it difficult for him to grow a thick sole, he is more comfortable in boots when ridden on rocky ground. Boots by Renegade®.

horse only needs boots for riding, they will add a couple of minutes to your prep time before each ride. If the horse needs them on for longer periods, you will have to check and clean them regularly to make sure they aren't rubbing or becoming unsanitary. There is also the consideration that for some people, dealing with hoof boots can be physically uncomfortable. If you have trouble bending or your hands are weak or painful, you may find putting boots on and pulling them off to be less than pleasant.

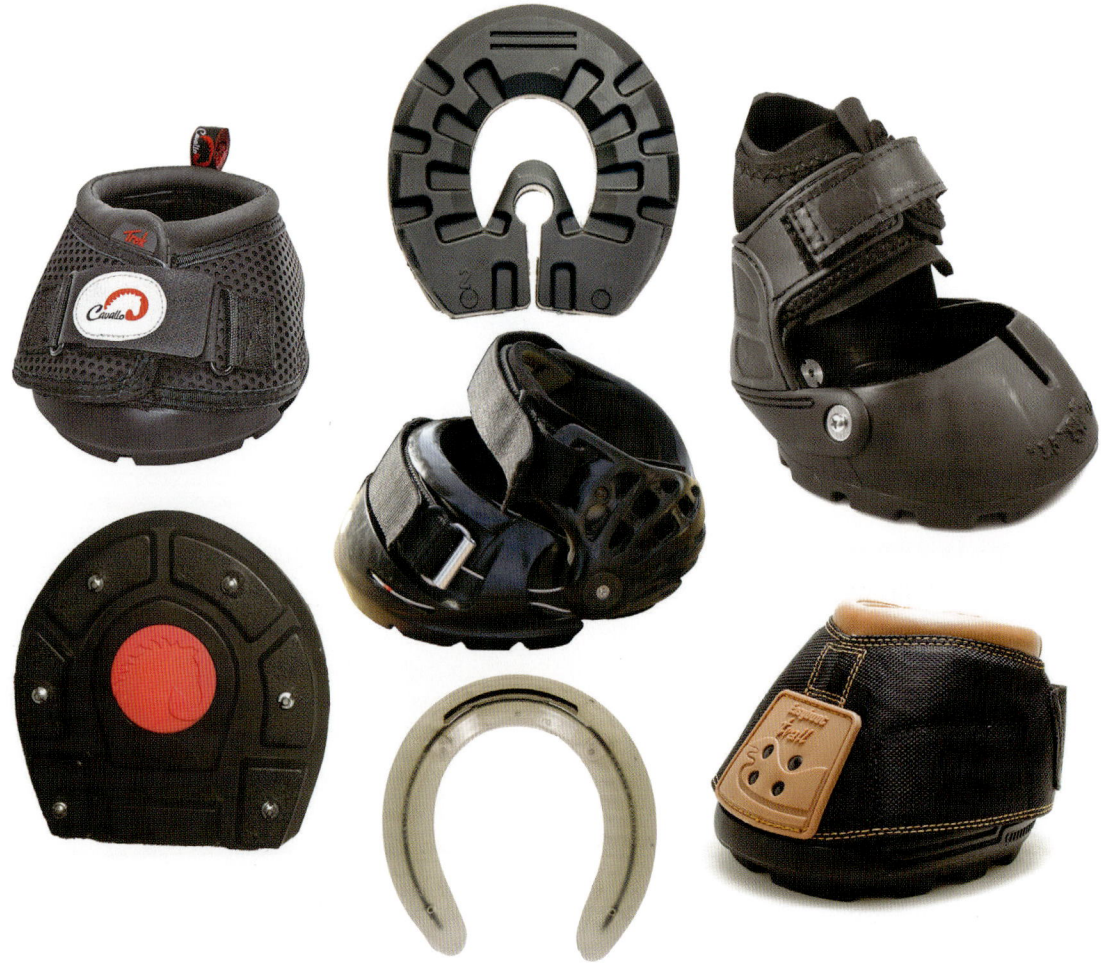

15.7 The explosion of interest in barefoot hoof care has prompted the development of an ever-expanding variety of boots and flexible shoes to suit many different needs.

Fortunately, there are so many different kinds of hoof boots on the market that most people can find something to work with. The variety of boots available, in terms of both styling and technology, has increased dramatically in recent years, and new boots are coming out on a regular basis (fig. 15.7). However, this abundance of choice can make selecting the best boot for your horse more complicated than simply looking for what is popular or what has the best price. Some boots are better than others for different disciplines, and some boots fit different hoof shapes better than others. Some boots are easier to put on and take off, and others perform better in specific types of terrain or are made to accommodate studs.

There are also many kinds of flexible shoes and cuffs, some of which are designed to be glued on and some that can be nailed. They offer a sort of middle ground between being shod and barefoot that some horses find very comfortable and which some owners find easier than dealing with boots. Because there is so much selection, it is an excellent idea to consult someone experienced in booting to help make the best choice for you and your horse.

3 *Is the terrain my horse lives on similar to what I want him to work on?*

In general, a horse that lives on footing similar to what he is expected to work on is going to have an easier time going barefoot. For example, a horse that lives in a soft environment or a stall is not going to have the toughest feet, but if he only gets ridden in a cushy, well-groomed arena, he may be able to sail from shod to barefoot with no boots and no difficulty, especially if his feet are healthy to start with. But take that same horse and expect him to go out and blast down rock-strewn trails every weekend, and he is probably going to need boots for those rides, possibly indefinitely (fig. 15.8). The feet of horses that live on forgiving terrain simply don't have the chance to get conditioned to hard and rocky surfaces, so you must have realistic expectations about what they are going to be capable of doing.

Even if horses do live on a firm, rocky surface, the extra weight we put on them can sometimes make a difference in how comfortable they are being ridden on demanding terrain. They may be perfectly sound carrying just their own weight, but add 200 pounds of rider and tack, and suddenly feet that are accustomed to carrying around 1,000 pounds are now carrying 1,200 pounds—a significant increase that can push some horses out of their comfort zone. Still, your best bet for creating rock-munching hooves is to turn your horse out in

as large an area as possible on firm ground that has some areas of rock or gravel. The size of the enclosure definitely makes a difference, as the more a horse moves, the stronger his feet are likely to become. Stalling horses or keeping them in small paddocks minimizes how much they can move, and, therefore, how much progress their feet can make.

4 *Is my hoof-care provider truly knowledgeable about barefoot trimming and hoof care?*

One of the most important factors, and one that can make or break your chances at barefoot success, is how much your hoof-care provider knows about barefoot hoof care. There are specific ways to trim the hoof to maximize barefoot comfort and

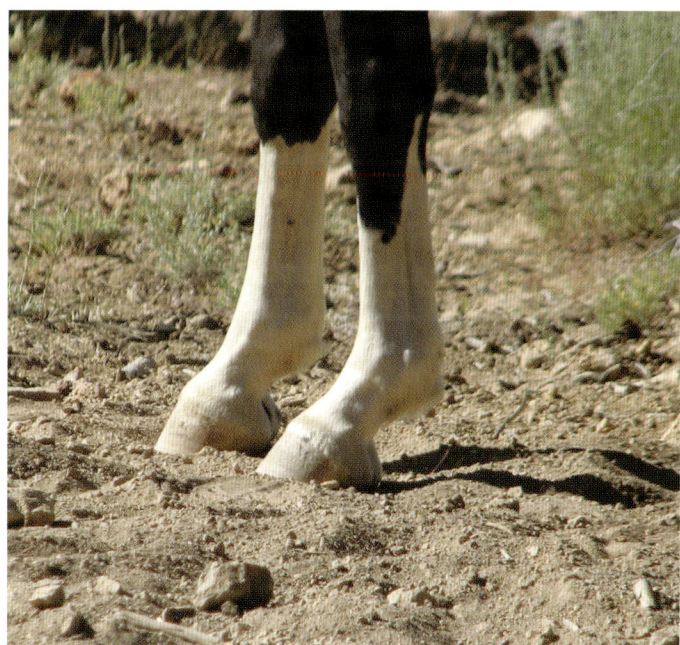

15.8 If you expect your horse to carry you over terrain like this, he will need well-conditioned feet used to dealing with rocks and uneven surfaces.

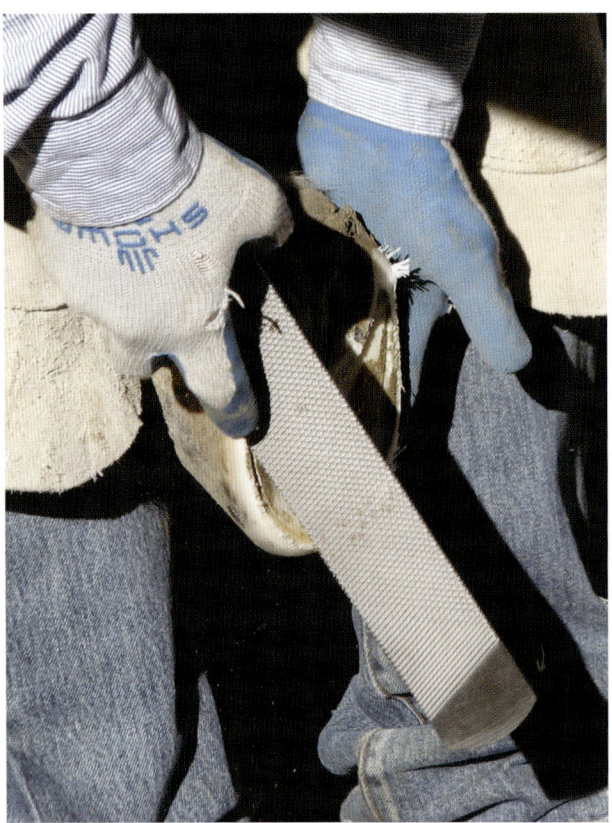

15.9 Whether they are barefoot specialists or farriers who also shoe horses, hoof-care providers who do the best work on barefoot horses understand the specific trimming requirements that allow barefoot horses to perform at their best.

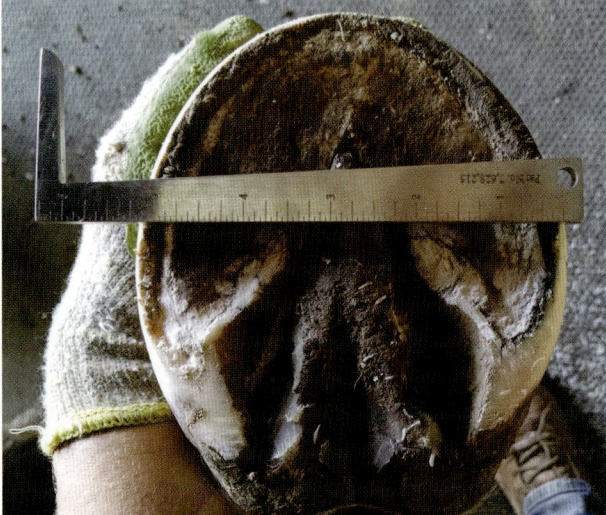

15.10 This foot is being measured for boots, but if a hoof-care provider starts taking various measurements and tells you that your horse's feet need to conform to specific angles, that is a clue that his methods may not be the best for your horse.

function, and these are often quite different from what is taught to many farriers (fig. 15.9). Barefoot specialist Pete Ramey, who started out as a farrier shoeing horses, tells a story about his early days, when he "proved" to himself that "barefoot doesn't work" by trimming a bunch of horses the traditional way he was taught and leaving their shoes off. The horses invariably got sore, so he put them back in shoes and thought that was that. Later on, however, Ramey met someone who taught him techniques

specific to barefoot trimming, and he discovered that these techniques made all the difference. This time, the horses did not get sore, and in fact, they were sounder and could work harder than they had when they were shod.

Your choice of trimmer can make all the difference for your horse, too, both short- and long-term. If you have the option to use someone who specializes in barefoot trimming, this may be a good bet. However, just as in everything else in life, not every barefoot trimmer is a good one. There are certainly some wonderful trimmers with the skills and understanding to help horses transition to barefoot successfully, but there are also some who should have their tools ripped from their hands and locked away where they will never find them. The saddest part is that many who fall into the latter category are very nice, well-meaning people who have simply been taught bad techniques.

So, how can you, as the horse owner, tell the difference? One dead giveaway is the trimmer's approach to the sole. As you learned earlier, paring into the live sole is almost always a big no-no and is very likely to make your horse sore and leave him vulnerable to bruising and abscesses. Trimmers who use such invasive techniques on the sole (and often on the bars, as well) will often say that soreness and abscessing are a "normal part of the healing process" as the foot recovers from the damage caused by shoes and "cleanses itself of toxins," but this is an absolute falsehood. Add to that the fact that aggressive trimming is often at least a contributing factor, and sometimes the direct cause, of the coffin bone penetrating through the sole, and you will understand why you really don't want such a trimmer working on your horse.

Another red flag is when trimmers have the idea that all feet should have the same specific angles, regardless of hoof conformation, current or past pathology, or how those angles relate to the rest of the limb. Such trimmers may carry around a collection of measuring devices to help them see what they need to do to force a horse's feet to conform to their preconceived ideals (fig. 15.10). A good trimmer, on the other hand, will assess a horse's feet based on the unique characteristics and challenges present in each individual foot, and then come up with a plan to help each foot get as close to *its own ideal* as possible.

It should also be noted that there are plenty of "regular" farriers out there who do a very good job working with barefoot horses. If you are trying to assess whether that might be the case with a farrier you know, ask him what his take is on barefoot hoof care, and whether or not he has many sound, actively ridden barefoot horses among his clientele. If you start hearing talk along the lines of, "Sure, I trim some barefoot horses, but they are pretty much pasture pets," or "Really, horses need shoes if you expect them to work," he is probably not the right person for the job.

Ultimately, judging the work of any hoof-care provider is very much a the-proof-is-in-the-pudding sort of situation. If your horse's feet are making good progress under your HCP's care, you can feel confident that he knows what he is doing. If progress is slow or nonexistent, it may or may not be the HCP's fault, depending on what is going on with the feet. However, if your HCP is consistently making your horse sore every time he works on his feet, or the feet are morphing in the wrong direction as a result of his techniques, *this is not okay*, and you may want to seriously consider switching to another professional.

5 *Is my horse's diet going to impede the transition to barefoot?*

Bare hooves are very honest, as there is nothing covering them to dull down or hide their problems. This is especially evident when it comes to diets that are too high in non-structural carbohydrates. When a horse is eating excessive amounts of sugar and/or starch, his body will experience low-grade inflammation that can easily cause foot soreness. Since a formerly shod barefoot horse is likely to have increased feeling in his feet due to improved perfusion, he is more likely to notice the effects of carb-related inflammation than he would have

15.11 Many people don't realize that carrots contain a fair amount of sugar, about half the amount found in apples. While this is a not a problem for most horses, it could contribute to foot soreness in sensitive individuals, especially if carrots are fed in significant amounts.

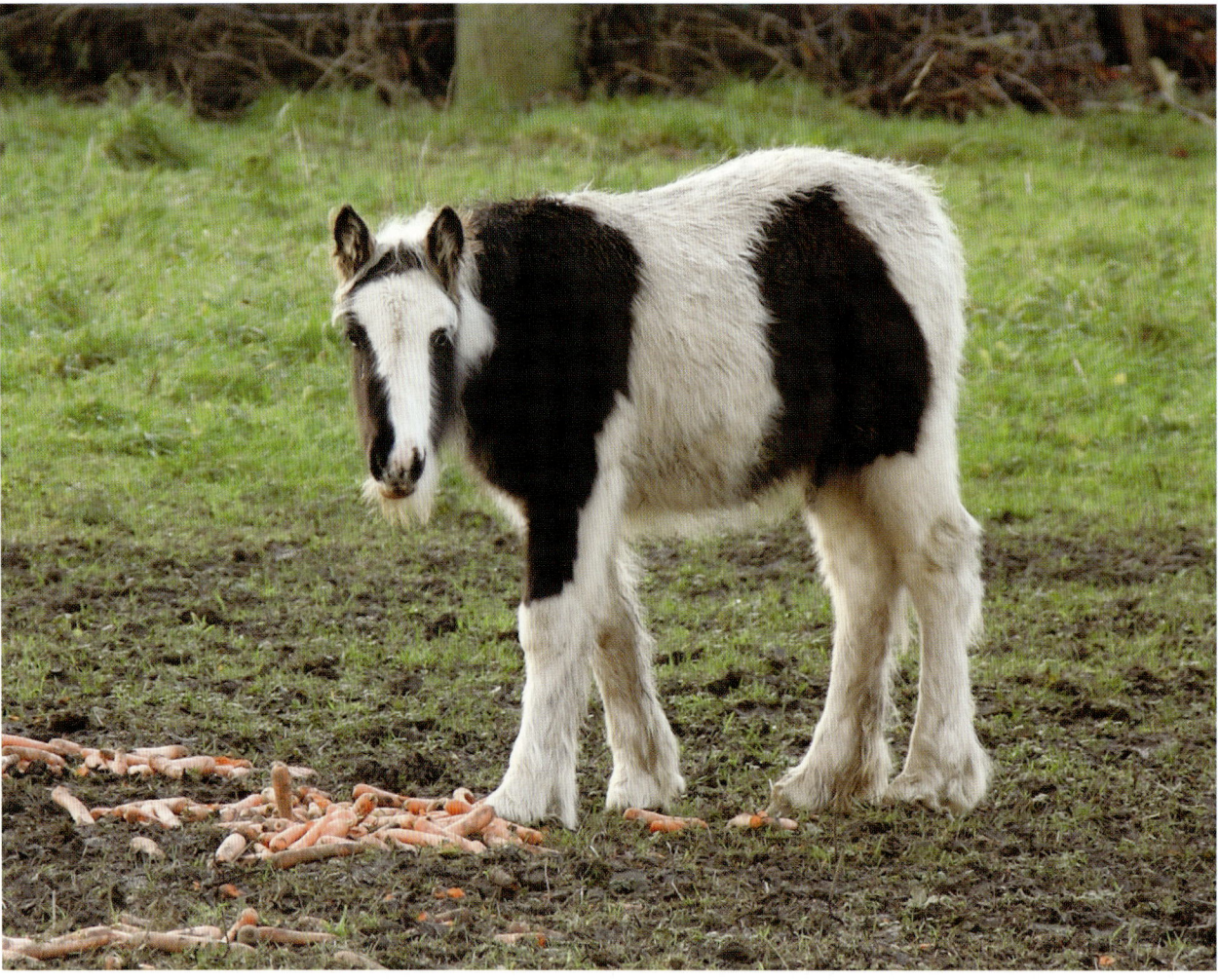

when he was in shoes. If this makes you think that maybe you should just go back to shoes so that your horse doesn't get sore like that, think again: Shoeing does not prevent inflammation—it just makes it so your horse can't feel it as easily, which means that all kinds of damage could be taking place and you wouldn't know a thing about it.

So, if your seasoned barefoot horse suddenly gets tender when turned out on grass, there's a

good chance that the sugars in the grass are not agreeing with his feet. Or, if your new-to-barefoot horse has reasonably good feet but isn't getting over being very tender after coming out of shoes, take a thorough look at what is going in his mouth to ensure there are no dietary triggers that may be perpetuating the tenderness (fig. 15.11). In addition, pay attention to anything else going into the horse's body, such as supplements, vaccines, medications, injections, and dewormers, as all of these can cause tender feet in some horses.

6 *Do I have the time to let my horse adjust?*

Even if a horse has fairly good feet, there may be an adjustment period while he gets used to being barefoot after being shod for an extended period. The foot will function a bit differently, the frog and soles may need to thicken up, and the horse may need to get used to feeling the ground in a new way. Sometimes this transition is almost instantaneous, but it can take weeks, months, or even longer when a horse has foot issues. Therefore, if you want to make the transition to barefoot, it is wise to plan for some possible down time while your horse's feet are toughening up. Don't pull the shoes the week before a big show or the day before a grueling trail ride, as this will just set you up for failure. For most people, it is easiest to start transitioning a horse to barefoot during the off season, when riding would already be at a minimum. The horse can then adjust without the pressures of competition schedules, heavy training, and so on.

One last note: When you start looking into the idea of going barefoot, you will undoubtedly hear stories from people who tried to take their horses barefoot but found that "it just didn't work." Take such stories with a grain of salt, as it is very easy to create a barefoot failure if you are not aware of all the components that go into creating a barefoot success, or if you don't have a trimmer with the right skill set. That said, there are a few horses out there that, for whatever reasons, are never able to adjust to being barefoot, even with the very best and most comprehensive care. So if you have made all the necessary lifestyle changes and tried every option at your disposal, but your horse is still sore without his shoes, do what you need to do to get him comfortable. If this means putting the shoes back on, that is okay. Barefoot is not for everyone, and ultimately, keeping your horse as sound and comfortable as he can be is what matters most.

16

A Few Notes on Mules, Donkeys, Minis, and Drafts

Some of our equine friends have feet that are a bit different than the typical horse due to their natural size or shape. Donkeys, mules, drafts, and Miniature Horses all fall into this category, and there are a few points that merit consideration when dealing with their hoof care.

Mules

Mules tend to have good, strong feet that are a little more on the upright side than the typical horse, but as mules are a cross between a donkey and a horse, their feet can resemble either one or be somewhere in between (figs. 16.1 A–C). A good rule of thumb

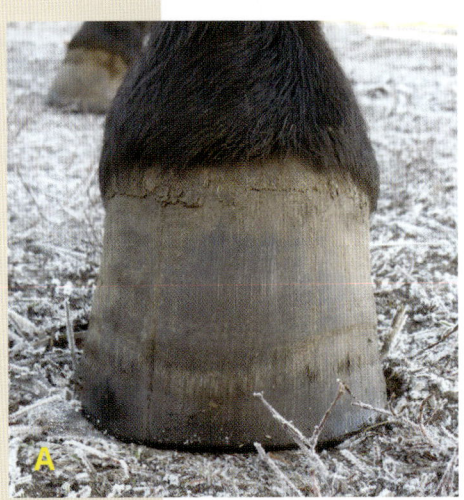 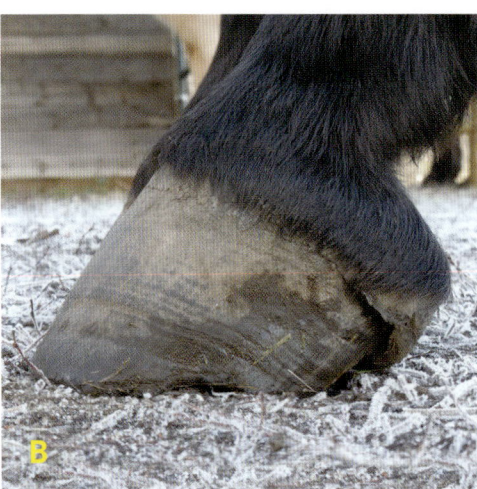 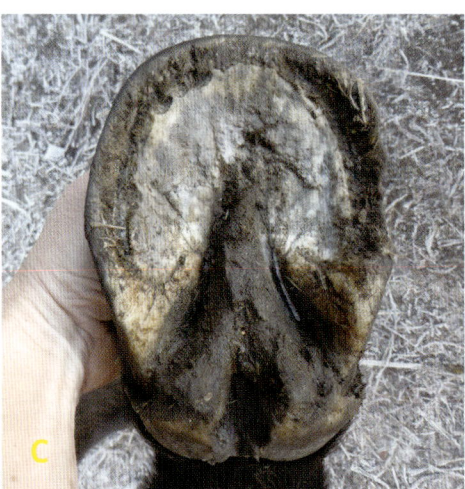

16.1 A-C This mule, like most of his kind, has solid strong feet whose shape are somewhere between a horse and a donkey. The front view of his hoof shows that his foot is a little less "cone shaped" than a typical horse, but not quite as upright as a donkey (A). In the side view, you can see the strong heel conformation that is part of what makes mule feet so tough (B). And the solar view really shows this animal's hybrid nature, as you see a horse-like frog paired with an oval (rather than round) foot shape (C).

for mules is to treat their feet according to which side of their parentage they most resemble. If the feet look horse-like, you can expect them to have the same needs as a horse's would. If, however, they are fairly donkey-like, they may have some different requirements (see below).

Donkeys

Donkeys' feet differ from horses' feet in quite a few ways:

Walls
• The wall is uniformly thick all the way around the hoof, whereas a horse has a thicker wall in the toe region.

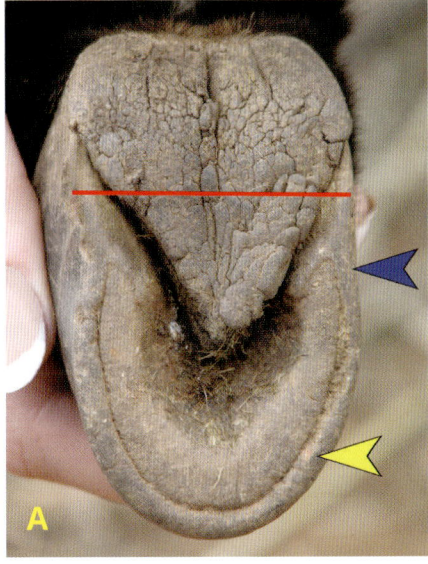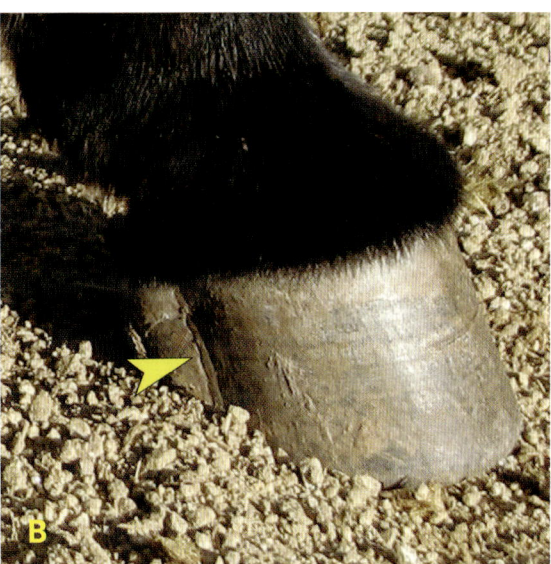

16.2 A & B This Miniature Donkey's foot shows a number of common characteristics (A): the relatively thick wall is of uniform thickness all around the foot (yellow arrow); the quarters pinch in slightly in front of the heels (blue arrow), though this can be more marked in some donkeys; the sole is U-shaped; the frog is wide and pie-shaped and extends well past the heel buttresses (back of buttresses marked by red line). The lateral view clearly shows the inward "pinch" of the quarters quite common in donkeys' feet (B).

• Overall, the walls are very thick relative to their size, and they don't break off easily, even when overgrown. As a result, a donkey's overgrown hoof can take on a variety of long, distorted shapes.

• The hoof wall in the quarters often has a slight inward bend or "pinch" with a corresponding flared shape to the heels.

• Heel buttresses are closer together than on a horse (figs. 16.2 A & B).

Sole
• Donkeys' soles are U-shaped, not round like a horse's and they often have a high degree of concavity.

• Their soles grow nearly as much as the walls and can grow overly thick if they don't get lots of movement on abrasive ground or don't get trimmed often enough. The soles, therefore, may need some paring down at times, which is almost never the case with a horse (fig. 16.3).

Frog
• The frog on a donkey is a big, pie-shaped, flattened wedge, angling sharply out from the apex to the heels.

• Normally in donkey feet, the frog goes just halfway toward the toe on the bottom of the hoof, but it extends well past the back of the heel buttresses (see fig. 16.2 A).

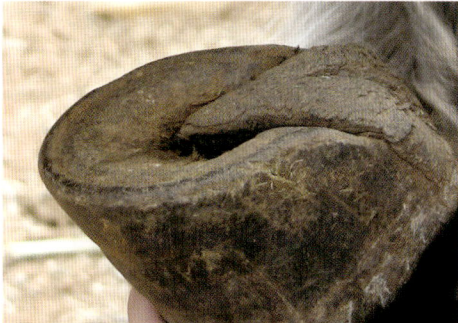

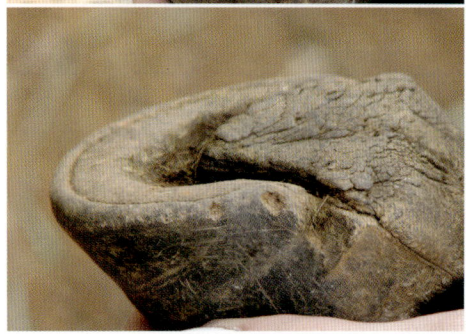

16.3 The soles on donkeys' feet are very thick and often very concave (above). However, the soles can grow in too thick and start to fill in the foot excessively (below), in which case they should be pared down.

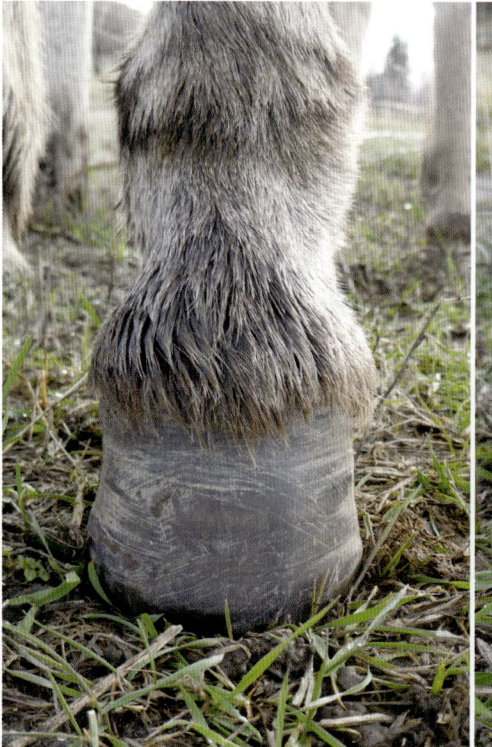

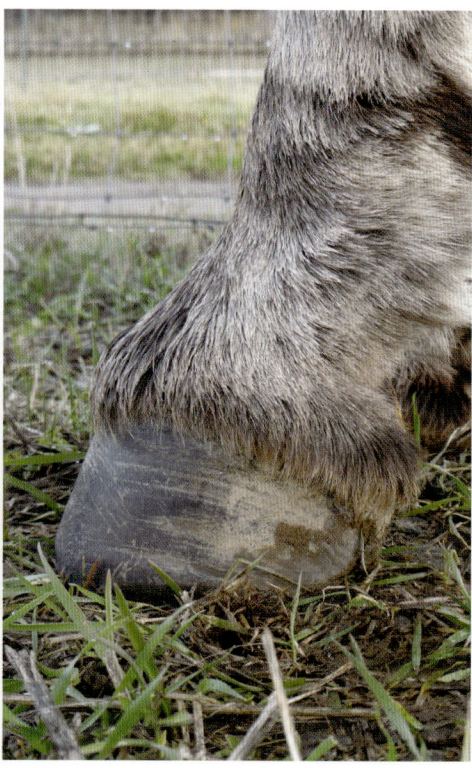

16.4 Though this upright foot would look problematic on a horse, it is just fine on a donkey.

Angles

• Donkeys' feet are quite upright from the side view, generally 5–10 degrees more so than the average horse. Viewed from the front, the walls are also more upright, with the foot resembling a tube more than a cone. This is quite normal and does not indicate contraction (fig. 16.4).

• The heels are relatively tall compared to a horse's, so the hairline is more parallel to ground when viewed from the side. A broken-forward axis (see fig. 6.3, p. 64) is not uncommon, though there is some debate as to whether this is actually okay or just a problem that is common enough to be considered within the range of normal.

In addition, donkeys were designed by nature to live on hard, dry, rocky ground, which makes them more susceptible to problems related to moisture. Soft, fluffy footing doesn't help their feet either, especially if they do not receive regular hoof care. Lastly, donkeys are *very* easy keepers, and are highly prone to obesity and laminitis due to overfeeding or inappropriate feeding. Letting them get overweight is asking for serious trouble, so be careful with their diet and try to give them plenty of exercise.

One last note on donkeys: Our long-eared equine friends tend to be extremely stoic and often do not show evidence of hoof-related pain when they have a problem. Therefore, it is easier to miss an issue in a donkey's foot than in a horse's, so donkey owners need to keep a diligent eye on their donkey's hooves to try to spot problems.

Draft Horses

Draft feet have a reputation for becoming hopelessly splayed, dinner-plate-sized pancakes with all manner of flares, splits, and cracks (fig. 16.5). While it is true that we do see that sort of thing far too often in draft horses' feet, the problem in most instances is not the feet, but rather the people entrusted with the care of those feet. In general, draft horses start out being well set up to have strong, healthy hooves. They tend to have thick hoof walls, robust frogs and digital cushions, and thick soles—all of which are definite positives (fig. 16.6).

The main reason why so many draft feet are in such bad shape is simple: not enough hoof care. In many instances, it comes down to money. Everything about caring for a draft horse costs more, from feed to tack, and hoof care is no exception. Working on a draft horse is significantly more labor for the farrier and often requires a different set of expensive tools. Additionally, many farriers don't want to (or flat out won't) work on drafts because of the damage a poorly behaved horse can inflict on their body. Working on draft horses' feet the size of passenger car tires is hard enough, but the job is made

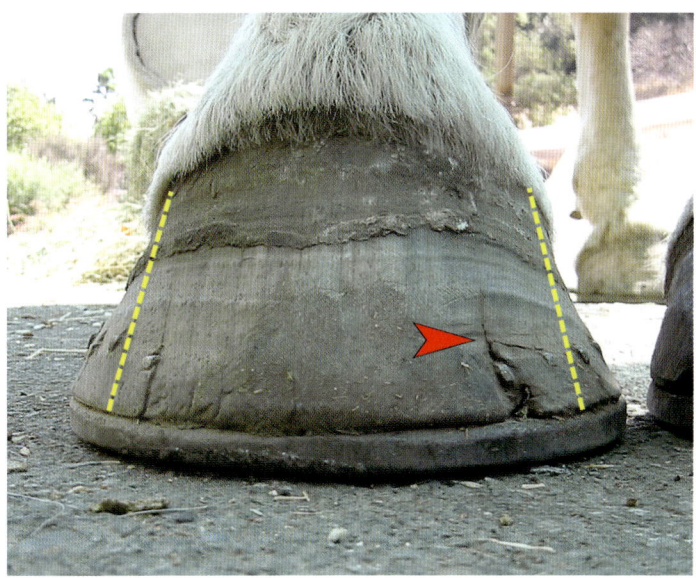

16.5 Flared walls (wall outside yellow lines) and cracks (red arrow) are far too common among draft horses—often much worse than what we see in this foot.

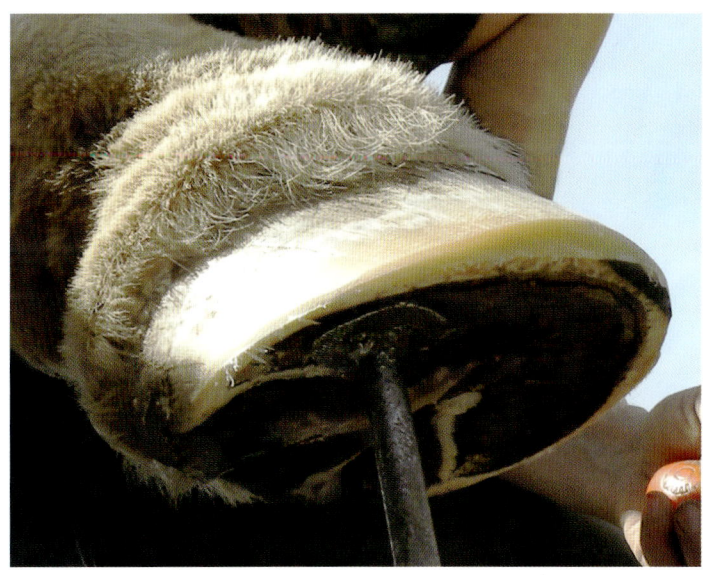

16.6 Draft horses by nature tend to have thick hoof walls, good frogs, and many other positive features, as this well-cared for foot illustrates.

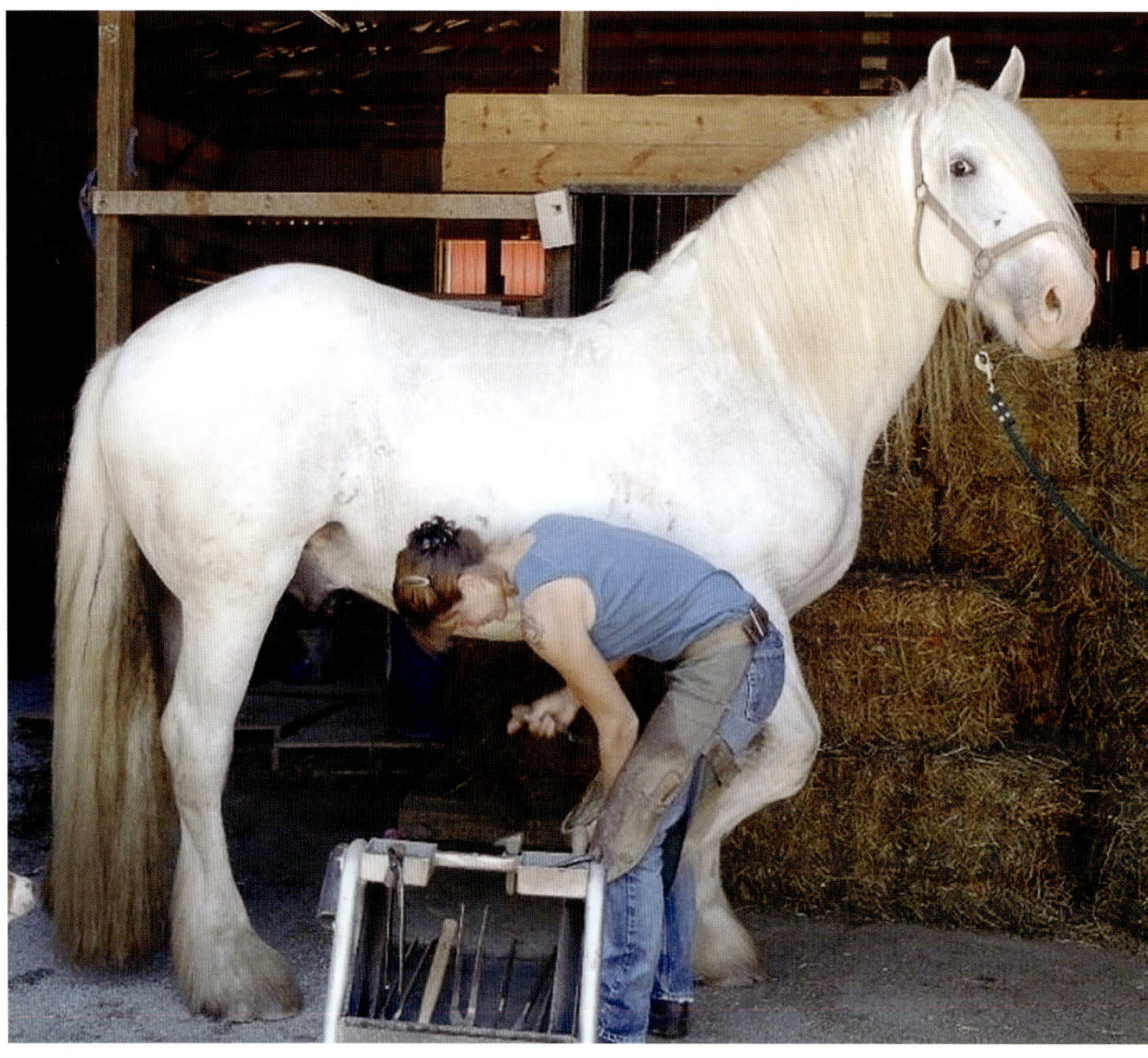

16.7 This lovely Shire stallion has been taught to stand nicely for the farrier, which is critically important for a draft horse, given the enormous power of these animals.

exponentially more difficult and dangerous if Baby Huey has no manners. This makes it even more critical for a draft horse to be trained to stand well for the farrier (fig. 16.7).

Because labor, equipment costs, and risk exposure are increased with draft horses, farriers typically charge significantly more to trim or shoe a draft horse than they would to work on a light horse. Because of this expense, many owners spread their hoof-care appointments too far apart for optimal hoof maintenance. Even if you have the world's best farrier, he cannot keep a horse's feet in good shape if he only works on those feet every three months. And to compound the situation, many drafts really should be on an even shorter hoof-care cycle than a lighter horse, as the weight of a draft makes any extra hoof wall growth flare, chip, or crack very quickly (fig. 16.8). Thus, if you own a draft horse or are thinking of acquiring one, budgeting for hoof care is vital.

Of course, draft feet can have pathologies too. They are more prone to developing sidebone and ringbone, due to the extra PSI they have coming down on each hoof with every step. The risk is even greater when a big, heavy draft is asked to do a lot of canter and jumping work: that is a boatload of weight coming down on the hoof. With the extra load they have to endure, the lateral cartilages have a greater tendency to ossify and become sidebone, and the coffin and pastern joints experience more wear and tear, which can lead to ringbone.

On the flip side, draft horses are typically less prone to palmar heel pain than light riding horses. Another positive is that even truly dreadful-looking draft feet can often bounce back if you can rid them of that all-too-common pathology: "lack of farrier disease."

Miniature Horses

The feet of Miniature Horses are not actually much different from those of regular-sized horses—they're just smaller, and as such, tend to have less of a cone shape. Unfortunately, many owners of Minis don't seem to realize that the feet of these wee equines need just as much care and maintenance as their larger brethren. The logic seems to

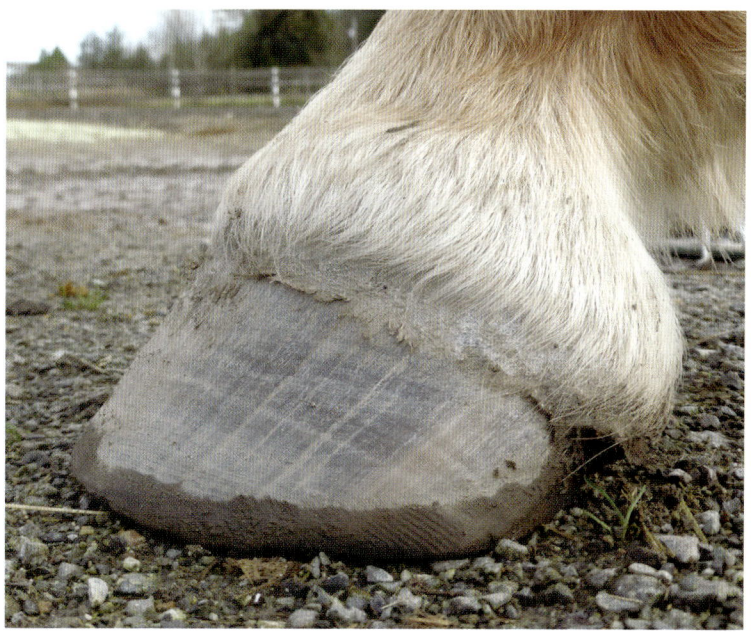

16.8 Draft feet like this one that are kept on an appropriate hoof-care cycle will do much better than those left too long between visits.

be that because Minis don't weigh much and don't get ridden, it doesn't really matter if their feet get unbalanced or overgrown. However, the reality is that Minis suffer just as badly as other horses when something is wrong with their feet.

While neglect is often a contributing factor when Minis have hoof issues, they are vulnerable to foot problems for a couple of other reasons. One is that Minis, like donkeys, are almost always very easy keepers, and because of their diminutive size, it is extremely easy to overfeed them. Here is why: the average adult mini weighs 150–250 pounds. If you were to feed a 175-pound Mini 1.5% of his body weight in hay per day, that is only about 2.6 pounds of hay—about half of a typical flake—*for the entire day*. Since obesity often goes hand in hand with the development of insulin resistance and increases the risk of laminitis, it is not surprising that Minis have an extremely high incidence of laminitis (fig. 16.9).

Minis also frequently have crooked legs due to a high incidence of genetic dwarfism, which can make their hooves have balance issues. While it is true that their small size and light weight puts less strain on the bones and soft tissues of a crooked limb than a full-sized horse with the same problem would experience, crooked legs and feet are still detrimental and should be addressed as early as possible.

A final note on Minis: Because they are so small and adorable, and because most are pets not expected to perform in any way, people often overlook the fact that Minis need to be trained. For their own sake, they must be as easy to handle as a large horse for daily care, veterinary examination,

16.9 This very overweight Mini is certainly enjoying being out in the pasture, but the rich clover in this field and her obesity put her at extreme risk of foundering. Judging by the dishing and rings on her hoof walls, she already has low-grade laminitis.

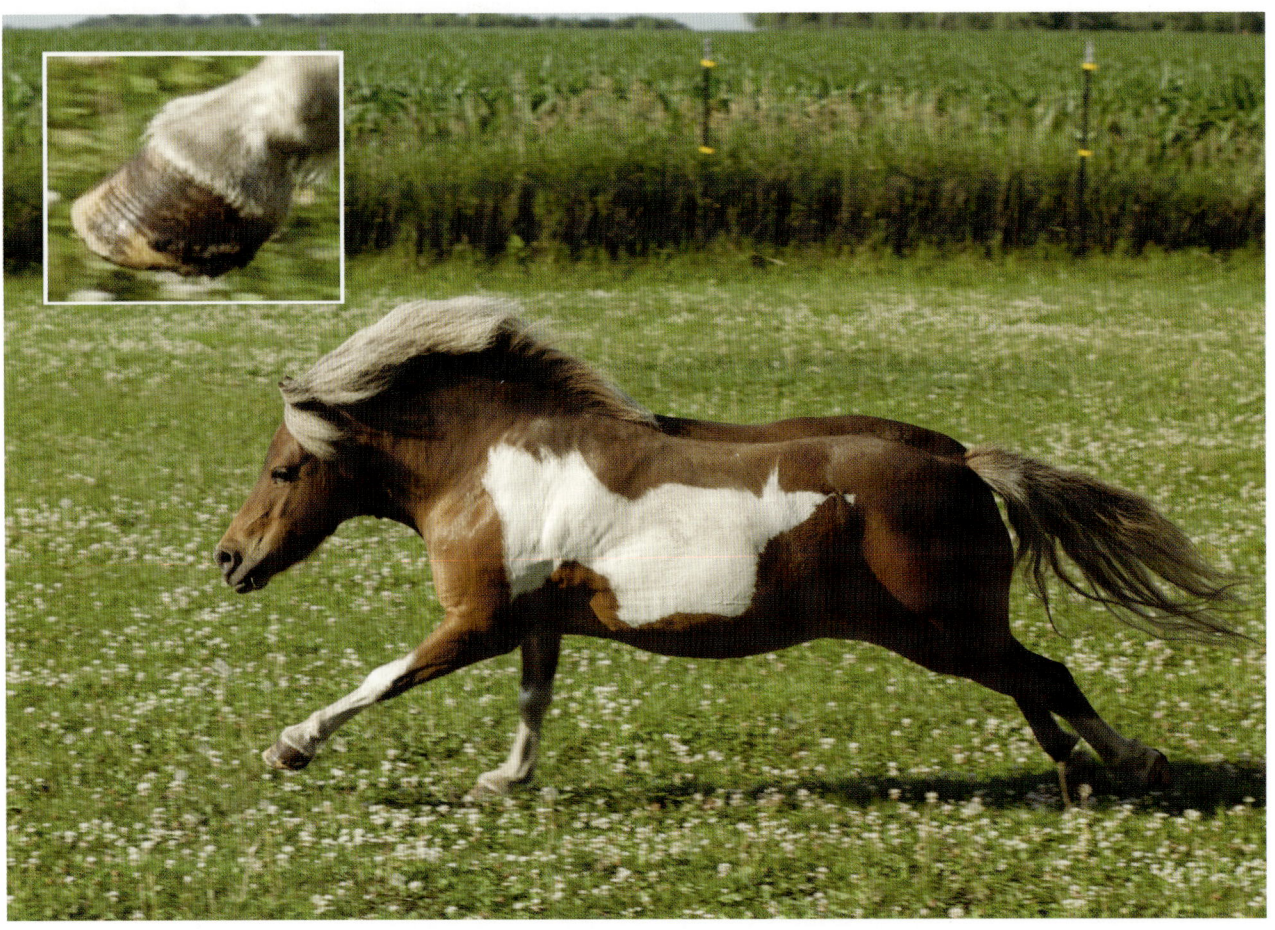

and hoof maintenance. This last aspect is so frequently neglected that many hoof-care providers truly dread trimming Minis, who can be unruly and surprisingly dangerous. Think about the fact that in order to trim these wee horses, an HCP has to get down very low, which can put his head and face at the perfect height for a hind leg to get a kick in. Losing an eye to a sharp little hoof is not something any HCP wants to experience. Many HCPs will also say that trimming Minis is harder on the body than trimming regular-sized horses, as the contortions they have to go through to get down low enough for those tiny equines' comfort is anything but comfortable for the trimmer (fig. 16.10).

So, please train your horses—whatever their size—to be good for hoof-care procedures. Your hoof-care provider will thank you, and so will your horses.

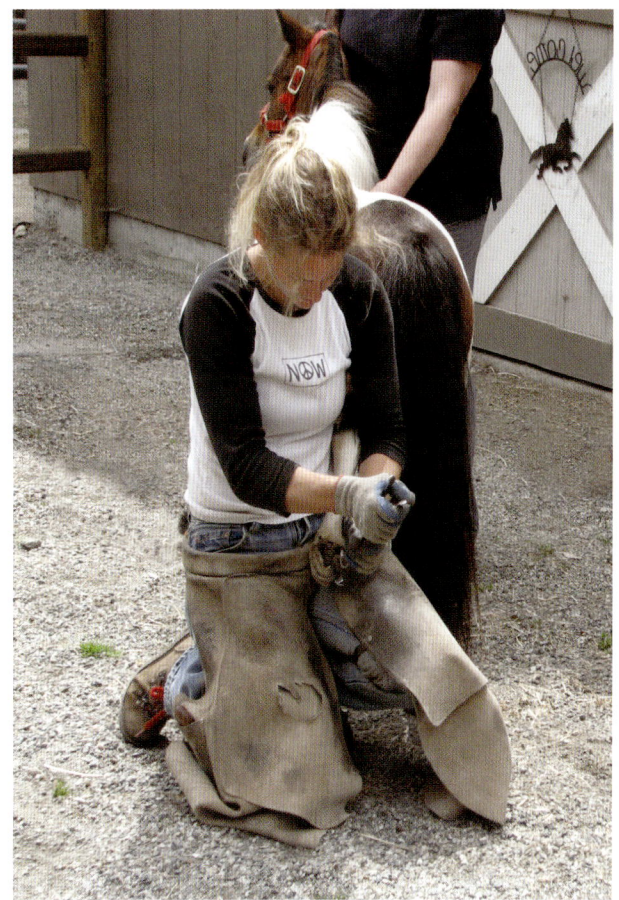

16.10 Trimming Minis requires that the hoof-care practitioner get down low to the ground, which can be hard on the back—or in this case, the knees.

Appendix

HOOF GROWTH CHART

For this hands-on activity, draw a short line with a permanent marker on the front center of each hoof wall just below your horse's coronets. Keep track of these lines and touch them up as necessary over time to keep them visible.

In the provided chart, measure how much each foot grows each month. For example, if the left front is ¼ inch down from the coronet at one month, write down, "¼ inch," in the appropriate space. If it is ¾ inch down from the coronet the following month, it has grown ½ inch, so put that in your chart. Keep doing this until an entire new hoof wall has grown down to the ground, then you can redraw the line at the top again so that you can chart a whole year of growth.

In the "Notes" column, keep track of any changes in diet, supplementation, activity, or health issues that may affect hoof growth. If you see any changes such as a prominent growth ring, look back at your notes to see what might have caused it.

HORSE:

MONTH	LEFT FRONT	RIGHT FRONT	LEFT HIND	RIGHT HIND	NOTES

For Further Information

There are many excellent websites where you can get additional information relevant to the equine hoof. We particularly recommend the following:

Master Farrier Gene Ovnicek's website: Ovnicek is widely respected by veterinarians, researchers, farriers, and barefoot trimmers the world over. He has great articles, videos, a shop for hoof-support products, and more at: *hopeforsoundness.com*

Dr. Ric Redden's website: R.F. Redden, DVM, is considered the father of modern equine podiatry, for good reason. His website contains many in-depth articles and educational videos on various aspects of hoof health. Some of these are more on the technical side, but definitely worth exploring. You can find them at: *nanric.com*

Pete Ramey's website: Ramey's books, videos, and online articles are invaluable to anyone interested in learning about barefoot hoof care, or who just wants to learn more about the function of the hoof in general. Even if you shoe your horses, Ramey's insights will help you take better care of your horse's feet. Visit him at: *hoofrehab.com*

Dr. Stephen O'Grady's website: Equine Podiatrist Stephen E. O'Grady, DVM, MRCVS, is a leading voice in therapeutic farriery. He has a number of informative articles, again tending toward the more technical but of great value, at: *www.equipodiatry.com/podiatry.html*

Equine Lameness Prevention Organization website: The E.L.P.O. is a non-profit group dedicated to preventing and treating lameness in horses. They offer training and education, and have made some of their excellent study materials available online. Check them out under the education tab at: *www.lamenessprevention.org*

Anatomy of the Equine website: This unique website provides detailed anatomical photos and information to help horse owners, hoof-care professionals, and veterinarians better visualize and understand the interrelationships between the hoof's many structures. Find this wonderful resource at: *anatomy-of-the-equine.com*

Equine Cushings and Insulin Resistance Group website: This website, as well as the ECIR web group, is a fabulous source of information for people dealing with horses with metabolic challenges and laminitis. Find the website and web group at: *ecirhorse.org* and *https://ecir.groups.io/g/main*

Katy Watts's website: Katy Watts is a forage researcher who has given us life-saving information on carbohydrates in grass and hay, and how that affects our horses. Her website contains a tremendous amount of valuable content for horse owners. Visit her at: *safergrass.org*

The American Association of Equine Practitioners (AAEP) website for horse owners: The AAEP has a website especially for horse owners where you can not only find many articles on equine health, but also use their "GET-A-DVM" feature to locate a veterinarian near you. They also have an "ASK-THE-VET" tab that takes you to the page where you can send in questions on this month's topic, and also see questions and answers from previously covered topics. Check them out at: *www.aaep.org/info/owners*

Equi-Analytical website: This forage analysis laboratory is the gold standard for the horse industry. On its website, you can learn more about forage testing, how to get a good hay sample, and how to interpret test results. You can also find nutritional profiles of common feeds that can be useful to get a general idea of what different hays are like. Find them at: *equi-analytical.com*

The Laminitis Site website: The Laminitis Site is a useful place to start if you are looking for additional information about Laminitis, Cushing's Disease (PPID), body condition scoring, Insulin Resistance/Equine Metabolic Syndrome, and equine obesity. They have many articles collected from a variety of sources, along with plenty of images to help you visualize the topics being discussed. Visit them at: *thelaminitissite.org*

The Horse Side Vet Guide website and app: Equine Veterinarian Doug Thal, DVM, Dipl. ABVP, has put together a great resource for horse owners, enabling them to get reliable information about their horse's health concerns through a searchable and ever-growing online database. What's more, he has created a mobile app that allows you to take that database right into the barn, to a show, out on the trail, or wherever you might need it. Take a look at: *horsesidevetguide.com*

Jaime Jackson's Paddock Paradise webpage: Barefoot pioneer Jaime Jackson has a number of books of great interest to anyone exploring the option of barefoot hoof care, but his Paddock Paradise concept is potentially of benefit to all horses, even if they are shod. You can find out more about it at: *www.aanhcp.net/pages/welcome-to-paddock-paradise*

About the Authors

Susan Kauffmann has been a professional in the horse industry for over three decades. The early part of her career was devoted to training and coaching, then in 2004, she branched out to become an equestrian journalist and photographer specializing in topics relating to equine health and welfare. She has been widely published in magazines such as *EQUUS, Trail Blazer*, and *Western Horse Review*, for whom she also served as Health Editor. In addition, Susan has written content for a number of courses for Michigan State's My Horse University program, gives educational classes and seminars for horse owners, and still trains horses and riders using a blend of classical and natural horsemanship philosophies.

Susan lives with her husband, three horses, a mini donkey and various cats and dogs in northern Nevada, where she is active in wild horse advocacy and rescue.

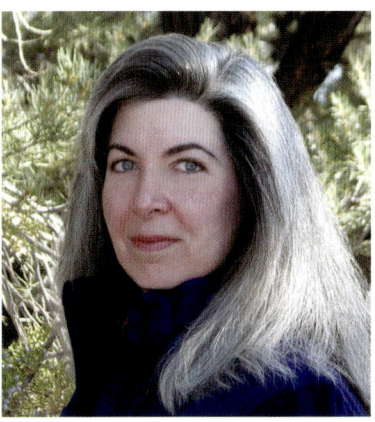

Susan Kauffmann

Christina Cline became a certified trimmer through the American Association of Natural Hoof Care Practitioners in 2004, and has trimmed full-time ever since. In her career, she has worked on thousands of hooves of every size and description. She is an instructor with the Equine Sciences Academy and a mentor with Pacific Hoof Care Practitioners. She has mentored directly with Pete Ramey, Cindy Sullivan, and Jaime Jackson, and has broadened her knowledge base by attending workshops with Dr. Robert Bowker, Dr. Debra Taylor, Dr. Brian Hampson, Dr. Kerry Ridgway, Katy Watts, Dr. Cindy Nielson, Dr. Tomas Teskey, and Dr. Deb Bennett, among others. She also received a certificate in Equine Massage from the Northwest School of Animal Massage in Redmond, Washington.

Christina lives with her seven horses, three dogs, and three cats in the Methow Valley of Washington State. When she is not working under a horse, she is often found backcountry riding in the North Cascades.

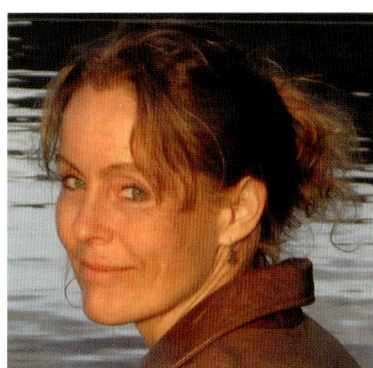

Christina Cline

Photograph and Illustration Credits

Fig I by Susan Kauffmann

Fig. II by Susan Kauffmann

Fig. III by Susan Kauffmann

Fig. IV by Susan Kauffmann

Fig. 1.1 by Susan Kauffmann

Fig. 1.2 A by Susan Kauffmann

Fig. 1.2 B by Susan Kauffmann

Fig. 1.3 by Susan Kauffmann

Fig. 1.4 by Susan Kauffmann

Fig. 1.5 by Susan Kauffmann

Fig. 1.6 by Christina Cline

Fig. 1.7 by Patricia Stiller

Fig. 1.8 by Christina Kusznir

Fig. 2.1 by Susan Kauffmann

Fig. 2.2 by Susan Kauffmann

Fig. 2.3 by Schools of Barehoof Strategy

Fig. 2.4 diagram by Susan Kauff-mann, photo by Christina Cline

Fig. 2.5 by Susan Kauffmann

Fig. 2.6 by Professor Chris Pollitt

Fig. 2.7 by The Glass Horse

Fig. 2.8 by Susan Kauffmann

Fig. 2.9 by Susan Kauffmann

Fig. 2.10 by Patricia Stiller

Fig. 2.11 by Christina Cline

Fig. 2.12 by Susan Kauffmann

Fig. 3.1 A by Susan Kauffmann

Fig. 3.1 B by Susan Kauffmann

Fig. 3.2 by Susan Kauffmann

Fig. 3.3 by Heike Bean (L) and Susan Kauffmann (R)

Fig. 3.4 by Heike Bean (L) and Susan Kauffmann (R)

Fig. 3.5 A by Gene Ovnicek

Fig. 3.5 B by Susan Kauffmann

Fig. 3.6 by Patricia Stiller (L) and Alicia Mosher (R)

Fig. 3.7 by Susan Kauffmann

Fig. 4.1 upper by The Glass Horse, lower by Dr. T.E. Rihll

Fig. 4.2 by The Glass Horse

Fig. 4.3 by The Glass Horse

Fig. 4.4 by Alicia Mosher

Fig. 4.5 by Alicia Mosher (top) and Sarah Williams (bottom)

Fig. 4.6 composite created by Susan Kauffmann from images by The Glass Horse (top) and Susan Kauffmann (bottom)

Fig. 4.7 composite created by Susan Kauffmann from an image by The Glass Horse

Fig. 4.8 by Susan Kauffmann

Fig. 4.9 by The Glass Horse

Fig. 4.10 by Dr. Alex zur Linden

Fig. 4.11 by The Glass Horse

Fig. 4.12 by The Glass Horse

Fig. 4.13 by Canadian Horse Journal

Fig. 4.14 by The Glass Horse

Fig. 4.15 by Christina Cline

Fig. 4.16 by Professor Chris Pollitt

Fig. 4.17 by Christina Cline

Fig. 4.18 by Heike Bean (top) and Susan Kauffmann (bottom)

Fig. 4.19 by Christina Cline

Fig. 4.20 by Susan Kauffmann

Fig. 4.21 A courtesy of Professor Chris Pollitt

Fig. 4.21 B by Schools of Bare-hoof Strategy

Fig. 4.21 C by Alicia Mosher

Fig. 4.22 by Professor Chris Pollitt

Fig. 4.23 by Professor Chris Pollitt

Fig. 4.24 from Merck

Fig. 4.25 by Paige Poss

Fig. 4.26 by Paige Poss

Fig. 4.27 by Paige Poss

Fig. 5.1 by Susan Kauffmann

Fig. 5.2 by Susan Kauffmann

Fig. 5.3 by José Reynaldo da Fonseca (https://commons.wikimedia.org/w/index.php?curid=727364)

Fig. 5.4 by Susan Kauffmann

Fig. 5.5 by Susan Kauffmann

Fig. 5.6 A by Susan Kauffmann (top) and Christina Cline (bottom)

Fig. 5.6 B by www.hoofhelpon-line.com

Fig. 5.7 by Christina Cline

Fig. 5.8 by Susan Kauffmann

Fig. 5.9 by Susan Kauffmann, from a photo by Christina Cline

Fig. 5.10 by Susan Kauffmann

Fig. 5.11 by Heike Bean

Fig. 5.12 by Heike Bean

Fig. 5.13 by Christina Cline

Fig. 5.14 by Christina Cline

Fig. 5.15 by Christina Cline

Fig. 5.16 by Susan Kauffmann

Fig. 5.17 by Schools of Barehoof Strategy

Fig. 5.18 by Susan Kauffmann

Fig. 5.19 by Susan Kauffmann

Fig. 5.20 by Susan Kauffmann

Fig. 5.21 by Christina Cline

Fig. 5.22 by Christina Cline

Fig. 5.23 by Susan Kauffmann

Fig. 5.24 by Professor Chris Pollitt

Fig. 5.25 by Schools of Barehoof Strategy

Fig. 5.26 by Schools of Barehoof Strategy

Fig. 5.27 by Schools of Barehoof Strategy

Fig. 5.28 by Schools of Barehoof Strategy

Fig. 5.29 by Schools of Barehoof Strategy

Fig. 5.30 by Wallace Liberman, DVM

Fig. 5.31 by Susan Kauffmann

Fig. 5.32 by Christina Cline

Fig. 5.33 by George Lager

Fig. 5.34 by Susan Kauffmann

Fig. 5.35 by Christina Cline

Fig. 5.36 by Susan Kauffmann

Fig. 5.37 by Schools of Barehoof Strategy (A and C), and Susan Kauffmann (B)

Fig. 5.38 by Schools of Barehoof Strategy

Fig. 5.39 by Susan Kauffmann

Fig. 5.40 by Susan Kauffmann, photos by Christina Cline

Fig. 6.1 by Susan Kauffmann

Fig. 6.2 by Christina Cline

Fig. 6.3 by Susan Kauffmann

Fig. 6.4 by Susan Kauffmann

Fig. 6.5 by Susan Kauffmann and Christina Cline

Fig. 6.6 A by Christina Cline

Fig. 6.6 B courtesy of J. Dikes

Fig. 6.7 by Christina Cline

Fig. 6.8 by Christina Cline (top), and Susan Kauffmann (bottom)

Fig. 6.9 by Christina Cline

Fig. 6.10 by Christina Cline

Fig. 6.11 by George Lager

Fig. 6.12 by Christina Cline

Fig. 6.13 by Alicia Mosher (L two) and www.hoofhelponline.com (R two)

Fig. 6.14 by Christina Cline

Fig. 6:15 by Susan Kauffmann

Fig. 6.16 by Susan Kauffmann

Fig. 6.17 by Christina Cline

Fig. 6.18 by Patricia Stiller (L) and Alicia Mosher (R)

Fig. 6.19 by Christina Cline

Fig. 6.20 by Susan Kauffmann from an image by The Glass Horse

Fig. 6.21 by Christina Cline

Fig. 6.22 by Alicia Mosher (L) and Christina Cline (R)

Fig. 6.23 by Christina Cline (L) and Alicia Mosher (R)

Fig. 6.24 by Susan Kauffmann

Fig. 6.25 by Alicia Mosher

Fig. 6.26 by Alicia Mosher

Fig. 6.27 by www.hoofhelp-online.com, lines by Susan Kauffmann

Fig. 6.28 by Susan Kauffmann

Fig. 6.29 by Christina Cline

Fig. 6.30 by Alicia Mosher

Fig. 6.31 by Susan Kauffmann, based on a photo by Gene Ovnicek

Fig. 6.32 by Gene Ovnicek

Fig. 7.1 by Susan Kauffmann

Fig. 7.2 by Christina Cline

Fig. 7.3 by Christina Cline

Fig. 7.4 by Susan Kauffmann

Fig. 7.5 by Susan Kauffmann

Fig. 7.6 by Susan Kauffmann

Fig. 7.7 A-D by R.F. Redden, DVM

Fig. 7.8 by R.F. Redden, DVM

Fig. 7.9 by R.F. Redden, DVM

Fig. 7.10 by Christina Cline

Fig. 7.11 by Chris Minick

Fig. 7.12 by www.hoofhelpon-line.com

Fig. 7.13 by Susan Kauffmann

Fig. 7.14 by Alicia Mosher

Fig. 7.15 by R.F Redden, DVM

Fig. 7.16 by Alicia Mosher (L) and Patricia Stiller (R)

Fig. 7.17 by Gene Ovnicek

Fig. 7.18 by Susan Kauffmann (top) and Patricia Stiller (bottom)

Fig. 7.19 by Susan Kauffmann

Fig. 7.20 by Susan Kauffmann

Fig. 7.21 by Gene Ovnicek

Fig. 7.22 by Susan Kauffmann

Fig. 7.23 by Susan Kauffmann (top) and Christina Kusznir (bottom)

Fig. 7.24 by Susan Kauffmann

Fig. 7.25 by Christina Cline

Fig. 7.26 by Susan Kauffmann

Fig. 7.27 by Susan Kauffmann

Fig. 7.28 by Christina Cline

Fig. 7.29 by Christina Cline

Fig. 7.30 by Susan Kauffmann

Fig. 7.31 by Susan Kauffmann

Fig. 7.32 by Susan Kauffmann

Fig. 7.33 by www.hoofhelpon-line.com

Fig. 7.34 by Agustin Almanza, DVM

Fig. 8.1 by Chris Minick

Fig. 8.2 by Pete Ramey

Fig. 8.3 by Susan Kauffmann

Fig. 8.4 by Susan Kauffmann

Fig. 8.5 by Horse Side Vet Guide–Equine Health Resource, www.horsesidevetguide.com

Fig. 8.6 by R.F. Redden, DVM

Fig. 8.7 by Chris Minick (top) and Gene Ovnicek (bottom)

Fig. 9.1 by Susan Kauffmann

Fig. 9.2 by Alicia Mosher

Fig. 9.3 by Susan Kauffmann

Fig. 9.4 by April Raine

Fig. 9.5 by Heike Bean (top L), Susan Kauffmann (top R), Mary Cotrill (bottom L), Susan Kauffmann (bottom R)

Fig. 9.6 by Christina Cline

Fig. 9.7 by Alicia Mosher

Fig. 9.8 by Susan Kauffmann

Fig. 9.9 by Susan Kauffmann and Alicia Mosher

Fig. 9.10 by Chris Minick

Fig. 9.11 by Susan Kauffmann

Fig. 9.12 by Susan Kauffmann

Fig. 9.13 by Christina Cline

Fig. 9.14 by Patricia Stiller (top) and www.hoofhelponline.com (bottom)

Fig. 9.15 A by Susan Kauffmann

Fig. 9.15 B by Schools of Barehoof Strategy

Fig. 9.16 courtesy of Pete Ramey, by Alex Sperandeo

Fig. 9.17 by Susan Kauffmann

Fig. 9.18 by Susan Kauffmann

Fig. 9.19 by Christina Cline

Fig. 9.20 by Susan Kauffmann

Fig. 9.21 by Susan Kauffmann

Fig. 9.22 by Christina Cline

Fig. 9.23 A by Susan Kauffmann

Fig. 9.23 B by Christina Kusznir

Fig. 9.24 by Christina Kusznir

Fig. 9.25 by Susan Kauffmann

Fig. 9.26 A by Christina Kusznir

Fig. 9.26 B by Heike Bean

Fig. 9.26 C by Susan Kauffmann

Fig. 9.26 D by Gene Ovnicek

Fig. 10.1 by Christina Cline

Fig. 10.2 by Christina Cline

Fig. 10.3 by Susan Kauffmann

Fig. 10.4 by Schools of Barehoof Strategy

Fig. 10.5 by R.F. Redden, DVM

Fig. 10.6 by www.hoofhelpon-line.com

Fig. 10.7 by www.hoofhelpon-line.com

Fig. 10.8 by Christina Cline

Fig. 10.9 by Susan Kauffmann

Fig. 10.10 by www.hoofhelpon-line.com

Fig. 10.11 by Christina Cline

Fig. 10.12 by www.hoofhelpon-line.com

Fig. 10.13 by Susan Kauffmann

Fig. 10.14 by Susan Kauffmann

Fig. 10.15 by Christina Kusznir

Fig. 10.16 by Schools of Barehoof Strategy

Fig. 10.17 by Schools of Barehoof Strategy

Fig. 10.18 by www.hoofhelpon-line.com

Fig. 10.19 by Gene Ovnicek

Fig. 10.20 by Susan Kauffmann

Fig. 10.21 by Chris Minick

Fig. 10.22 by April Raine

Fig. 10.23 by Wallace Liberman, DVM

Fig. 10.24 by Javier Donatelli, DVM

Fig. 10.25 by Wallace Liberman, DVM

Fig. 10.26 by April Raine

Fig. 10.27 by Gene Ovnicek

Fig. 10.28 by Christina Kusznir

Fig. 10.29 by Christina Cline

Fig. 10.30 by Javier Donatelli, DVM

Fig. 10.31 by Wallace Liberman, DVM

Fig. 10.32 by Wallace Liberman, DVM

Fig. 10.33 by Alicia Mosher

Fig. 10.34 by Alicia Mosher

Fig. 10.35 by Javier Donatelli, DVM

Fig. 10.36 by Steinbeck Country Equine Clinic

Fig. 10.37 by Javier Donatelli, DVM

Fig. 10.38 by Wallace Liberman, DVM

Fig. 10.39 A by Wallace Liber-man, DVM

Fig. 10.39 B by Wallace Liber-man, DVM

Fig. 10.40 by Wallace Liberman, DVM

Fig. 11.1 by Professor Chris Pollitt

Fig. 11.2 by Wallace Liberman, DVM

Fig. 11.3 by Schools of Barehoof Strategy

Fig. 11.4 by Wallace Liberman, DVM (top) and The Laminitis Site (bottom)

Fig. 11.5 (A) by Susan Kauffmann

Fig. 11.5 (B) by Anna Gamsgaard Frederiksen

Fig. 11.6 by Vxla, Creative Com-mons License: https://creative-commons.org/licenses/by/2.0/legalcode

Fig. 11.7 by Susan Kauffmann

Fig. 11.8 by Alicia Mosher

Fig. 11.9 courtesy of Professor Chris Pollitt

Fig. 11.10 by Sammy L. Pittman, DVM

Fig. 11.11 by Susan Kauffmann

Fig. 11.12 by Susan Kauffmann

Fig. 11.13 by Susan Kauffmann

Fig. 11.14 by Christina Cline

Fig. 11.15 A by Susan Kauffmann

Fig. 11.15 B by Paige Poss

Fig. 11.16 by The Laminitis Site

Fig. 11.17 by Schools of Bare-hoof Strategy

Fig. 11.18 by Alicia Mosher

Fig. 11.19 by The Laminitis Site

Fig. 11.20 by Schools of Bare-hoof Strategy

Fig. 11.21 by Schools of Bare-hoof Strategy

Fig. 11.22 by Wallace Liberman, DVM

Fig. 11.23 by Gene Ovnicek

Fig. 11.24 by Alicia Mosher

Fig. 11.25 by Gene Ovnicek

Fig. 11.26 by Alicia Mosher

Fig. 11.27 by Pete Ramey

Fig. 11.28 by Pete Ramey

Fig. 11.29 by Pete Ramey

Fig. 11.30 by Paige Poss

Fig. 11.31 by Paige Poss

Fig. 11.32 by Paige Poss

Fig. 11.33 by Susan Kauffmann

Fig. 11.34 by Susan Kauffmann

Fig. 11.35 by Susan Kauffmann

Fig. 11.36 by Susan Kauffmann

Fig. 11.37 A by Donald Walsh, DVM

Fig. 11.37 B by Donald Walsh, DVM

Fig. 11.37 C by Donal Walsh, DVM

Fig. 11.38 by Gene Ovnicek

Fig. 11.39 by George Lager

Fig. 11.40 by Pete Ramey (top), and The Laminitis Site (bottom)

Fig. 11.41 by The Laminitis Site

Fig. 11.42 by The Laminitis Site

Fig. 11.43 by Susan Kauffmann

Fig. 11.44 by The Laminitis Site

Fig. 11.45 by The Laminitis Site

Fig. 11.46 by Gretchen Fathauer, www.naturalhorsetrim.com

Fig. 11.47 by Sammy L. Pittman, DVM

Fig. 11.48 by Gretchen Fathauer, www.naturalhorsetrim.com

Fig. 11.49 (A) by Anvil Brand, (B) by RGM, (C) by Michel Vaillant, www.euroforgesupplies.com, (D) R.F. Redden, DVM

Fig. 11.50 by Gene Ovnicek

Fig. 11.51 by Gene Ovnicek

Fig. 11.52 courtesy of Equicast Inc.

Fig. 11.53 courtesy of Equicast Inc.

Fig. 11.54 courtesy of Easycare

Fig. 11.55 by Gene Ovnicek

Fig. 11.56 by The Laminitis Site

Fig. 11.57 by The Glass Horse

Fig. 11.58 by Judit Somogyi

Fig. 12.1 by Wallace Liberman, DVM

Fig. 12.2 by The Glass Horse

Fig. 12.3 by Hallmarq

Fig. 12.4 by Hallmarq

Fig. 12.5 by Hallmarq

Fig. 12.6 by Schools of Barehoof Strategy

Fig. 12.7 by Stephanie Travers

Fig. 12.8 by Susan Kauffmann, based on an image from The Glass Horse

Fig. 12.9 by Gene Ovnicek

Fig. 12.10 by Susan Kauffmann

Fig. 12.11 A by Gene Ovnicek

Fig. 12.11 B by Gene Ovnicek

Fig. 12.12 by Pulse Veterinary Technologies

Fig. 12.13 by Schools of Bare-hoof Strategy

Fig. 13.1 by Alicia Mosher

Fig. 13.2 by Patricia Stiller

Fig. 13.3 by Susan Kauffmann

Fig. 13.4 by Christina Cline

Fig. 13.5 by Alicia Mosher

Fig. 13.6 by Alicia Mosher

Fig. 13.7 by Susan Kauffmann

Fig. 13.8 by https://commons.wikimedia.org/wiki/File:W-CLV07f.JPG

Fig. 13.9 by Wallace Liberman, DVM

Fig. 14.1 by Susan Kauffmann

Fig. 14.2 by Schools of Barehoof Strategy

Fig. 14.3 by Jen Reid

Fig. 14.4 by Susan Kauffmann

Fig. 14.5 by Susan Kauffmann

Fig. 14.6 by Nilfanion https://commons.wikimedia.org/wiki/File:Dartmoor_pony_foal_2.jpg

Fig. 14.7 by Susan Kauffmann

Fig. 14.8 by Susan Kauffmann

Fig. 14.9 by Jill Willis, AANHCP

Fig. 14.10 by Christina Kusznir

Fig. 14.11 by Sini Merikallio https://commons.wikimedia.org/wiki/File:Finnhorse_stallions_lunch_time.jpg

Fig. 14.12 by Susan Kauffmann

Fig. 14.13 by Susan Kauffmann

Fig. 14.14 by Susan Kauffmann

Fig. 14.15 by Francisco M. Marzoa Alonso https://commons.wikimedia.org/wiki/File:ErcinaLakeHorse2.JPG

Fig. 14.16 by Murry Ranch, Reno, NV

Fig. 14.17 by Susan Kauffmann

Fig. 14.18 by Susan Kauffmann

Fig. 14.19 by Susan Kauffmann

Fig. 14.20 by Paige Poss

Fig. 14.21 by Susan Kauffmann

Fig. 14.22 by Patricia Stiller

Fig. 14.23 by Patricia Stiller (top) and Paige Poss (bottom)

Fig. 14.24 by Paige Poss

Fig. 14.25 A by Schools of Barehoof Strategy

Fig. 14.25 B by Stephen Mowbray

Fig. 14.26 photo by Christina Cline

Fig. 14.27 by © 1971markus@wikipedia.de https://commons.wikimedia.org/wiki/File:Windschutzscheibe,_gesplittert_(1).jpg

Fig. 14.28 by Susan Kauffmann

Fig. 14.29 by Alicia Mosher

Fig. 14.30 by Gene Ovnicek

Fig. 14.31 by Gene Ovnicek

Fig. 14.32 by Chris Minick

Fig. 14.33 by Alicia Mosher

Fig. 14.34 by Susan Kauffmann, photo from Schools of Barehoof Strategy

Fig. 14.35 by April Raine

Fig. 14.36 by Susan Kauffmann

Fig. 14.37 by Susan Kauffmann

Fig. 14.38 by Christina Cline

Fig. 14.39 by Susan Kauffmann

Fig. 14.40 by Susan Kauffmann

Fig. 15.1 by Susan Kauffmann

Fig. 15.2 photo by Nicolas Mariton, courtesy of Sandra Gaspar Carreira

Fig. 15.3 by Lora Thorson

Fig. 15.4 A courtesy of Houston Police Department Mounted Patrol

Fig. 15.4 B courtesy of Houston Police Department Mounted Patrol

Fig. 15.5 by Patricia Stiller

Fig. 15.6 by Susan Kauffmann

Fig. 15.7 courtesy of Cavallo Hoof Boots—The Trusted Authority (L two); Renegade Hoof Boots (Center, photo by Susan Kauffmann), EasyCare Inc. (top and bottom; R two)

Fig. 15.8 by Susan Kauffmann

Fig. 15.9 by Susan Kauffmann

Fig. 15.10 by Alicia Mosher

Fig. 15.11 by Phil Sangwell https://commons.wikimedia.org/wiki/File:Someone_likes_carrots_(6337708908).jpg

Fig. 16.1 A–C by Christina Cline

Fig. 16.2 A–B by Susan Kauffmann

Fig. 16.3 by Susan Kauffmann

Fig. 16.4 by Christina Cline

Fig. 16.5 by Chris Minick

Fig. 16.6 by Sandy Zeigler

Fig. 16.7 by Sandy Zeigler

Fig. 16.8 by Christina Cline

Fig. 16.9 by Peter Markham https://commons.wikimedia.org/wiki/File:Miniature_Horse_Runs_Through_the_Pasture.jpg

Fig. 16.10 by Susan Kauffmann

Acknowledgments

Putting together a book of this scope is a daunting task, but we were fortunate to be helped and encouraged at every stage by a number of world-class researchers, exceptional veterinarians, and leading hoof-care experts who were incredibly generous in sharing their expertise and experience. Some have been our teachers and mentors for years, inspiring us and guiding us as we sought to increase our understanding of the equine hoof. They and many others made this project possible by taking the time to answer questions, clarify critical details, review materials, and contribute invaluable information and illustrations, all of which gave this book a depth and breadth it could not otherwise have had. We are also deeply indebted to the pioneers who continue to push forward the boundaries of what we know about the hoof, providing learning opportunities for us all through the publication of their discoveries. In alphabetical order, we offer our sincerest thanks to:

Robert Bowker, VMD, PhD; Dan Brown, BVSc, ACIM; Hilary Clayton, BVMS, PhD, DACVSMR, MRCVS; Jaime Jackson; Eleanor M. Kellon, VMD; Wallace H. Liberman, DVM; Stephen E. O'Grady, DVM, MRCVS; Gene Ovnicek, GPF, RMF; Chris Pollitt, BVSc, PhD; Pete Ramey; RF (Ric) Redden, DVM; Debra R. Taylor, DVM, MS, DACVIM-LA; Kathryn Watts, BS

We also want to thank the many other veterinarians, hoof care professionals, and others who allowed us to use their photographs or photograph their horses' feet. Your contributions also enriched this book immeasurably.

The authors also wish to express their gratitude to the entire team at Trafalgar Square Books. They are an amazing group of women who work incredibly hard to bring important works to the equestrian community. Their dedication and professionalism is second to none, and we feel blessed that *The Essential Hoof Book* came through their capable hands.

Lastly, Susan Kauffmann would like to thank Christina Cline: *She was my entrée into the fascinating world of the horse's hoof many years ago and has always been there for me as both friend and educator. Without her unflagging patience, incomparable kindness, priceless sense of humor, and tremendous knowledge, this book never would have happened.*

Index

Page numbers in *italics* indicate illustrations.

over-trimming of, 251
puncture wounds, 156
width, 72, *73*
Hemodynamic flow. *See* Blood flow
Henneke scale, 242, *242*
High/low syndrome, *65*, 82–84
Hind feet, vs. front feet, 81–82, *82*
Hindle, Emma, 266
Hoof angle
assessment of, 63–68, *63–67*, 103, *103*
in donkeys, *277*, 278
standardized, trimming to conform to, *272*, 273
Hoof boots
in barefoot hoof care, 269–271, *269–270*
therapeutic uses, 145, 159, 185, 200–201, *200*, 218
Hoof care. *See also* Barefoot hoof care; Shoeing
cleaning/picking, 19–20, 21, 116, 117, 264
general guidelines, 125–26
physiologically correct, 247–253, *248*, *258*
Hoof care providers, 260–64, 271–73, *272*
Hoof casts, 141, 199–200, *199–200*
Hoof characteristics
color, 10, 11, *11*, 15–16
common not always healthy, 39
developmental considerations, 46, *46*, 87, *87*, 233–34, *235*
environmental factors, 42–43, *43*, 49, 76, 237
of healthy feet, generally, 233
misrepresentation of, in models, 108
shape, 45–47, *45–47*, 212 (*see also* Club feet; Tall feet)
size, 41–44, 147, 214
Hoof dressings, 135
Hoof mechanism, 45, 253–55, *253*

Hoof testers, *177*
Hoof wall
anatomy, 9–12, *9–12*, *15*
in donkeys, 277, *277*
growth of, 49, 137
injuries to, 143–44, *144*, *155*
regions of, 12–13, *12*
separation of, 57
solar view, 15–16
weaknesses in, 51–54
"Hoof-bound." *See* Contracted heels
Hoof-pastern alignment, 64–68, *64–67*
Horn tubules, 10, *10*, 48, *48*, *51*
Hospital plates, *158*, 159
Houston Police Mounted Patrol Unit, 267, *268*
Hyperlipidemia, 206

Ice ball formation, 146–47
Icing. *See* Cryotherapy
Imbalances, 104–6, *104–6*, 142, 145, 212, 258. *See also* Balance
Impar ligament, 26, 28–29, *29*, 96
Infections. *See also* Thrush
from cracks, 138
flares and, 100
from puncture wounds, 156–160, *159*
in retained sole, 129
in septic osteitis, 227
white line disease, 57–58, *57*, 155
Inferior check ligament, 88
Inflammation, 51, 223, 273–74, *274*
Insulin levels, 168–69
Insulin resistance, 100, *101*, 243
Interfering, 110, *110*, 147
Inulin, 243
Isoxuprine, 217

Jackson, Jaime, 237–38
Joint injections, 216, 224
Joints
fusion of, 223, 224

ringbone and, 221–26
torque effects on, 14

Knock knees, 60, *60*, 106, *106*

"Lack of Farrier Disease." *See* Overgrowth
Lactic acid buildup, 168
Lamellar corium, *37*, 38
Lamellar wedge, 182, *182*, 184–85
Laminae
anatomy, 16, 34–37, *35–36*
connection to coffin bone, 24, 26
damage to, 137, *171*, 249
Laminitis
overview, 163–65, 170–71
abscesses and, 148, *148*
acute phase, 165, 170–71, 176–79, *177–79*, 187–190
chronic, 50, 171, 179–183, *179–182*
developmental phase, 170, 171–74, 176, 189–190
diet and, 240, 243
effects of, 23, 37, 100, *100*, 147, *147*, *184–86*
emergency treatment of, 187–191, *187–190*
examples of, *88*, *101*, *232*
in miniature horses, 282
ongoing care, 197–204
reversal of, 183–87
signs of, 61
subacute phase, 171
subclinical, 165, *165*
triggers, 167–170
Landing patterns
contracted heels and, 75
heel-first, 49, 177, 213–15, *214*
toe-first, 65, *136*, 137, 213–15, *214*, 255
Lateral, defined, 7, *7*
Lateral cartilages, 30, *30*, 212, 220–21
Lateral symmetry, 81